Collective Behavior of Magnetic Micro/Nanorobots

Collective Behavior of Magnetic Micro/Nanorobots: Control, Imaging, and Applications reviews recent advances in the design and construction of magnetic collective micro/nanorobot systems, and promotes the bridging of the gap between their theoretical investigation and practical applications.

By summarizing the recent progress in control, imaging, and biomedical applications of collective micro/nanorobots, the authors show the big picture of micro/nanorobotics and the roadmap of collective micro/nanorobots. They then discuss the control, imaging, and biomedical applications of collective micro/nanorobots, respectively, demonstrating the state-of-the-art techniques and ideas for designing systems of collective micro/nanorobots that can help researchers have a better understanding and further stimulate the development of such an exciting field.

This book is suitable for scientists, engineers, and students involved in the study of robotics, control, materials, and mechanical/electrical engineering.

Qianqian Wang is a professor at Southeast University, Nanjing, China. He received his Ph.D. from the Chinese University of Hong Kong, Hong Kong, China. Dr. Wang's research interests lie in collective behaviors, wireless control, and medical applications of small-scale robots.

Jiangfan Yu is an assistant professor at the Chinese University of Hong Kong, Shenzhen, China. He received his Ph.D. from the Chinese University of Hong Kong, Hong Kong, China. Dr. Yu's research interests lie in micro/nanorobotics and medical robotics.

Collective Behavior of Magnetic Micro/Nanorobots

Control, Imaging, and Applications

Qianqian Wang and Jiangfan Yu

CRC Press
Taylor & Francis Group
Boca Raton London New York

CRC Press is an imprint of the
Taylor & Francis Group, an **informa** business

Designed cover image: © Astibuag

First edition published 2024
by CRC Press
2385 NW Executive Center Drive, Suite 320, Boca Raton FL 33431

and by CRC Press
4 Park Square, Milton Park, Abingdon, Oxon, OX14 4RN

CRC Press is an imprint of Taylor & Francis Group, LLC

ISBN: 978-1-032-66548-1 (hbk)
ISBN: 978-1-032-66582-5 (pbk)
ISBN: 978-1-032-66578-8 (ebk)

DOI: 10.1201/9781032665788

Typeset in Latin Modern font
by KnowledgeWorks Global Ltd.

To the Visionaries, Innovators, and Explorers of the Micro/Nanorobotics World.

Contents

Preface

Micro/nanorobots have emerged as a captivating field of research, particularly in the realm of biomedical applications. The limitations posed by the size and surface area of individual tiny robots make it challenging to address certain problems, such as targeted drug delivery and material manipulation. However, by drawing inspiration from collective behavior observed in nature, such as ants collaborating in food transportation and birds migrating in unison, we can introduce the concept of collective behavior into microrobots and utilize microrobot swarms to tackle complex tasks, thereby significantly enhancing efficiency and task completion rates.

This book aims to explore the integration of collective behavior into micro/nanorobots and delve into the formation, transformation, and navigation of collective micro/nanorobots. It covers various control strategies and algorithms employed to drive and manipulate these swarms. Previous research has demonstrated the remote control of microrobots by leveraging interactions among microrobots and their environment, enabling the adaptation to diverse environments and the execution of versatile tasks. Given that microrobots often operate within opaque environments, the integration of imaging systems with microrobot control systems becomes essential. This enables visual manipulation of microrobot swarms through imaging systems, image processing, and motion tracking algorithms.

The five sections of this book aim to provide readers with a comprehensive understanding of micro/nanorobots, stimulate research interest in this field, and serve as a valuable reference. Section 1 introduces the collective behavior of micro/nanorobots, including the driving modes of swarms and their biomedical applications. Section 2 delves into swarm control, elucidating how the adjustment of driving field parameters, combined with motion and obstacle avoidance algorithms, leads to effective control of collective patterns and motion. The feasibility and effectiveness of these control mechanisms are demonstrated through simulations and experimental results. Section 3 explores the achievement of formation, localization, and navigation of collective micro/nanorobots in invisible environments through image processing aided by imaging systems. In Section 4, readers gain insights into the applications and fundamentals of micro/nanorobot swarms within the field of biomedicine. Lastly, the book concludes with a summary of the current development status of micro/nanorobots, while highlighting the forthcoming opportunities and challenges that researchers in this field are likely to encounter.

The book is written with the kind help of many organizations and individuals. The authors would like to acknowledge support from the National Natural Science Foundation with project Nos. 52205590 and 62103347; the Natural Science Foundation of Jiangsu Province with project No. BK20220834; the start-up Research Fund of Southeast University (SEU) with project No. RF1028623098; Shenzhen Science and Technology Program with Grant No. RCBS20210609103155061; Guangdong Basic and Applied Basic Research Foundation with project Nos. 2023A1515012973 and 2022A1515110499; and the start-up funding of CUHK, Shenzhen with project No. UDF01001929.

We are very grateful to Prof. Bradley Nelson from ETH Zurich, Switzerland; Prof. Yangsheng Xu, President of the Chinese University of Hong Kong (CUHK) Shenzhen; Prof. Li Zhang from CUHK; Prof. Yu Sun from the University of Toronto; Prof. Zhonghua Ni and Prof. Yunfei Chen, Co-directors of Jiangsu Key Laboratory for Design and Manufacture of Micro-Nano Biomedical Instruments, SEU; Prof. Yong-Ping Zheng from the Polytechnic University of Hong Kong, and the other collaborators, as well as the colleagues from the School of Mechanical Engineering at SEU and the School of Science and Engineering at CUHK Shenzhen, for their long-term guidance and generous support to our group's research on collective micro/nanorobots. We appreciate all the lab ex- and current members, and many other researchers for contributing their excellent research work to this book, including Dr. Dongdong Jin, Dr. Xingzhou Du, Dr. Ben Wang, Dr. Tony Chan Kai Fung, Dr. Shijie Wang, Dr. Fengtong Ji, Dr. Neng Xia, Dr. Mingxue Cai, Dr. Tiantian Xu, Dr. Zhaoxin Lao, Hui Chen, Qian Zou, Junhui Law, Kathrin Schweizer, Qinglong Wang, and we would also like to thank Guangjun Zeng, Ying Cao, Yuanbiao Ma, Yimin Sun, and Shihao Yang for their assistance in editing and proofreading. The editorial and production staff of Taylor & Francis are gratefully acknowledged for the kind arrangement in writing this book that enables its publication. Thanks to the great and fascinating efforts achieved by numerous researchers all over the world, the continuous discoveries keep pushing the forefront of collective micro/nanorobots, and we sincerely hope that this book enhances readers' comprehension of micro/nanorobots and inspires further exploration in this exciting area of research. May the contents within these pages provide valuable references and inspire new perspectives for researchers venturing into this domain.

Finally, we would like to take this chance to send our best greeting for celebrating the 121st anniversary of the Southeast University and the 60th anniversary of the Chinese University of Hong Kong in 2023.

I

Introduction

CHAPTER 1

Introduction to Collective Behaviors of Micro/Nanorobots

1.1 INTRODUCTION

There is a very common phenomenon of collective behavior in the biological world. Numerous biological individuals can come together through communication, and gathered individuals can demonstrate different forms of cooperation [1, 2, 3]. Each aggregated swarm can migrate as an entity, and its shape can be significantly changed according to environmental stimulation or meeting the requirements of specific tasks: the collective stability can be improved by the swarms through positively changing their structure and morphology [4]. Ants connect their bodies into rafts in order to survive the flood and move large foods in a state of gathering [5, 6]. Diverse swarming intelligence and emergent behaviors have inspired the design of artificial robot systems, which can adjust their collective behaviors as needed to perform coordination tasks that are difficult to achieve with a single agent [7, 8].

The rapid development of nanotechnology and manufacturing makes it possible to reduce the size of remote control machines, and they can perform tasks as required. As a small machine, micro/nanorobot can navigate in various physiological environments in a controllable way through external energy [9, 10, 11, 12, 13, 14], self-propulsion [15, 16, 17, 18], and hybrid propulsion [19, 20, 21, 22]. Recent achievements on fabrication, actuation, and functionalization have provided a variety of capabilities for micro/nanorobots with more biocompatibility and biodegradability [23, 24, 25, 26]. The potential for a variety of biomedical applications such as targeted delivery [27, 28, 29, 30], biosensing [31, 32, 33, 34, 35], micromanipulation [36, 37, 38], and minimally invasive surgery [39, 40, 41] are offered by these micro- and nanoscale robots.

There are several key steps that should be studied before applying microrobot swarms to practical applications. When the building blocks have different energy inputs, their interactions play an important role in pattern formation and control,

DOI: 10.1201/9781032665788-1

including collective formation and motion control under different conditions. Collective movement and transformation give it the ability to adapt to different environments. In practical application, pattern positioning is needed, and the imaging system must be compatible with the control system. Finally, based on the basic understanding of different types of microrobotic swarms with the integration of imaging model, the imaging-guided delivery can be designed based on the application site and delivery objects.

In the first half of this chapter, the active substance swarm is developed from the perspective of robot delivery, and the collective behavior of micro/nanorobots driven by external power, and its application in imaging-guided delivery are summarized and discussed. Firstly, the swarm formation under the external field (magnetic field, light, sound field, electric field, and hybrid fields) is summarized and discussed, including the basic interaction between building blocks and the agent-boundary interaction. Then the collective motion and pattern navigation of microrobot swarms are introduced, and it includes the interaction between swarms and the surrounding environment. In order to locate the swarm in biological and opaque environment, in this chapter, the swarm location in different imaging modes is summarized and compared, and the integration of control system and imaging technology is discussed. Finally, the research work of image-guided micro/nanorobot swarm delivery is summarized, which shows the research progress of remote-driven micro/nanorobot swarm. Then the second half of this chapter focuses on how micronanoswarms are utilized in typical biomedical scenarios, that is, targeted drug delivery, hyperthermia, imaging and sensing, and thrombolysis, which are strongly required in healthcare.

1.2 EXTERNAL FIELD-DRIVEN PATTERN FORMATION AND NAVIGATION

The collective behaviors observed in micro/nanorobots stem from the fundamental interactions among individual units. These interactions can be adjusted to facilitate swarm formation, navigation, and pattern transformation in various environments. In this section, we begin by summarizing the interactions between micro/nanorobots that are induced by external fields such as magnetic fields, light, acoustic fields, and electric fields. We also briefly touch upon interactions resulting from hybrid fields, which involve combinations of magnetic and acoustic fields. Furthermore, we summarize and compare the mechanisms of swarm formation and navigation in response to different field inputs.

1.2.1 Magnetically Driven Microswarms

Under the action of external magnetic field, the interaction between magnetic agents enables themselves to form various patterns dynamically. Magnetic agents usually refer to ferromagnetic and paramagnetic materials strongly influenced by external magnetic fields. As can be seen from the magnetization curve of ferromagnetic materials (such as Fe, Co, Ni), the hysteresis phenomenon indicates that ferromagnetic materials remain magnetized after external field magnetization [42]. When a relative weak magnetic field is applied, the magnetic moment usually aligns with the external magnetic field. When the external magnetic field is removed, the magnetism of paramagnetic substances will additionally disappear. One of the typical materials is iron-oxide nanoparticles, and they are used in microrobotic operation and targeted delivery procedures [43, 44]. Paramagnetic particles have mutually adjustable interactions that provide a mechanism for organizing them into complex patterns. According to the formation mechanism of magnetic field-driven microrobots, they are divided into three types: magnetic interaction-induced swarm, hydrodynamic interaction-induced swarm, and weakly-interacted swarm.

(1) Magnetic Interaction-Induced Swarm. The magnetic agent-agent interactions govern the formation of the magnetic interaction-induced, and the magnetic agent-agent interactions can be controlled by the input magnetic field. For a single magnetic agent, its induced magnetic moment $\mathbf{m}$ and the field gradient $\nabla\mathbf{B}$ determine the subjected magnetic force $\mathbf{F}$, as

$$\mathbf{F} = \nabla(\mathbf{m} \cdot \mathbf{B}) \tag{1.1}$$

where the materials and volume of the agent determine the magnetic moment $\mathbf{m}$, as

$$\mathbf{m} = \frac{3V}{\mu_0}\left(\frac{\mu - \mu_0}{\mu + 2\mu_0}\right)\mathbf{B} \tag{1.2}$$

where μ is the magnetic permeability, μ_0 is the permeability of free space, and V is the volume of the magnetic materials. In the process of swarm formation, multiple agents gradually gather, and each agent is subjected to magnetic forces from other magnetic agents [54]. By simplifying two agents into two magnetic dipoles ($\mathbf{m}_i$, $\mathbf{m}_j$ located at $\mathbf{P}_i$ and $\mathbf{P}_j$), the magnetic force between them is

$$\mathbf{f}_{ij} = \frac{3\mu_0}{4\pi\|\mathbf{r}_{ij}\|^4}\left((\hat{\mathbf{r}}_{ij}^T\mathbf{m}_j)\mathbf{m}_i + (\hat{\mathbf{r}}_{ij}^T\mathbf{m}_i)\mathbf{m}_j + (\mathbf{m}_i^T\mathbf{m}_j - 5(\hat{\mathbf{r}}_{ij}^T\mathbf{m}_i)(\hat{\mathbf{r}}_{ij}^T\mathbf{m}_j))\hat{\mathbf{r}}_{ij}\right) \tag{1.3}$$

where $\mathbf{r}_{ij} = \mathbf{P}_i - \mathbf{P}_j$, and $\hat{\mathbf{r}}$ is the unit vector between the two dipoles.

Rotating magnetic fields have been applied to introduce interactions between agents. A typical in-plane rotating field is expressed as $\mathbf{B}(t) = B[\cos(2\pi ft)\hat{\mathbf{x}} - \sin(2\pi ft)\hat{\mathbf{y}}]$, where B is the field strength and f is the frequency. During the actuating process, the magnetic force $\mathbf{f}_{ij}$ between microrobots changes, *i.e.*, becomes maximally attractive when $\mathbf{m}_i$, $\mathbf{m}_j$ are parallel to $\mathbf{r}_{ij}$ while repulsive with the two moments normal to $\mathbf{r}_{ij}$. From the point of view of average time, the interaction becomes attraction, resulting in the aggregation of magnetic microrobots (Figure 1.1a) [45]. The paramagnetic particles can self-assemble into a circular rotating pattern when a rotating magnetic field is present [55]. When the external magnetic field is removed, the dipole-dipole interactions will disappear, which will lead to the disassociation of the assembled pattern. In addition to the direct interactions between particles, the microrobotic pattern formed by the interaction between particle chains under the action of precession magnetic field has been confirmed (Figure 1.1b) [46]. The magnetic attraction between particles forms particle chains (Eq. (1.3)), and balancing the magnetic dipolar attraction and multipolar repulsion between particle chains forms the swarm. The precession angle of input field plays an important role in regulating

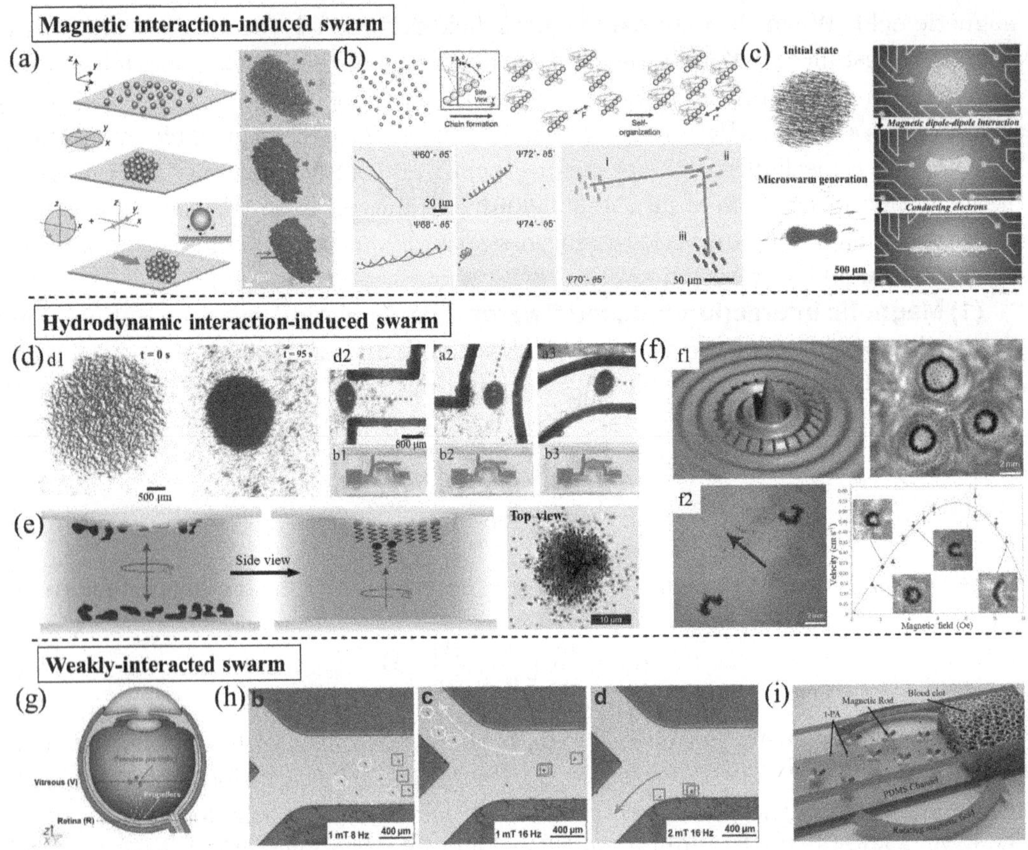

Figure 1.1 Magnetically driven microrobotic swarms. (a) A rotating magnetic field propels a colloidal carpet magnetically. Reproduced with permission from reference [45]. (b) Formation and navigation of a self-organized mobile microswarm driven by a precessing magnetic field. Reproduced with permission from reference [46]. (c) Ant bridge-shaped microswarm of conductive nanoparticles actuated under an oscillating field. Reproduced with permission from reference [47]. (d) Vortex-like rotating microswarm, which are formed by hydrodynamic interactions between nanoparticle chains, and it sails in a semicircular channel. Reproduced with permission from reference [48]. (e) At the air-liquid interface, helical microrobots form a circular pattern. Reproduced with permission from reference [49]. (f) (f1) The self-induced circular standing waves at the liquid-liquid interface with an alternating magnetic field form magnetic asters. (f2) Swarm navigation is realized by adding a static field in the plane. Reproduced with permission from reference [50]. (g) In vitreous fluid driving of helical robots. Reproduced with permission from reference [51]. (h) The surface coating realizes the selective control of two groups of helical microrobots. Reproduced with permission from reference [52]. (i) A swarm of magnetic rods moves toward the blood clot in a PDMS channel. Reproduced with permission from reference [53].

the magnetic dipole interaction. The mean interaction between $\mathbf{m}_i$ and $\mathbf{m}_j$ over a cycle is expressed as [56]

$$\mathbf{F}_m = -\frac{3\mu_0 \mathbf{m}_i \mathbf{m}_j}{4\pi \|\mathbf{r}_{ij}\|^4}\left(\frac{3\cos^2\varphi - 1}{2}\right) \tag{1.4}$$

where φ is the precession angle to the rotating axis. Eq. (1.4) indicates that the magnetic interaction can be both repulsion ($0° < \varphi < 54.7°$) and attraction ($54.7° < \varphi < 90°$). When $\varphi = 54.7°$ (magic angle), the average dipolar interaction is zero. In Figure 1.1b, when the φ is adjusted in a range of 68° to 72° to obtain attraction between particle chains, where the pairwise distance converges to a dynamic stability range. When $\varphi < 61.5°$, in addition to the dipole-dipole interaction, the dipole-hexapole interaction dominates the repulsive multipole interaction, which results in long-range attraction and short-range repulsion [57].

Nanometer-scale magnetic building blocks can also be aggregated into swarm states. The interaction between nanoparticle chains forms a banded microswarm driven by the oscillating field (Figure 1.1c) [47, 58]. The input parameters affect the magnetic chain-chain interactions, *i.e.*, field strength, frequency, and field ratio. Field ratio is defined as the ratio between the alternating and the constant fields. The main two torques are magnetic torque Γ_m and hydrodynamic drag torque Γ_d from viscous fluids. By balancing them, we can form an actuated particle chain in a low Reynolds number regime. The total magnetic moment applied to the center of the chain is calculated by adding the torques of adjacent particles, and the chain is composed of N particles with radius a, as

$$\Gamma_m = \frac{3\mu_0 m^2(t)}{4\pi}\sin(2\theta)\sum_{i=1}^{N/2}\left(2r_i \sum_{j=1,i\neq j}^{N/2}\frac{1}{r_{ij}^4}\right) \tag{1.5}$$

where r_i is the distance between ith particle and center of the chain and $m^2(t)$ represents the induced dipole moment of a particle. The viscous resistance of a chain with angular velocity $\omega(t)$ is estimated as [59]

$$\Gamma_d = \frac{8\pi a^3}{3}\frac{N^3}{\ln(\frac{N}{2}) + \frac{2.4}{N}}\eta\omega(t) \tag{1.6}$$

where η is the viscosity of the surrounding fluid. Mason number is defined as the ratio between the two torques ($R_T = \Gamma_d/\Gamma_m$) and is applied to estimate the length of chains. If $R_T < 1$, the chain is stabilized by the stronger magnetic torque. If beyond unity, fragmentation will occur due to the strong viscous drag. By considering a critical situation that the two moments balance each other before the chain breaks ($R_T = 1$), the length of the chain can be calculated ($L = 2Na$). In the process of swarm formation, through time-dependent chain-chain interactions, the nanoparticle chains are actively assembled, disassembled, and gathered. Finally, we obtain a ribbon-like swarm pattern which contains millions of nanoparticles (Figure 1.1c).

(2) Hydrodynamic Interaction-Induced Swarm. The interaction of fluid dynamics plays an important role in the formation of microrobotic systems. Driving building blocks can disrupt the surrounding fluid and deform interfaces (such as air-liquid interface, and liquid-liquid interface), further affecting collective states and pattern-environment interactions. Based on interaction exerted through the medium (*e.g.*, hydrodynamic flow and interface), the microrobotic swarms are formed, and they are categorized as hydrodynamic interaction-induced swarms. In a low-Reynolds-number environment, there is a vortex generated around a rotating nanoparticle. It can produce a long-range attraction to adjacent chains and shortens the distances between chains. The two vortices rotate coaxially and merge after reaching a critical distance, resulting in the aggregation of nanoparticles. After reaching the equilibrium state, the circular pattern is gradually obtained (Figure 1.1d1) [48]. The vortex-based analysis can also be used to study the collective state within the swarm. In the core area of the swarm, the vorticity will not decay because of the driving of the external rotating magnetic field [60]. So the vorticity (ξ_z) and velocity (u_θ) distributions inside the vortex core become

$$\xi_z = \frac{\Gamma_0}{\pi R^2} \quad (r < R) \tag{1.7}$$

$$u_\theta = \frac{\Gamma_0 r}{2\pi R^2} \quad (r < R) \tag{1.8}$$

where Γ_0 is the circulation of the vortex, and R is the radius of the vortex core. Because of the viscosity of the fluid, the vorticity attenuates with the distance to the core. In the range of low-Reynolds-number, the inertia forces can be ignored. Outside the vortex core, the vorticity and velocity distributions become

$$\xi_z(r,t) = \frac{\Gamma_0}{4\pi\nu t} \exp\left(\frac{-r^2}{4\nu t}\right) \quad (r > R) \tag{1.9}$$

$$u_\theta = \frac{\Gamma_0}{2\pi r}\left(1 - \exp\left(\frac{-r^2}{4\nu t}\right)\right) \quad (r > R) \tag{1.10}$$

where ν is the kinematic viscosity of fluid. Therefore, the inner interactions between the core region and nanoparticles decide the size of a vortex-like swarm. The particle chains rotate from the self-center and run around the swarm center at the same time. This swarm induced by hydrodynamic interaction is very different from that controlled by magnetic interaction, although both of them are produced under the control of a rotating magnetic field. Because of the strong magnetic attraction between building blocks, the swarm controlled by magnetic interaction plays the role of a rolling disk. The velocity distribution can be estimated as $u_i = 2\pi f R_{ci}$, where R_{ci} is the distance between the ith particle and the center of the pattern. A set of helical microrobots driven by a rotating magnetic field swim upwards, reaching the top air-liquid interface and forming a co-rotating swarm pattern (Figure 1.1e). Here, the rotation–translation coupling dominates the hydrodynamic effect [61], which is similar to the dynamic self-assembly of spherical particles [62]. By tuning the hydrodynamic interactions, the collective state can be tuned. The strong hydrodynamic repulsion between the rotating chains of ferromagnetic microparticle chains leads to the formation of dynamic lattices rather than a high-concentrated aggregated state [63]. From an alternating magnetic field, the vortices can also be induced, in which the particle density of assembly pattern is adjusted by adjusting the field parameters

[64]. The special place for the formation of swarms is the interface, in which capillary interaction plays an important role [65]. Actuated with the aid of an alternating magnetic field, microparticles form dynamic asters at a liquid-liquid interface (Figure 1.1f1) [50]. The formation of asters depends on the induced hydrodynamic streaming flows and the magnetic repulsion between chains. The chains respond in the external field and oscillate periodically, and a circular wave excited by the chain leads to the formation of chains in a radially ordered form. These chains are distributed on different slopes of the same wave, forming a pattern similar to that of an aster. Compared with swarm formation at the air-liquid interface, the existence of the liquid at the top greatly changes the internal hydrodynamic interactions and force balance, resulting in a very different dynamic pattern [66].

(3) Weakly-Interacted Swarm. If the interactions between agents are too susceptible, and they cannot have an effect on the movement of one another, then the agent in a microswarm will go independently. We classified the swarm as a weakly-interacted swarm. A group of helical microrobots which are driven by a rotating magnetic field move through the vitreous fluids (Figure 1.1g) [51]. Because the separation distance between microrobots is large, neither the magnetic nor hydrodynamic interactions are enough to affect the motion behavior of other robots. The robots move independently and gradually reach the retina. The surface coating can affect the motion of a group of helical microrobots (Figure 1.1h) [52]. Driven by a rotating field below the step-out frequency, robots with different coatings (including hydrophobic and hydrophilic) move at the same speed ratio. At this time, they show different motion behaviors. By increasing the frequency to make it higher than the step-out frequency, robots with different surface coatings can be selectively controlled. A set of magnetic rods moves independently toward the fluid-clot interface in order to enhance the mass transfer (Figure 1.1i) [53]. The use of collective nanorods can increase the rate of thrombolysis mediated by tissue plasminogen activator (tPA) by a factor of two, suggesting that collective mircroreagents can increase individual function.

(4) Swarm Navigation Under Magnetic Field. This part studies the controlled movement of the swarms to perform target navigation and material delivery. One of the swarm locomotion mechanisms depends on the excitation near a boundary (such as substrate and sidewall) because the drag coefficient increases as an object approaches a wall [67]. The different hydrodynamic interactions between different parts of swarming agents and a boundary lead to the force asymmetry, resulting in movement [68]. Driven by a rotating magnetic field, rotating nanoparticles in the XZ-plane are coupled to the substrate hydrodynamically, converting the rotation into translational motion (Figure 1.1a). In the process of the locomotion, the attractive dipole interactions induced by the field along Y-direction avoid the separation of particles, and the whole swarm pattern as an entity can be actuated. The above-mentioned motion can be realized by using the radiation force induced by the sound field to migrate the rotating particle swarm to the channel wall [55]. Except for the rotation of the particles, all the particles rotate around the center of the pattern. So the rotation of the entire pattern breaks the symmetry of movement, which leads to translational motion. The movement of building blocks may affect their adjacent building blocks. The fluid asymmetry between the two ends of the chain leads to the movement of the chain. At the same time, the pairwise movement of chains is mainly influenced by the fluid from other precession chains (Figure 1.1b). For the two-dimensional swarm pattern in the in-plane dynamic field, the motion can be induced by increasing the out-of-plane static field component (Figure 1.1c, d). The rotation/oscillation plane of the nanoparticle chains in the swarm is inclined to the substrate by a small angle (pitch angle), which leads to the translational motion of the chains. Meanwhile, the interaction of magnetic force and hydrodynamic force between chains enables pattern navigation to be carried out in a controlled manner (Figure 1.1d2).

In addition to boundary-enabled locomotion, breaking the symmetry of pattern-induced flow enables swarm navigation. The balance between magnetic interactions and chain-induced flows determines the shape of an axisymmetric aster. Therefore, the flow is symmetric and the observed motion can be ignored. Adding an in-plane static magnetic field has broken the hydrodynamic symmetry (Figure 1.1f2). The opening of pattern causes the breakdown of the axial symmetry of hydrodynamic flow, where the pattern locomotion is controlled by the direction of the in-plane field. The in-plane field strength leading to different open states determines the motion speed. Pattern deformation increases with increasing field strength (0–10 Oe), which results in higher actuation speeds. However, due to the fully open pattern (10–22 Oe), the flow becomes symmetric and the velocity gradually decreases to zero. For the non-axisymmetric swarm pattern, the non-magnetic beads are placed on one side of the swarm pattern, which can break the symmetry of the flow [69]. This method can also introduce motion into the swarm pattern. However, the direction of movement is difficult to control. Navigation of weakly interacting swarms depends on the movement of building blocks. The helical microrobots display its motion by generating non-reciprocating motion under rotating magnetic fields. One advantage of helical microrobots is that it does not need boundary conditions and can move in three dimensions (Figure 1.1e, g). The density of helical microrobots significantly affects the collective state. High concentrations lead to stronger interactions between them and dynamically stable patterns can be obtained. Magnetic collections can also occur within swarms [70]. In contrast, helices with relatively low concentrations show independent motion (Figure 1.1h). For building blocks that have no propulsion ability or control the driving direction, such as a swarm of rotating nanorods, magnetic field gradients can be applied to guide the movement (Figure 1.1i).

1.2.2 Light-Driven Microswarms

Light has been used to drive photoresponsors because it provides adjustable radiation energy for wireless and long-distance transmission. In order to introduce interactions between agents, light-driven building blocks rely on photoactive materials. The light induces a solute concentration gradient in specific directions around photoactive substances, such as AgCl and TiO_2 particles, TiO_2/Pt and TiO_2/Au Janus particles.

(1) Homogeneous Building Blocks. When exposed to ultraviolet (UV) light, 1 μm-diameter AgCl particles with a diameter of 1 μm in DI water move at a speed of up to 100 μm/s because of the asymmetric photolysis [71]. This asymmetric rate creates an electrolyte gradient around the particles, resulting in self-diffusiophoresis similar to the diffusiophoretic movement of particles, as

$$4\,\mathrm{AgCl} + 2\,\mathrm{H_2O} \xrightarrow{hv,Ag+} 4\,\mathrm{Ag} + 4\,\mathrm{H^+} + 4\,\mathrm{Cl^-} + \mathrm{O_2}. \tag{1.11}$$

Electrolyte gradient is caused by the production of H^+ and Cl^-, and it leads to the motion of AgCl particles. The particles gather gradually, but the physical contact between particles is avoided because of short-range repulsion of electrostatic interaction (Figure 1.2a1). By adding SiO_2 particles into the system, the long-range attraction diffusion swimming interaction is studied experimentally. In this system, the passive SiO_2 particles are gathered round the AgCl particles and showcase predator–prey-like conduct (Figure 1.2a2). Janus particle is a special kind of particle, and its surface has two or more different physical properties. Their asymmetric structure or functionalization enables them to drive and behave collectively under external fields. Driven by laser (wavelength 532 nm), graphite/SiO_2 Janus particles showed propulsive force in the mixture of water and 2,6-lutidine [72]. The carbon coating hemispheres absorb light and undergo local delamination because of the thermal effect, in which the delamination-induced electrophoretic force pushes particles. In this quasi-two-dimensional suspension, low particle densities form clusters, phase transitions to larger clusters, and diluted gas phases occur at higher densities. Clusters are formed through a self-trapping mechanism: particles are blocked by head-on collisions because of the persistence of their orientations. The probability of collisions between the cluster and other particles increases with a higher driving speed, resulting in larger cluster sizes (Figure 1.2b). By controlling the UV radiation, a reversible gather-spreading behavior of a group of SiO_2/TiO_2 Janus particles is proved (Figure 1.2c) [73]. A similar behavior is observed in a system composed of pure SiO_2 and TiO_2 particles, in which SiO_2 component acts as a surface pump to repel the TiO_2 particles. However, it is not easy to control the colloidal patterns of these swarming in a controllable way. In a monovalent salt solution (concentration gradient: ∇c), the particle velocity (U) driven by the electrolyte gradient is expressed as [78]

$$\begin{aligned} U =& \frac{\nabla c}{c_0}\left[\left(\frac{D_c - D_a}{D_c + D_a}\right)\left(\frac{k_{\mathrm{B}}T}{e}\right)\frac{\epsilon(\xi_p - \xi_w)}{\eta}\right] \\ &+ \frac{\nabla c}{c_0}\left[\left(\frac{2\epsilon k_{\mathrm{B}}^2 T^2}{\eta e^2}\right)\left(\ln(1-\gamma_w^2) - \ln(1-\gamma_p^2)\right)\right] \end{aligned} \tag{1.12}$$

where c_0 is the bulk concentrations of ions, D_c and D_a are the diffusion coefficients of the cation and anion, k_{B} and T are Boltzmann constant and absolute temperature, respectively. e is the charge of an electron. ϵ is the dielectric permittivity of the solution, η is the viscosity, and ξ_p, ξ_w are the zeta potentials of the particle and wall, respectively. The above analysis shows that it is difficult to control the motion direction of a self-diffusiophoresis particle. The use of a patterned substrate and moving light spot (source) facilitates the swarm navigation. Sagués *et al.* have proved that the use of functional substrates makes the formation of light-driven swarms and controllable navigation possible [74]. The photosensitive azo-silane monomolecular is *cis*-configuration (planar) and *trans*-configuration (homeotropic) under UV and

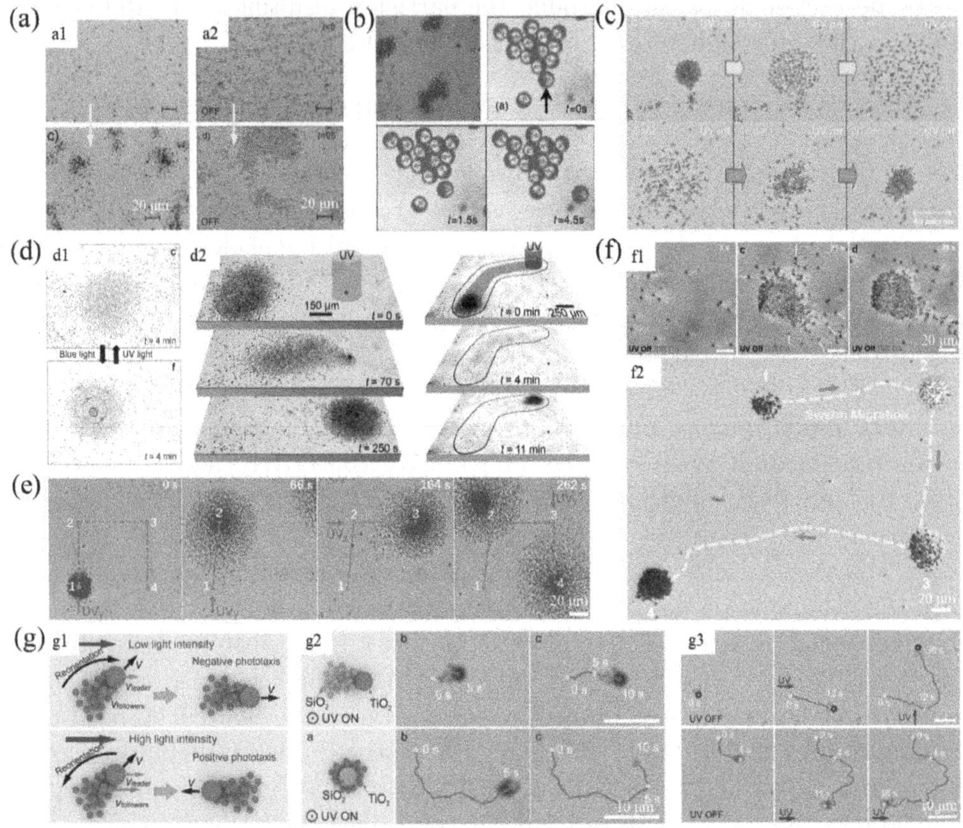

Figure 1.2 Light-driven microrobotic swarms. (a) (a1) The previous deionized water had AgCl particles in it, and then it was subjected to 90 seconds of ultraviolet radiation. (a2) Predator–prey behavior of AgCl particles (darker objects) and silica spheres under UV light. Reproduced with permission from reference [71]. (b) Assembly of active Janus particles under laser light. Reproduced with permission from reference [72]. (c) Reversible collective behaviors of SiO_2/TiO_2 Janus particles in water. Under ultraviolet irradiation, the particles repel each other, and under no ultraviolet irradiation, the particles tend to merge. Reproduced with permission from reference [73]. (d) Formation of polystyrene microparticle-based swarm: (d1) colloidal aster and vortex driven by light and alternating electric field. (d2) Navigating the swarm by changing the positions of the UV spots. Reproduced with permission from reference [74]. (e) A swarm of TiO_2 micromotors travels along the designed path under pulsed ultraviolet radiation. Reproduced with permission from reference [75]. (f) Formation and navigation of a swarm of TiO_2/Pt Janus particles under NIR irradiation. Reproduced with permission from reference [76]. (g) Light-driven microswarms with similar master-slave structures. Reproduced with permission from reference [77].

blue light, respectively. Under the action of an alternating electric field, polystyrene (PS) particles form aster- and vortex-like swarm patterns between the photosensitive plate and the non-photosensitive plate (Figure 1.2d1). Due to the switchable *trans* and *cis* isomers, the conversion between the two patterns is performed by changing the radiation type (UV, blue light). There are two ways to guide the swarms, one is to change the position of the light spot, and the other is to move the irradiation area along the pre-designed path (Figure 1.2d2). Particles move to new positions in a leader-follower way, not as a strongly interacting whole.

In addition to adjusting the position of the light spot, swarm navigation can also be performed by programming light radiation [75]. When UV light is applied laterally, the TiO_2 particles tend to move in the same direction in the spreading state. When the lights are turned off, the motion stops and becomes a random Brownian motion. The scattered particles then move away from the light source and gather into a circular pattern centered on the new position (Figure 1.2e) [75]. So, pulsed UV light with repetitive on-off cycles can be used to drive the swarm along a straight line with a diffusion-reaggregation state. With UV irradiation in different side directions, the pattern shows the expansion-aggregation behavior that the center moves to X or Y direction. In addition to UV light-driven collective motion, Deng *et al.* also proposed that near-infrared (NIR) light-induced convection can induce swarm formation and navigation [76]. The temperature in the liquid medium exposed to NIR increases, resulting in convective flow through exposed and unexposed areas. The TiO_2/Pt particles are resisted in this flow and move toward the center of the exposed region (Figure 1.2f1). The formation of particle swarms is controlled by the electrostatic attraction between particles and the repulsive force of diffusion electrophoresis. Navigating the swarm pattern by tracking the exposed area can be achieved by applying the positive phototaxis behavior (Figure 1.2f2). The movement speed of UV light source will also affect the aggregation state of silica particles [79]. If the speed of the light source is lower than the critical value, the particles follow the UV spot at a constant speed. Because the response of particles with different components and diameters is different, this method can be used to extract particles from mixed ensemble.

(2) Heterogeneous Building Blocks. Light-driven hierarchical microswarms are formed by multiple types of building blocks, and they show multi-responsiveness and have the potential to construct synergistic micromachines. Driven by an alternating current electric field, dielectric particles with different sizes and dielectric properties form leader-follower-like swarm patterns, and these dielectric microparticles are controlled by the electrohydrodynamic flow [77]. TiO_2 microparticles form microswarms with diameters of 2 μm (large) and 0.5 μm (small), which show switchable phototaxis, that is, negative and positive phototaxis with low (4 mW/cm^2) and high (500 mW/cm^2) lateral UV intensities, respectively (Figure 1.2g1). The particles are exposed to UV radiation, and then the particles show negative phototaxis by non-electrolyte self-diffusion electrophoresis [80]. Under the low UV intensity, the asymmetric photocatalytic reactions on the particle surface make the particle swarm pattern far away from the light source. The larger particle shows a higher phototaxis and becomes the leader of the pattern. The gathered small particles have a higher phototaxis speed due to increasing the light intensity. The electrohydrodynamic flows stabilize the whole pattern, and it tends to be consistent with the direction of light. So, swarm navigation can be carried out by adjusting the direction of light. By using different particles to form patterns, different collective light responses are displayed. Under vertically irradiated UV light, the small SiO_2 particles follow the large TiO_2 particles because of the negligible UV response (Figure 1.2g2). Due to the repulsion of diffusion between particles, the pattern becomes symmetrical by changing the diameters of two particles. Under this condition, the movement is controlled by switching on/off UV rays, and the two patterns show opposite phototaxis by applying lateral UV irradiation (Figure 1.2g3).

1.2.3 Acoustic Wave-Driven Microswarms

The use of acoustic waves to drive tiny agents in micro/nanoscale provides a wireless, non-contact method for the implementation of microrobotic drive and micromanipulation tasks [84, 85]. In recent research, piezoelectric sensors generate acoustic waves. Micrometer-scale particles in the acoustic field are subjected to the force of acoustic radiation [86]. Because the force of standing waves on the object is much greater than that of traveling waves, the current research mainly focuses on the actuating and micromanipulation driven by standing waves [87]. The acoustic force on an object can be expressed as [88]

$$F_a = -\left(\frac{\pi p_0^2 V \beta_w}{2\lambda}\right) \Phi(\beta, \rho) \sin(2kd) \tag{1.13}$$

where p_0 is the pressure amplitude, V is the volume of the object, λ is the wavelength, k is the wave number, and d is the distance between the particle and the node or the belly of the wave. $\Phi(\beta, \rho)$ represents the relationship between the density and compressibility between the object and the medium, which is $\Phi(\beta, \rho) = (5\rho_c - 2\rho_w)/(2\rho_c + 2\rho_w) - \beta_c/\beta_w$, where ρ_c and ρ_w are the density of object and medium, β_c and β_w are the compressibility of the object and medium, respectively. The expression shows that objects whose size is less than the wavelength are difficult to control because the acoustic force is proportional to the size of objects.

Under the action of acoustic waves, Au-Ru microrods are suspended to the middle plane. In the plane where the standing wave is formed by ultrasound (US), that is, the nodal plane, the microrods show switchable aggregation and random motion, which leads to a dispersed state with an annular pattern (Figure 1.3a) [81]. A single rod rotates around the chain axis at a frequency of kilohertz and moves along the chain at the same time. After the acoustic power is turned off, the swarm pattern is dispersed and microrods move in a disordered trajectory. The reversible collective behaviors of Pt-Au nanowires in hydrogen peroxide solution have also been proved [82]. The catalytic nanowires show autonomous motion in solution, which proves the diffusion state induced by electrophoretic propulsion (Figure 1.3b1). The standing waves are generated by the acoustic field, and they can form high-density patterns. At the same time, the pressure gradient drives the Pt-Au nanowires to move to the low-pressure region. The acoustic force is divided into two forces: the primary radiation force and secondary radiation force, in which the secondary radiation force is caused by the acoustic waves re-scattered by the nanowires, and it increases with the decrease of the distance between inter-agents [89]. The formation of circular nanowire patterns is mainly driven by the horizontal components of primary radiation force and secondary radiation force. The agent-agent interaction caused by secondary radiation force can be attractive or repulsive [90]. Therefore, by turning on and off ultrasonic waves, the aggregation and diffusion of nanowires can be controlled (Figure 1.3b2). By adjusting the acoustic frequency, the position of the pressure node can be changed, and the change of the position of the pressure node can further realize the movement of the swarm pattern. The swarm pattern moves to a new location at a speed of about ~45 μm/s. At the same time, the swarm pattern keeps the circular shape because of the secondary radiation force (Figure 1.3b3). However, it is difficult to navigate the swarm pattern along a pre-designed path, because it is difficult to directly define the low-voltage area by adjusting the input frequency. The acoustic collection effect is also reflected in the formation of liquid metal microswarm. The stripes of EGaIn nanorods are formed at a frequency of 730 kHz. By modulating the frequency to 728 kHz, these stripes gradually merged into larger stripes, and a dandelion-like pattern is observed (Figure 1.3c1) [83]. Finally, Decreasing the frequency to 680 kHz can disperse the swarm pattern. The patterns of sound pressure field vary with the input frequency, which represents the distribution of primary acoustic radiation forces caused by the standing waves. The nanorods in the node plane are subjected to the force along the acoustic energy gradient, which results in different mobile frequency-dependent patterns (Figure 1.3c2).

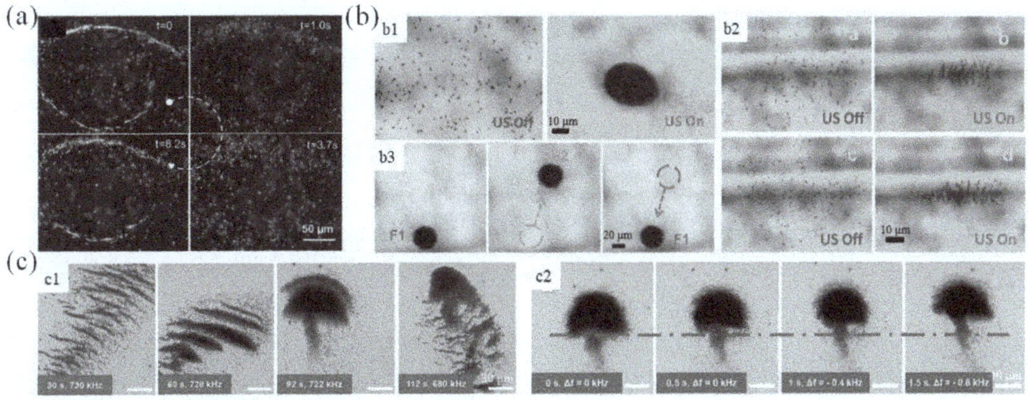

Figure 1.3 The swarm and collective behavior of microrobot under sound field. (a) The reversible aggregation and diffusion collective behavior of a set of Au–Ru microrods on the acoustic nodal plane (ultrasound off at t = 0 and on at t = 3.7 s). Reproduced with permission from reference [81]. (b) (b1) The diffusion and aggregation behavior of Au-Pt nanowires driven by sound field, and (b2) the reversible aggregation and diffusion of Au-Pt nanowires by turning on and off the sound field. (b3) moving the swarm pattern by adjusting the input frequency of the sound field. Reproduced with permission from reference [82]. (c) The formation (c1) and motion (c2) of an acoustically driven EGaIn nanorod swarm. The movement of the swarm can be realized by adjusting the input frequency. Reproduced with permission from reference [83].

1.2.4 Electric Field-Driven Microswarms

According to the interaction between components based on electrostatic force and field-induced electrohydrodynamics (EHD), we divide the microrobot swarms driven by electric field into two types. The attraction or repulsion force is mainly determined by the charge of the agent as well as the distance between them, and the repulsion force can be realized by inducing EHD flow. The electrostatic imbalance on the building blocks provides a basic mechanism for different collective behaviors to realize the microswarm induced by electrostatic force. Yan *et al.* reported a strategy to adjust the collective states of Janus particles by adjusting the frequency of the input electric field [91]. The local field-induced ion flows near the particle surface have different orders of magnitudes in two hemispheres, that is, a hemispheric silica sphere coated with metal (Figure 1.4a). Via the charge-induced electrophoresis in the gas state, these Janus particles initially exhibit self-propulsion [94]. Due to the negligible dipole interactions and strong ion shielding effects between them, the particles move isotropic [95]. With the increase in frequency, the stronger dipole interaction affects the collective behavior, in which the repulsion between the metal hemispheres dominates the formation of patterns (swarm state). By further increasing the input frequency, the opposite dipoles of the two hemispheres (metallic and dielectric) produce attractive interactions between particles, which is similar to the particle chain formation in the magnetic field drive system (active chain state) [96]. In addition

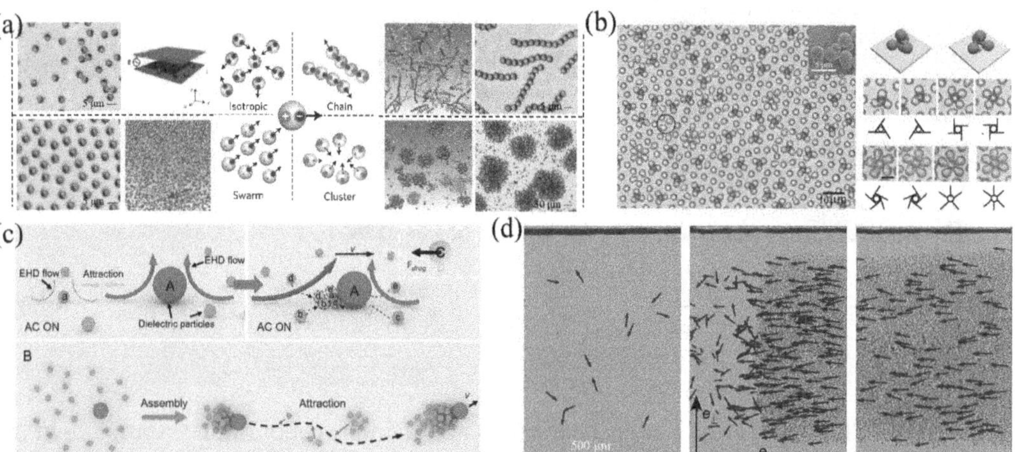

Figure 1.4 The swarm and collective behavior of microrobot under electric field. (a) Collective behaviors of Janus colloidal spheres which have unbalanced, off-centered charges. Reproduced with permission from reference [91]. (b) Chiral colloidal structures formed by asymmetric dimers under AC electric fields. Reproduced with permission from reference [92]. (c) Schematic diagram of the assembly, motion, and growth of a graded microswarm of electrohydrodynamic interactions induced by an AC electric field. Reproduced with permission from reference [77]. (d) The collective motion of rolling particles, from isotropic gas to propagation zones and uniformly polar liquid. Reproduced with permission from reference [93].

to regulating the frequency-dependent dipole interactions, the dipole interaction is regulated by adding salt to the medium to achieve the particle aggregation (cluster phase). Under the action of the electric field, the particle polarization with geometric asymmetry provides different collective states. Colloidal dimers with different geometric ratios form chiral and achiral structures, which are determined by the in-plane dipole repulsion between petals and out-of-plane attraction between central dimer and surrounding petals (Figure 1.4b) [92]. The assembled structure could be affected by the number of dimers and the ratio between lobe radii. Most dimers with more than five are achiral structures, and all structures with four or fewer petals are chiral. But as the radius ratio approaches 0 or 1, the chirality disappears. The rotational propulsion of assembled structures relies on the imbalance hydrodynamics generated by cluster-based chirality.

Driven by an alternating current electric field, the induced directed EHD flow around particle leads to the self-assembly process. Yeh and colleagues showed the EHD-driven assembly to form ordered colloidal aggregrates [97]. The velocity around a dielectric particle with radius R and polarization coefficient K is expressed as [98]

$$U_{EHD} \sim \frac{C}{\mu}\left(\frac{K' + \varpi K''}{1+\varpi^2}\right)\left(\frac{3(r/R)}{2\left[1+(r/R)^2\right]^{5/2}}\right) \tag{1.14}$$

where $C = \epsilon\epsilon_0(E_p/2H)^2\kappa H$, H is the separation distance between electrodes, E_p is the amplitude and ϖ is the frequency. $\epsilon\epsilon_0$ is permittivity and μ is viscosity of medium, and r is the distance between particle and the affected region. The above analysis shows that the types of particles have a great influence on U_{EHD}, and this indicates that the combination of different particles may lead to unbalanced EHD flows and particle propulsion. As Guan *et al.* reported, they applied microparticles of different sizes and dielectric properties to form electric field-driven hierarchical microswarms (Figure 1.4c) [77]. The particles with the same size and dielectric properties tend to aggregate each other, while the clustered clusters do not show propulsion because of the symmetric EHD flow. If new particles of different sizes or dielectric properties are added to the system, this symmetry will be broken, which will lead to the net propulsion of the newly formed microswarm. In the process of movement, the swarm attracts and absorbs new particles through EHD and shows coordinated movement. Hydrodynamic interaction between agents can also be introduced into the electric field. The charge distribution on the surface of particles is disturbed because an electric field is applied to the insulating particles inside the conductive fluid [93]. The particles are driven to rotate in random directions by the electrostatic torque showing various collective states (Figure 1.4d). The rolling particles show a random rotation direction at the same speed, and form an isotropic gaseous phase at low density. By increasing the particle fraction above the critical value, a macroscopic band is formed and propagates through the isotropic phase at a constant speed, and this is independent of the particle velocity and the amplitude of the external field. By further increasing the particle fraction, a homogeneous polar liquid phase is observed where the heads of the propagating bands catch up to their own tails. The above results indicate that hydrodynamic interactions enable a single particle to perform the directional collective motion.

1.2.5 Hybrid Fields-Driven Microswarms

Microrobotic swarm responding to double stimuli and controlled by mixed external powers is classified as microrobotic swarms driven by mixed field. With more controllability they can adapt to more complex environments. The hybrid power-enabled control strategies usually include an external power to initiate interactions for pattern formation, and another power for pattern navigation or conversion based on the mission requirements and application locations. Combined with magnetic field and acoustic field, the microrobotic swarms driven by hybrid field show switchable collective behaviors (Figure 1.5a) [99]. By controlling the field input, three aggregation states of nanorods are demonstrated, that is, the aggregation of rotational pattern, translational motion, and no stable pattern under hybrid field, magnetic field, and acoustic field. The aggregation behavior induced by the acoustic field can use a similar mechanism [82]. The the attractive interactions between nanorods and the driven torque of pattern rotation are provided by the rotating magnetic field. Thus, the swarm pattern is governed by the relationship between the magnetic and acoustic forces. At the boundary of an equilibrium swarm, the magnetic and acoustic forces are equal, forming a circular-pattern swarm. The secondary radiation force causes the further gathering effect. The switchable and reversible behavior shows that the hybrid driving method can provide new swarm patterns and navigation methods, and is also beneficial to the delivery of goals in different environments. As Ahmed *et al.* reported, a rotating swarm of magnetic microparticles formed under a rotating magnetic field, and the particles are moved to the boundary bt the acoustic radiation force on the swarm [55]. The boundary allows the conversion from the rotation to translation, and the pattern can move along the boundary (Figure 1.5b). A small (10 V_{pp}) acoustic force is difficult to affect the whole pattern, in which the weak contact between the microparticles and the wall will lead to drifting motion. Increasing the swarm-boundary contact (20 V_{pp}) and the rotating frequency input will lead to a higher translation speed. This hybrid actuation methods may be suitable for movement in the vascular system where the delivery tasks could be performed in a controlled manner.

In addition to the magnetic-acoustic hybrid control strategy, the collective behaviors of Janus microrobots can also be induced by the combination of acoustic power and light illumination (Figure 1.5c) [100]. Driven by the acoustic field, the second-order sound flow generated by the oscillating edge causes the outward motion of the bowl-shaped TiO_2/Au microrobot [104]. Therefore, this motion has nothing to do with the materials (position of the TiO_2 and Au layers). Different from the acoustic driving motion, the self-prediction motion driven by UV light depends on the material, that is, the microrobot moves to the TiO_2 side. Actuated by the acoustic pressure gradient, two groups of Janus microrobots gather at the low-voltage nodes with the outer side facing to the center of the pattern. When the UV light is turned on, the two patterns made up of Janus microrobots with opposite TiO_2 and Au layers show different behaviors: pattern expansion and pattern contraction with the outer layers of Au and TiO_2, respectively. In addition, this optical-modulated aggregation can be controlled by turning the UV light on/off. Palacci and co-workers have shown

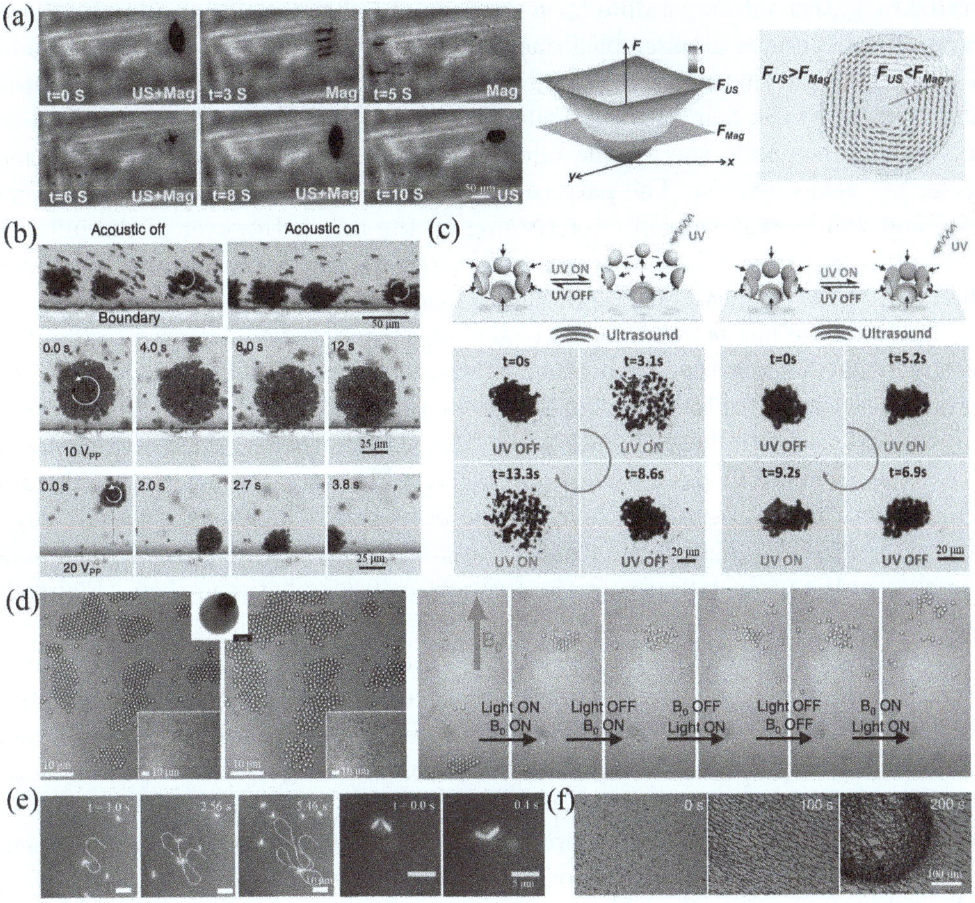

Figure 1.5 Swarm formation and collective motion of microrobots driven by hybrid power. (a) Collective behaviors of magneto-acoustic hybrid microrods under magnetic and acoustic fields. Reproduced with permission from reference [99]. (b) The combined patterns of microparticles migrate to the wall under acoustic field. Reproduced with permission from reference [55]. (c) Optical modulation collective behavior of TiO_2/Au (left) and Au/TiO_2 (right) Janus microbowls under acoustic field. Reproduced with permission from reference [100]. (d) Collective formation and motion of polymer microparticles encapsulated by hematite cubes driven by blue light and mixed light/static magnetic field. Reproduced with permission from reference [101]. (e) Bimetallic nanorods demonstrate assembly and propulsion under acoustic field (left) and magnetic field guidance (right). Reproduced with permission from reference [102]. (f) Collective behavior of magnetic peanut-shaped microparticles under blue light irradiation. Reproduced with permission from reference [103].

hybrid light/magnetic-controlled collective behavior [101]. The polymer microrobot is wrapped with hematite cube, which is partially exposed to the hydrogen peroxide. Under blue light irradiation, due to the decomposition of H_2O_2, a chemical concentration gradient with osmotic and phoretic effects is produced. These microrobots gradually gather into crystallite structures. In the absence of light illumination, the crystallite structures disassembled due to thermal diffusion (Figure 1.5d). By adding a static field (strength: ~1 mT), the rotation diffusion is suppressed, because the arrangement of the hematite cube tilts the direction of the microrobots. Driven by mixed light/magnetic energy, the microcrystal structure remains stable and moves along the field direction. The pattern is decomposed under the drive of a magnetic field and will be reassembled after turning on the lights. However, if the initial separation distance exceeds the critical value, the microrobot will move alone in the direction of the magnetic field and will no longer form a pattern.

The intrinsic magnetic moments of building blocks have been used to induce collective behaviors together with other external powers. The assembly of Au-Ru-Ni nanorods is controlled by the magnetic interactions between the Ni segments without an external magnetic field (Figure 1.5e) [102]. Under the hybrid acoustic/magnetic drive, the assembly mode is warned and behaves like a structure with flexible hinges. This structural changes affect the direction of motion, which leads to a circular trajectory. Under blue light irradiation, peanut-shaped hematite particles are banded together in H_2O_2 solution due to the frequent collisions between them (Figure 1.5f) [103]. The magnetic attraction between particles further stabilizes the ribbon because of the intrinsic magnetic moments. These two researches show that the inherent moment can be used to assist the formation of patterns and even change the mode of collective motion. A recent study by Cui *et al.* shows that the residual magnetization of nanomagnets can be adjusted by a series of magnetization processes [105]. Assembly of modular units with encoded magnetization enables to show complex behaviors. Building blocks with programmable magnetization can be obtained by applying this strategy, especially for building blocks with structural anisotropy. The microrobotic swarms composed of these 'smart agents' can obtain more controllability and complex behaviors under the magnetic field-hybrid control method and show better adaptability to complex environments.

1.3 SWARM TRANSFORMATION UNDER DIFFERENT DRIVEN FIELDS

In the context of navigation within confined environments, swarm transformation plays a crucial role. It enables enhanced adaptability and the ability to reconfigure formations in narrow and restricted conditions. By adjusting the input field, the interactions between building blocks or the interactions between the agents and the surrounding medium can be fine-tuned. This adjustment allows for greater control and optimization of the swarm's behavior in order to navigate effectively in constrained spaces. As reported by Yu *et al.*, input frequency of the rotating field can significantly affect the collective state of a nanoparticle swarm [48]. Increasing the frequency above a critical value results in particle chains within the vortex-like microswarm exhibiting a step-out behavior. This step-out behavior is characterized by decreased vortex inward forces. Consequently, the pattern of the swarm becomes unstable and transitions into a spreading state (Figure 1.6a). This spreading state can be utilized to introduce interactions between multiple microswarms. However, when there is a relatively large distance between two swarms, the interaction may be

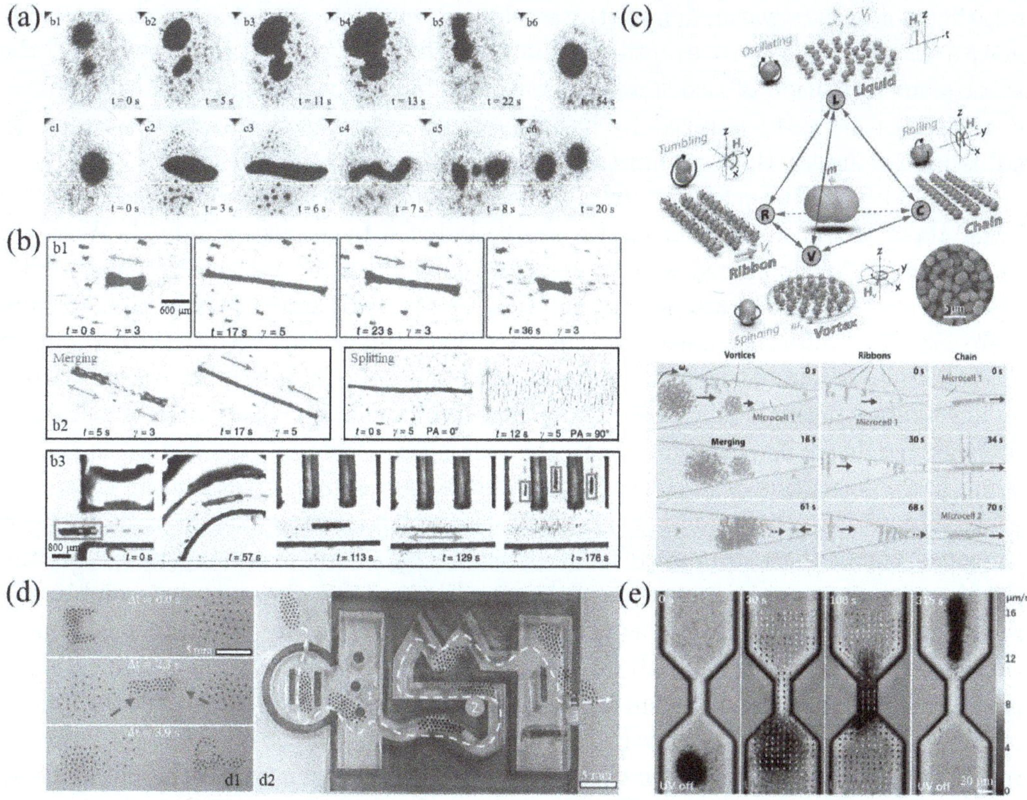

Figure 1.6 Active and passive pattern transformation. (a) Spreading and merging of nanoparticle-based vortex-like microswarm under different input frequencies. Reproduced with permission from reference [48]. (b) Transformation and navigation of a nanoparticle microswarm. (b1) Reversible elongation under different field ratio γ. (b2) Merging and splitting of the microswarm. (b3) Navigation in a semi-circular channel. The microswarm exhibits transformation and splitting to access the target region. Reproduced with permission from reference [58]. (c) Four collective states of peanut-like microparticles and their transformation under different external magnetic fields. Collective states are affected by the boundary. Reproduced with permission from reference [106]. (d) A two-dimensional swarm of ferromagnetic microrobots. (d1) Reconfiguring formations driven by coordinating three external magnets. (d2) Collective navigation in a cluttered environment. Reproduced with permission from reference [107]. (e) Passive elongation of TiO_2 microparticle microswarm through a narrow channel. Reproduced with permission from reference [75].

insufficient to drive the merging process effectively. During the spreading state, a connecting band gradually expands, bringing the swarms into contact with each other. Eventually, through this contact, a new vortex-like swarm is formed. This formation is achieved by reducing the field frequency, which helps maintain a stable inward force necessary for the stability of the newly formed swarm. Moreover, the pattern transformation can be reversibly applied. Under the influence of an elliptically rotating field, the swarm demonstrates elongation. However, due to the unstable inward force, the pattern eventually splits, leading to a splitting process and the subsequent formation of two separate swarms. This study highlights that the collective state of a swarm induced by hydrodynamic interactions can be controlled by adjusting the interactions within the inner medium.

By modifying the magnetic interactions among constituent units, one can also bring about a transformation in the swarm induced by a magnetic field. When an oscillating field is combined with an in-plane constant field and an alternating field, a swarm resembling a ribbon is generated, as $\mathbf{B} = B_x \sin(2\pi f t)\hat{\mathbf{x}} + B_y\hat{\mathbf{y}}$ (Figure 1.6b) [58]. The initial formation of nanoparticle chains is followed by the estimation of their time-dependent lengths, accomplished through the utilization of the torque balance-based method (Eqs. (1.5), (1.6)). The dynamic fragmentation and reassembly of nanoparticle chains, combined with the magnetic attraction between these chains, result in the formation of intricate patterns. The internal magnetic interaction can be effectively modified by adjusting the field ratio, which is defined as the ratio between the strengths of the two applied fields ($\gamma = B_x/B_y$). The reversible elongation and contraction of the swarm pattern are a consequence of the dynamic disassembly and reconfiguration of particle chains (Figure 1.6b1). Through the simultaneous elongation of two microswarms and the coordination of their orientations, a connection is established between them, resulting in the emergence of a new microswarm following the merging process. Conversely, the splitting process is initiated by inducing magnetic repulsion between the chains, leading to the expansion of the pattern and covering a larger area (Figure 1.6b2). The controllable pattern transformation facilitates the implementation of an advanced swarm control strategy. When navigating through a narrow channel, the microswarm demonstrates the ability to elongate, split, and reassemble into multiple sub-swarms, enabling it to reach different branches (Figure 1.6b3). Furthermore, the application of swarm transformation can be extended to include conductive building blocks. By incorporating an Au layer on the particle surface, the microswarm gains conductivity and acquires the unique ability to repair and connect microcircuits, resembling a bio-mimicking structure [47].

The investigation focuses on the pattern transformation between microswarms based on magnetic interactions and hydrodynamic interactions. By applying various dynamic fields, the interactions among magnetic microparticles are adjusted, resulting in the emergence of liquid, chain, vortex, and ribbon collective states (Figure 1.6c) [106]. The collective states observed in the system are governed by the interplay between magnetic and hydrodynamic interactions. These interactions play crucial roles in shaping and determining the behavior of the microswarms. When a vertically oscillating field is applied ($\mathbf{B}(t) = B\sin(\omega t)\hat{\mathbf{z}}$), the particles repel each other due to the magnetic repulsion between them. After switching to a rotating field in the XZ-plane ($\mathbf{B}(t) = B[\cos(\omega t)\hat{\mathbf{x}} - \sin(\omega t)\hat{\mathbf{z}}]$), particle chains are formed because of the magnetic and hydrodynamic attraction between particles. Similar mechanism is applied to form a vortex-like swarm under an in-plane rotating field ($\mathbf{B}(t) = B[\cos(\omega t)\hat{\mathbf{x}} - \sin(\omega t)\hat{\mathbf{y}}]$) [48]. The collective behavior switches to ribbon-like state when the input field changing to a precessing field ($\mathbf{B}(t) = B_x\hat{\mathbf{x}} + B_i[\cos(\omega t)\hat{\mathbf{z}} - \sin(\omega t)\hat{\mathbf{y}}]$). This pattern transformation offers advantages for collective manipulation within specific constraints and facilitates transmission across diverse channels. The boundary conditions also influence the pattern transformation. In a narrowed channel, two vortex swarms have a tendency to combine and form a new microswarm. Additionally, the decreasing separation distance between multiple ribbons results in flow being exerted on them by their neighboring elements (Figure 1.6c). The categorization of such transformation, assisted by boundaries, as passive transformation is well established. Sitti *et al.* have effectively showcased a control strategy that enables switching between active and passive pattern transformation, as demonstrated in their work [107]. The dynamic alteration of a design is regulated through the programming of the external magnetic potential energy, *i.e.*, specifically by arranging the configuration of modular permanent magnets (Figure 1.6d1). The interplay between multiple magnetized patterned modules facilitates the reconfiguration, transformation, and formation of various shapes. When navigating through a restricted channel, the passive transformation of the collective is induced by direct contact with the surrounding boundaries. The robust interaction between the modules, characterized by strong repulsion forces, ensures pattern stability while also granting the swarm great adaptability. Throughout the navigation process, the swarm functions as a flexible miniature robot, adjusting its formation morphology through interactions with the environmental boundaries (Figure 1.6d2). The utilization of light as a driving force has demonstrated the ability of microswarms to undergo passive transformations [75]. As the swarm of TiO_2 particles approaches the entrance of a constricted channel, a portion of the particles enter the channel, resulting in the elongation of the swarm to match the shape of the channel's boundaries. This elongation continues as the swarm progresses toward the outlet of the channel (Figure 1.6e). The swarm navigation with pattern transformation has been successfully employed for transporting a cargo of SiO_2 particles within a narrow environment.

1.4 BIOMEDICAL APPLICATIONS OF MICROSWARMS

The potential of micronanoswarms to revolutionize minimally invasive treatments has been widely recognized. Numerous research studies have explored various applications for these swarms, resulting in significant advancements. As a result, the distance between fundamental research and practical clinical therapy has significantly decreased.

1.4.1 Targeted Drug Delivery

In the realm of targeted therapy, micronanoswarms have emerged as highly effective platforms. By transporting therapeutic drugs to inaccessible areas, they can enhance the concentration of drugs in localized regions and minimize negative impacts on the body [108]. Moreover, these swarms offer a range of benefits in terms of targeted drug delivery, such as the ability to control release rates and accommodate high drug loads.

(1) *In Vitro* Delivery. For precise delivery of therapeutic drugs to specific regions of the body, micronanoswarms require certain capabilities, including on-demand generation, navigational mobility, and precise control. swarm through the use of paramagnetic nanoparticles [109]. By utilizing the swarm, it is possible to gather and transport a batch of cargos to a specific area. Additionally, the research team developed a technique to generate ribbon-shaped swarms *in vitro* through the use of oscillating magnetic fields. As shown in Figure 1.7a, The swarms were set into translational motion by introducing a pitch angle to the magnetic field, which enabled them to move in a specific direction. Subsequently, it was confirmed that a vortex-shaped swarm could move as a cohesive entity with remarkable targeting efficiency through tight channels (Figure 1.7b) [48]. Apart from spherical nanoparticles, magnetic nanoparticles with other morphologies are also investigated to form micronanoswarms for targeted delivery. By using peanut-shaped hematite colloidal particles, Xie *et al.* developed a chain-like microswarm under rotating magnetic fields [110]. The swarm demonstrated a remarkable ability to undergo reversible assembly and disassembly, achieved respectively through the application of rotating and oscillating magnetic fields. In addition, the swarm's ability to navigate with high precision through branched and curved channels was demonstrated through visual tracking (Figure 1.7c). The same research team also reported generating four types of microswarms, including liquid, chain, vortex, and ribbon swarms, which can be transformed between different states by adjusting the applied fields [106]. Furthermore, the swarm's ability to pick up and release micro-objects was also demonstrated (Figure 1.7d). Additionally, functionalizing micronanoswarms can enhance the accuracy of targeted drug release and targeting ability [111, 112].

Recent research has shown that magnetic silk fibroin nanoparticle swarms loaded with curcumin can accelerate the release rate of curcumin by reducing the pH value. Moreover, Figure 1.7e shows that cancer cells cultured with curcumin-loaded swarms exhibited stronger fluorescence intensity, indicating improved curcumin absorption by cancer cells using the proposed swarming technique. A curcumin-loaded nanoparticle swarm with varying numbers of alginate and chitosan layers was also developed (Figure 1.7f) [115] ,with curcumin release rate increasing as the number of layers decreased. Ghezeli *et al.* generated chitosan-modified nanoparticle swarms to deliver imatinib to tumors [122]. *In vitro* experimental results have demonstrated that these swarms exhibit cytotoxicity on tumor cells, suggesting their potential as a drug delivery platform. In addition to their ability to suppress cancer cell development, the biocompatibility of swarms is crucial to protect non-targeted tissues and organs. Magnetic nanoparticle swarms were designed for doxorubicin delivery to kill cancer cells. With the biocompatibility of these swarms enhanced by coating with mesoporous silica to reduce unexpected cytotoxic effects. Dukenbayev *et al.* developed magnetic particle swarms loaded with carborane borate [116]. In Figure 1.7g, *in vitro* experimental results demonstrated that the viability of mouse embryonic fibroblasts cultured with the proposed swarm was higher compared to the other two groups, suggesting an improvement in biocompatibility.

In addition, living and hybrid swarms represent active platforms for targeted drug delivery. Certain bacteria have a natural swimming tendency, such as phototaxis, chemotaxis, and magnetotaxis, which allows them to autonomously propel themselves toward target sites based on the external environmental conditions.

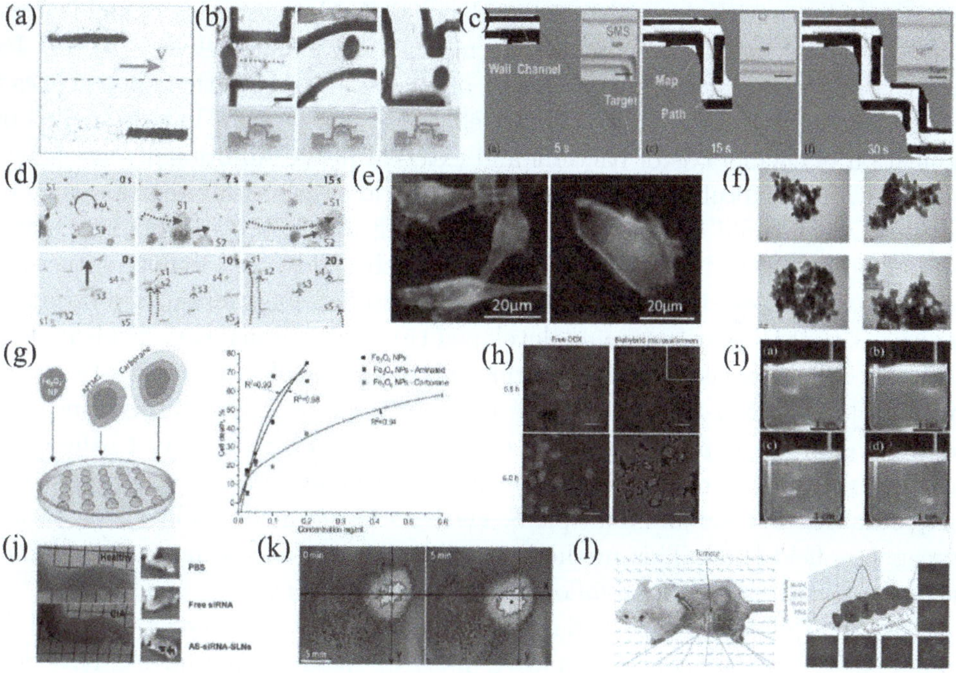

Figure 1.7 Targeted delivery using micronanoswarms. (a) The translational locomotion of a ribbon-like magnetic swarm. Reproduced with permission from reference [113]. (b) Movement of a vortex swarm in a branched microchannel. Reproduced with permission from reference [48]. (c) Navigation of a snake-like swarm in unknown environment. Reproduced with permission from reference [110]. (d) Manipulation of cargos by vortex and ribbon-like swarms. Reproduced with permission from reference [106]. (e) Cancer cells incubated with curcuma and curcuma-loaded microswarms for 4 h. Reproduced with permission from reference [114]. (f) Nanoparticle swarms with various number of chitosan and alginate layers (1, 5, 8, 9). Reproduced with permission from reference [115]. (g) Cytotoxic test: Mouse cells incubated with carborane-loaded swarms and control groups. Curves indicate cell death rate vs. swarm concentration. Reproduced with permission from reference [116]. (h) Cancer cells incubated with free drugs and drug-loaded swarms. Reproduced with permission from reference [117]. (i) Aggregation and locomotion of a magnetotactic bacteria swarm in a glass vial. Reproduced with permission from reference [118]. (j) The comparison of the siRNA distribution in mice with arthritis between experimental and control groups. Reproduced with permission from reference [119]. (k) Movement of an ABF swarm in the intra peritoneal cavity of a mouse. Reproduced with permission from reference [120]. (l) MTB swarm penetration in tumor: Left image - peritumoral injection, green insets - bacteria swarm distribution in transverse tumor sections via fluorescence imaging. Reproduced with permission from reference [121].

However, it is important to note that phototaxis and chemotaxis typically operate in a short-range with relatively large signal gradients [123]. Therefore, there is promise in using micronanoswarms comprised of bacteria and magnetic material as the platform for next-generation autonomous targeted drug delivery. By combining long-distance magnetic guidance with short-distance guidance through the sensing of ambient environments, these swarms hold potential for more effective drug delivery [20, 19]. Park *et al.* developed microswarms that consist of E. coli and magnetic nanoparticles capable of delivering doxorubicin to cancer cells [117]. The swarms were propelled by a combination of chemotaxis of bacteria and external fields. Additionally, as shown in Figure 1.7h, the doxorubicin delivered by the hybrid swarm exhibited slower absorption rates, which could enable long-term treatment and improve anticancer efficacy. Injection is one method for swarm delivery into the body, and remote gathering of injected swarm agents is essential to ensure controlled locomotion of swarms as a cohesive entity [124]. Lanauze *et al.* developed time-varying magnetic fields to enable remote three-dimensional (3D) aggregation and migration of a magnetotactic bacteria swarm [118]. As demonstrated in Figure 1.7i, this technique allowed the living swarm to aggregate on the upper left portion of a glass vial and then move to three other positions. In addition, remote motion control of a biohybrid swarm comprised of a superparamagnetic bead and multiple *S. marcescens* was achieved by slowly rotating the magnetic field [125]. This method significantly reduced the motion randomness of the swarm and enabled it to follow pre-designed trajectories.

(2) *In Vivo* Delivery. Animal trials have been conducted to develop targeted drug delivery platforms that can be deployed *in vivo*. *In vivo* experiments have investigated artificial micronanoswarms, such as lipid-based and polymeric nanoparticle swarms. For instance, a liposome swarm functionalized with siRNA and doxorubicin was presented, which demonstrated the capability of delivering drugs to the targeted tumor region and suppressing tumor growth [126]. Aldayel *et al.* proposed solid-lipid nanoparticle swarms to deliver tumor necrosis factor alpha siRNA to inflamed tissues, which were validated to effectively deliver the siRNA to the desired mouse feet for arthritis treatment (Figure 1.7j) compared to control groups [119]. Additionally, nanoparticle swarms loaded with docetaxel and cetuximab have been developed.76 The *in vivo* experiment showed that these targeting micronanocarriers were able to effectively inhibit tumor growth. In addition, ABF swarms have been tested *in vivo*, and Servant *et al.* reported successfully navigating an ABF swarm, which was functionalized with NIR dye, into the peritoneal cavity of a mouse using an external rotating magnetic field (Figure 1.7k) [120]. The real-time locomotion of the swarm was observable through fluorescence imaging. Furthermore, targeted drug delivery using bacteria swarms has been demonstrated *in vivo*. Felfoul *et al.* reported that magnetotactic bacteria swarms were able to deliver drug-loaded nanoliposomes to targeted tumor regions [121]. Using a magnetic field, the bacteria were able to penetrate the tumor and autonomously move to hypoxic regions, demonstrating their potential capability for targeted drug delivery. In a mouse model, the bacteria successfully reached hypoxic and necrotic regions of the tumor (Figure 1.7l).

The micronanoswarms were proposed as a potential active targeted delivery method, but in experiments, they did not effectively take drugs. Loading drugs onto swarm agents could alter swarm features, such as particle size and surface properties, which may impact swarm formation and delivery efficiency. Therefore, it is necessary to investigate the targeted delivery capability of drug-loaded swarms. Currently, most delivery strategies are studied in stable environments, but *in vivo* environments are dynamic, such as the flow in blood vessels and the peristalsis of intestines. Thus, investigating delivery methods in a dynamic environment is necessary to enhance the environmental adaptability of micronanoswarms.

1.4.2 Hyperthermia

Therapeutic hyperthermia involves exposing pathological tissue to high temperatures. By employing well-designed methods, only the local areas surrounding micronanoswarms are heated above physiological temperature. Consequently, this treatment can eliminate tumor cells with minimal side effects on normal tissues. Photothermal therapy (PTT) and magnetic hyperthermia (MH) are the two primary heating methods that have been extensively studied in recent years.

(1) Photothermal Therapy. Photothermal therapy (PTT) is a therapeutic method that utilizes near-infrared (NIR) radiation. Light-absorbing materials are employed to convert light energy into heat, thereby increasing temperature. Gold nanoparticles (AuNP) have emerged as effective photothermal agents owing to their exceptional features, including high photothermal conversion and light absorption capabilities [134, 135]. An AuNP swarm that can be photo-cross-linked was utilized for tumor PTT, as reported in a study [127]. This swarm was shown to be effective for cancer treatment through the comparison of changes in tumor sections in mice (Figure 1.8a). Additionally, a micronanoswarm composed of small AuNPs was developed for PTT of breast tumors under NIR laser irradiation (Figure 1.8b) [128]. The effectiveness of the tumor PTT using the swarm was demonstrated through the achieved regression of tumor volume.

In order to enhance the photothermal conversion efficiency for tumor PTT, researchers have developed various morphologies of AuNP swarms, such as nanorods, nanoshells, nanostars, and nanocages. For instance, Seo *et al.* developed gold nanorod swarms to improve the efficacy of PTT therapy [129], which was demonstrated through a gradual decrease in the viability of live and dead cancer cells with increasing irradiation time using the swarm as a hyperthermia agent (Figure 1.8c). Similarly, Wang *et al.* investigated gold nanoshell swarms that can generate heat for effective PTT and doxorubicin release under NIR laser irradiation [130]. Figure 1.8d illustrates that the drug can be released and dispersed in the tumor over time using the gold nanoshell swarm. It has also been confirmed that PTT utilizing the nanoshell swarm has an inhibitory effect on tumor growth, but the combined treatment was found to be more effective. Other morphologies of AuNP swarms, such as nanostar-like and nanocage-like structures, have also been developed to improve light absorption capability for tumor PTT [136, 137]. Additionally, the photothermal conversion efficiency can be enhanced by changing the size of nanoparticles. For example, Jiang *et al.* developed AuNPs with various diameters [138]. When subjected to a green laser, the heating efficiency decreased with increasing nanoparticle size. Moreover, *in vitro* assembly of AuNPs has also been shown to increase the photothermal conversion efficiency. For instance, a microswarm composed of AuNPs and a nanotube ring was realized *in vitro*, and was able to effectively decrease the tumor volume in a mouse after PTT (Figure 1.8e).

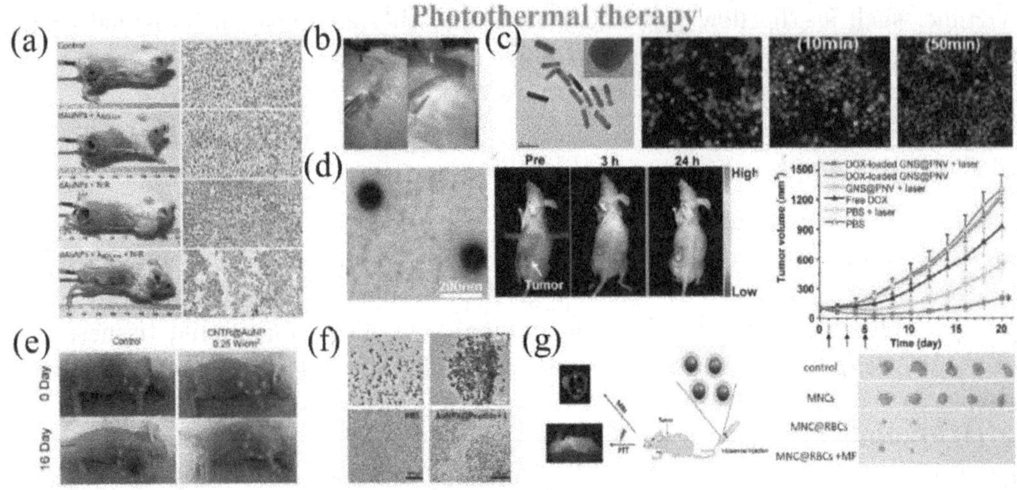

Figure 1.8 Photothermal therapy using micronanoswarms. (a) *In vivo* tumor detection in mice using experimental swarms and control groups. Reproduced with permission from reference [127]. (b) Thermographic image during photothermal therapy (PTT). Reproduced with permission from reference [128]. (c) Viability of cancer cells with different PTT durations using gold nanorod swarms. Reproduced with permission from reference [129]. (d) *In vivo* results of PTT using gold nanoshell swarms. Reproduced with permission from reference [130]. (e) Tumor changes in mice before and after PTT. Reproduced with permission from reference [131]. (f) Therapeutic results of *in vivo* swarm assembly for PTT. Reproduced with permission from reference [132]. (g) PTT results using nanoparticle swarms with red blood cells. Reproduced with permission from reference [133].

In vivo formation of nanoparticle swarms based on environmental stimuli could also be an effective method to adaptively perform hyperthermia. Yang *et al.* developed peptide modifified AuNP swarms that can be triggered by alkaline phosphatase to form a large swarm in a tumor region (Figure 1.8f) [132]. The retention of the swarm in tumor tissues was enhanced, and the tumor growth was inhibited effectively by observing tumor sections after PTT. The self-assembly of AuNPs can also be triggered by pH [139]. The micronanoswarm consisting of AuNPs functionalized with 11-mercaptoundecanoic acid and trimethylammonium bromide was proposed for cancer PTT [140]. The pH sensitivity was obtained by adjusting the ratios of the two ligands. Therefore, the agents can be aggregated rapidly into a swarm with increased size after reaching the acidic tumor region, and the retention time and treatment efficiency can be improved. Metal nanoparticles, including Fe, Mn, and Zn, have been utilized for photothermal therapy (PTT) besides AuNP swarms. To exemplify, Ren *et al.* designed an iron oxide magnetic nanoparticle swarm, which was enclosed by red blood cell membranes, as demonstrated in Figure 1.8g [133]. This biomimetic approach prolonged the blood retention time and subsequently enhanced tumor accumulation efficiency of the swarm. The effectiveness of the swarm for tumor PTT was confirmed by comparing dissected tumors from various groups. Another proposal was a micronanoswarm that combined NIR dye and Mn, demonstrating effective tumor homing and photothermal conversion [141]. Nanoparticle swarms combining zinc oxide with berberine were also developed [142]. The swarm can be applied for lung cancers treatment under NIR irradiation, supported by the experimental results in mice.

(2) Magnetic Hyperthermia. Compared to PTT, magnetic hyperthermia (MH) may present some advantages. For instance, the use of AuNPs for PTT can potentially cause cytotoxicity on normal cells, and they may not be biodegradable. Conversely, the swarm building blocks for MH, such as iron oxide nanoparticles, have been reported to be biodegradable in some cases, and the released iron ions can be absorbed by the human body. Additionally, MH exhibits better tissue penetrability under an external alternating magnetic field (AMF), as the magnetic nanomaterials can convert electromagnetic energy to heat [150]. Therefore, if magnetic agents are delivered to tumors, the internal temperature can be elevated to kill cancer cells with an AMF. Mondal *et al.* developed iron oxide nanoparticle swarms for MH-mediated cancer therapy [143]. As demonstrated in Figure 1.9a, which showed that the

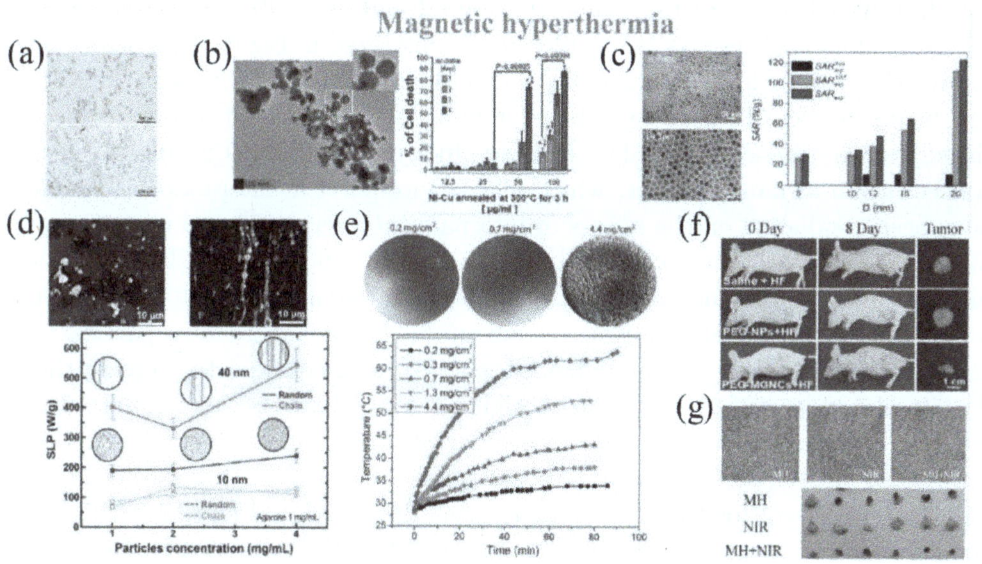

Figure 1.9 Magnetic hyperthemia using micronanoswarms. (a) Tumor cells without and with nanoparticle swarms after magnetic hyperthermia (MH). Reproduced with permission from reference [143]. (b) MH result using Ni-Cu nanoparticle swarms. Reproduced with permission from reference [144]. (c) Treatment efficiency of MH using nanoparticles of different diameters. Reproduced with permission from reference [145]. (d) Treatment efficiency of MH using randomly distributed and chain-like swarms. Reproduced with permission from reference [146]. (e) MH efficiency using swarms with different concentrations. Reproduced with permission from reference [147]. (f) Tumor changes in mice before and after MH. Reproduced with permission from reference [148]. (g) Comparison of results using MH, PTT, and both methods. Reproduced with permission from reference [149].

viability of osteosarcoma cells incubated with the proposed swarm under MH was lower than that of the control group. Efficient micronanoswarms that consisted of iron oxide nanoparticles doped with cobalt and manganese were also proposed [151]. Animal experiments confirmed that the swarm could accumulate in the tumor region and increase the temperature to kill cancer cells under AMF. Additionally, Ni-Cu nanoparticle swarms were developed for MH of cancer [144]. As displayed in Figure 1.9b, it indicated that the death rate of breast cancer cells increased with the concentration of nanoparticles and incubation time.

Extensive research has been conducted to investigate the magnetic properties of micronanoswarms, such as particle size, shape, and anisotropy, to enhance their heating capacity under an AMF [152, 153]. In the context of magnetic hyperthermia, magnetic nanoparticles ranging in size from 5 to 20 nm were synthesized (Figure 1.9c) [145]. The bar chart showed that 20 nm nanoparticles exhibited the highest specific absorption rates under an AMF. The impact of different shapes on heating was studied by comparing the experimental results using three distinct nanoparticle morphologies, namely sphere, cube, and ellipsoid [154]. It was confirmed that spherical building blocks were more effective at achieving better temperature distribution. The heating efficiency of randomly distributed and chain-like swarms composed of magnetic nanoparticles was also explored, as illustrated in Figure 1.9d, which demonstrated that the chain swarms had a more pronounced effect. Moreover, the MH effect can be strengthened or weakened under weak and strong anisotropy, respectively, through clusterization [155]. The heating efficiency of swarms is influenced by the concentration of nanoparticles, which affects interparticle interaction [156]. Studies have been conducted on the effects of interparticle interaction and concentration on heating [157, 158]. It was found that the heating efficiency increased with an increasing concentration of nanoparticles. Based on this observation, Wang *et al.* proposed a method to enhance local MH using reconfigurable ferromagnetic nanoparticle swarms [147]. Under a rotating magnetic field, the swarm can contract to increase the areal density of nanoparticles, leading to a higher temperature rise, as illustrated in Figure 1.9e. Moreover, the therapeutic efficiency of MH has been demonstrated *in vivo.* Jeon *et al.* developed iron oxide nanoparticle-based swarms that were coated with polyethylene glycol for tumor MH *in vivo*, as displayed in Figure 1.9f. The results showed that the tumor growth was suppressed after the swarms were heated under MH, as evidenced by the differences in tumor volume in mice.

Although MH and PTT are effective tumor therapy strategies, they have some limitations. MH requires a high concentration of magnetic agents to achieve the desired results, while PTT requires a high laser irradiation dose that decreases rapidly with depth, resulting in a relatively shallow effective range. To address these issues and provide a high synergistic effect, the combination of MH and PTT has been investigated [159, 160, 161]. Lu *et al.* studied magneto-photothermal therapy using micronanoswarms composed of iron oxide and gold magnetic nanoparticles, as demonstrated in Figure 1.9g. The results of glioma tumor sections and changes in tumor volume indicated that the apoptotic and inhibitory rates of cancer cells were significantly higher under the combined strategies. Another synergistic swarm made up of graphene quantum dots and magnetic mesoporous silica nanoparticles was developed

[162], which showed better efficacy in treating breast cancer compared to individual MH or PTT.

Numerous factors have been examined to enhance the heating efficiency for cancer hyperthermia, such as the characteristics of nanoparticles. Nevertheless, the applied magnetic fields also play a crucial role in the heating performance of MH, and the form of fields should be studied, despite the fact that some scientists have explored the effects of strength and frequency. Additionally, the aggregation and distribution of nanoparticle swarms at the tumor site have a critical impact on the hyperthermia effect. Active targeted techniques can be potentially employed in hyperthermia platforms to improve the aggregation and distribution of nanoparticles at the tumor site.

1.4.3 Imaging and Sensing

To precisely navigate and manipulate micronanoswarms, efficient imaging modalities are required to observe their position in real time. Moreover, after the swarms reach a targeted location, they can serve as sensing probes for desired signals.

(1) Imaging. *In vivo* imaging has several limitations, such as tissue thickness and interference from blood flow, which make it challenging to effectively observe the position and motion information of individual agents. However, micronanoswarms can provide better imaging contrast to enhance imaging effects due to their high agent concentration [176]. Numerous imaging methods have been studied recently to observe microswarms, including fluorescence imaging, magnetic resonance imaging (MRI), US imaging, and multimodal imaging.

(2) Fluorescence Imaging. Fluorescence is a well-known luminescence phenomenon that occurs naturally. Micronanoswarms can be designed with luminescent properties, enabling their imaging feedback *in vivo*. If multiple targeted objects are dyed with different colors, they can be easily identified with high sensitivity against the dark background [177]. A biohybrid micronanoswarm that combines microalgae organisms with magnetic nanoparticles was developed, which enables the swarm to be monitored non-invasively *in vivo* due to the intrinsic fluorescence properties of the organisms, as shown in Figure 1.10a. Wang *et al.* developed a five-pole magnetic platform by combining four fixed coils with one mobile coil to generate a rotating magnetic field, facilitating accurate navigation and control of a swarm coated with fluorescent dye in this workplace, as illustrated in Figure 1.10b.

(3) Magnetic Resonance Imaging. Here is the corrected version: MRI is an efficient imaging modality that can be used to examine body conditions, providing excellent imaging contrast on soft tissues without exposing biological tissues to ionizing radiation, which sets it apart from other imaging methods [27, 176]. The imaging results mainly rely on two parameters: longitudinal relaxation time (T1) and transversal relaxation time (T2). Micronanoswarms serving as T1 or T2 contrast agents are typically formed by magnetic nanoparticles [178]. Zhao *et al.* developed octagonal iron oxide nanoparticle swarms with a high transverse relaxivity value [179], which are experimentally validated to be effective T2 contrast agents with better imaging quality than conventional spherical magnetic nanoparticles. Moreover, a

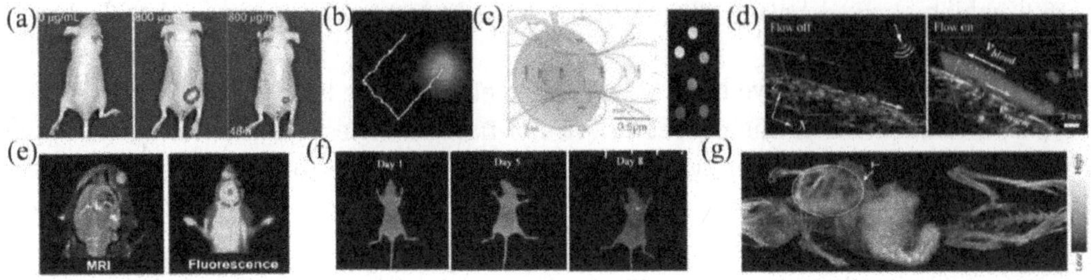

Figure 1.10 Imaging and sensing using microswarms. (a) Fluorescence at varying swarm concentrations and time. Reproduced with permission from reference [163]. (b) Position control of magnetic swarms using fluorescence. Reproduced with permission from reference [164]. (c) MRI imaging of magnetotactic bacteria swarms. Reproduced with permission from reference [165]. (d) Navigation of microswarms under US imaging with and without flowing blood. Reproduced with permission from reference [166]. (e) MRI and fluorescence imaging of a tumor labeled by swarms. Reproduced with permission from reference [167]. (f) Fluorescence imaging of a labeled tumor in a mouse. Reproduced with permission from reference [168]. (g) Distribution of tumor cells in a mouse. Reproduced with permission from reference [169].

medical platform that employs magnetotactic bacteria swarms was developed [165], as shown in Figure 1.10c. The magnetosomes chain was found in bacteria, and various concentrations of bacteria swarms were detected using MRI, indicating that the swarm can be used as an active drug delivery platform.

(4) US Imaging. US imaging provides the advantage of obtaining real-time position information for micronanoswarms, and it enables high penetration depth for deep tissue imaging, which sets it apart from other imaging methods [27]. Wang *et al.* proposed a strategy to actively navigate a nanoparticle swarm for endovascular delivery under US imaging [166], as depicted in Figure 1.10d. The swarm can be guided to move with and without flowing blood and has the capability of moving upstream and downstream near the boundary of vessels. Moreover, the magnetic navigation of a micronanoswarm has been investigated under US guidance [180]. Imaging experiments at different depths were conducted, and the minimal concentration of swarms at the corresponding depth was studied.

(5) Multimodal Imaging. While each imaging technique has its own benefits, there are also critical limitations that cannot be ignored. Fluorescence imaging has a relatively shallow imaging depth and may use dyes that are not biocompatible. MRI is an expensive and time-consuming technique, and image artifacts caused by the magnetic material may hinder accurate tracking of the target. In US imaging, bone and air pockets in living bodies may lead to imaging artifacts, and the low signal noise ratio may bring noise. To overcome these limitations, multimodal imaging that combines multiple imaging methods can provide better and comprehensive imaging outcomes to achieve more accurate diagnosis and treatment. Shen *et al.* developed nanoparticle swarms loaded with drugs for glioma treatment, which could be detected in the tumor region of a mouse under MRI and fluorescence imaging, indicating their potential to accumulate in the tumor [181], as shown in Figure 1.10e. Magnetic nanoparticle swarms functionalized with NIR dye were developed for multimodal imaging and photodynamic therapy, with the high stability of the dye enabling long-term observation [182]. Microswarms consisting of cobalt ferrite nanoparticles were also synthesized to serve as contrast agents in multimodal imaging methods, enabling metastases detection of cancer cells in mice under MRI and fluorescence imaging [183].

(6) Sensing. Micronanoswarms have shown significant potential to implement sensing applications based on various imaging modalities. For example, the metastasis of target cells can be transmitted by binding them with agents, and the concentration of interest can be sensed according to the imaging intensity of swarms [35]. Micronanoswarms have demonstrated promising capabilities in implementing sensing applications.

(7) Tumor Sensing. Micronanoswarms have the potential to sense the therapeutic effect of tumors and provide valuable pathological data for adjusting treatment schedules in a timely manner [181]. A microswarm composed of organic nanoparticles with photosensitizers was proposed [168]. Through fluorescence imaging, the position of a labeled tumor can be sensed for an extended period in *in vivo* experiments (as shown in Figure 1.10f). Zhao *et al.* proposed the use of AuNP swarms to detect cancer biomarkers [169]. As showed in Figure 1.10g, the tumor in a mouse model was labeled by the swarm and the information about the progression and metastasis of tumors can be effectively sensed using single photon emission computed tomography. Additionally, micronanoswarms can monitor drug release by detecting strength changes in imaging signals. Fan *et al.* developed peptide nanoparticle swarms capable of sensing the release of loaded doxorubicin [170]. The fluorescence intensity of doxorubicin was enhanced after incubating human carcinoma epithelial cells with the swarm for a long time, as shown in Figure 1.11a. Multifunctional nanoparticle swarms loaded with drugs and photosensitizer have been developed [184]. Following injection, the swarm was observed within the tumor, with the added benefit of real-time detection of drug release through signal amplification.

(8) pH Sensing. The stability of biologically active macromolecules in cells and tissues can be affected by the pH value, which is considered a critical physiological factor [185]. Therefore, real-time monitoring of pH is crucial. To achieve this, nanoparticle swarms containing NIR dye were developed for pH sensing [171]. In citrate buffer solutions with varying pH values, it was demonstrated that the photoacoustic signals of the swarm decreased significantly using an 810 nm laser and slightly with a 680 nm laser, respectively (Figure 1.11b). Based on this finding, the corresponding wavelength ratio curve can be plotted to sense pH. Furthermore, Yue *et al.* developed Janus nanoparticle swarms by encapsulating AuNPs and carbon dots into the two hemispheres for pH sensing [172]. In experiments, blue fluorescence was observed in the hemispheres containing carbon dots. As the pH values in Britton-Robinson buffer solutions increased, the size of the building blocks increased while the fluorescence intensity decreased (Figure 1.11c).

(9) Oxygen and Glucose Sensing. Maintaining oxygen homeostasis is crucial for regulating biological balance, including metabolism, as some diseases such as tumors and pathogenic infections are also linked to oxygen levels. Therefore, monitoring and

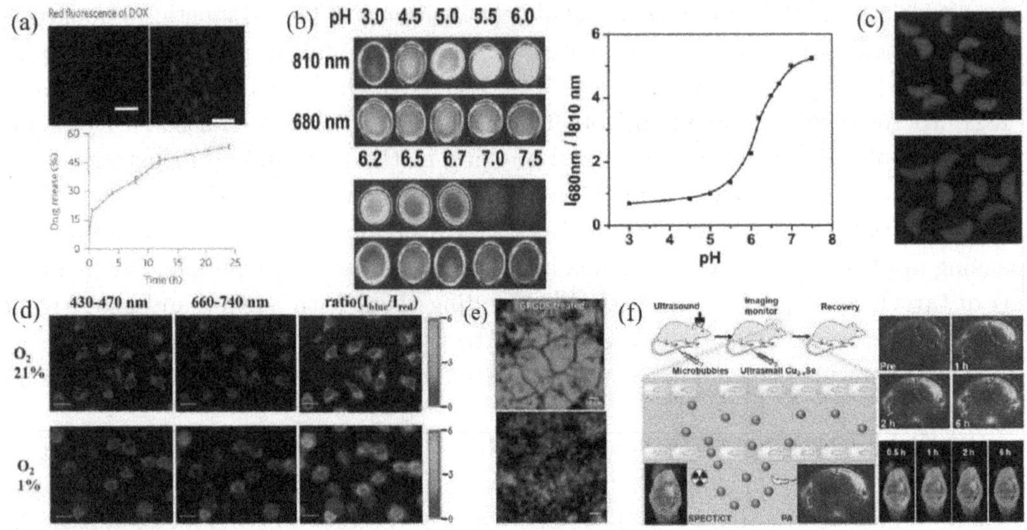

Figure 1.11 Imaging and sensing using microswarms. (a) Fluorescence imaging of drug release. Reproduced with permission from reference [170]. (b) Photoacoustic imaging of swarms in citrate buffers with varying pH. Reproduced with permission from reference [171]. (c) Brightness and size changes of a Janus nanoparticle swarm with the increase of pH. Reproduced with permission from reference [172]. (d) Fluorescence images of living cells cultured with swarms under different oxygen concentrations. Reproduced with permission from reference [173]. (e) NIR imaging of liver clots with swarms in ranges of 640–720 nm and 660–665 nm. Reproduced with permission from reference [174]. (f) Photoacoustic and CT imaging of mice brain over time. Reproduced with permission from reference [175].

sensing oxygen levels is essential, and micronanoswarms have emerged as effective and non-invasive probes for this purpose. Huang *et al.* developed polymer nanoparticle swarms for hypoxia sensing. Hypoxia sensing can be achieved by collecting blue and red fluorescence signals in different oxygen levels within living cells, and analyzing the ratio values of these signals (Figure 1.11d) [173]. Silica nanoparticle swarms loaded with perfluorocarbon have also been studied for oxygen sensing under MRI [186]. The T1 value decreases as the oxygen concentration increases, allowing for the sensing of oxygen levels. Additionally, changes in glucose levels can be detected by monitoring oxygen levels. As glucose is oxidized into gluconic acid, local oxygen is consumed, leading to changes in imaging feedback contrast [187]. Polymeric nanoparticle swarms for glucose sensing have been developed based on fluorescence imaging by Pandey *et al.* [188]. An enhanced fluorescence signal can be observed with an increase in oxygen concentration. For glucose sensing, alginate microparticle swarms have been proposed [189]. When deployed in simulated interstitial fluid and deionized water, it was observed that the ratio of fluorescein isothiocyanate and tetramethyl rhodamine isothiocyanate increased with glucose concentration.

(10) Sensing of Bleeding. The localization of internal bleeding is challenging without invasive procedures. If minimally invasive techniques can be developed to track the bleeding source, blood loss and bleeding time can be reduced. Gkikas *et al.* synthesized polymeric nanoparticle swarms for the treatment and position sensing of internal bleeding [174]. By labeling the swarm with NIR dye, it can be observed within the range of 660-665 nm, where the dye shows maximum emission (Figure 1.11e), allowing for the injury site to be sensed.

(11) Blood-Brain Barrier Sensing. In some cases, the delivery of therapeutic drugs for the treatment of brain diseases may be hindered by the blood-brain barrier (BBB), particularly in the case of drug molecules with large sizes. Therefore, it is necessary to sense the opening and recovery of the BBB in order to improve drug delivery efficiency. Zhang *et al.* developed nanoparticle swarms as dual-modal imaging contrast agents for BBB sensing [175]. After the BBB was opened using US, photoacoustic and computed tomography imaging were used to observe the positions of the swarms. As shown in Figure 1.11f, the signal increased at 2 hours after applying US, indicating that the swarm was able to move across the barrier and produce a strong signal, allowing for the sensing of the opening and recovery of the BBB.

Imaging and sensing trials in small animals have been extensively conducted, and a portion of the results have been satisfactory. However, challenges arise when applying imaging trials to the human body. One of the main problems is that human tissues are significantly thicker than those of small animals, and therefore, the penetration of imaging modalities needs to be improved to meet the requirements of treatment. In addition, contrast agents of different imaging methods can potentially be combined with swarm actuation strategies to increase the agent's areal concentration.

1.4.4 Thrombolysis

A thrombus refers to a local clotting phenomenon that increases with platelet aggregation until a complete blockage of a blood vessel is formed. This can result in the damage of organs leading to necrosis or even death [196]. Therefore, effective thrombolysis strategies are indispensable.

The usage of thrombolytic drugs is an efficient method to dissolve blood clots, with tissue plasminogen activator (tPA) being one of the widely used drugs *in vivo* [197]. However, some of the drawbacks of tPA cannot be neglected, such as short half-life, bleeding complications, and allergic reactions [198]. Therefore, to reduce the side effects and improve the targeting rate of thrombolytic drugs, many scientists have been attracted to develop methods by combining micronanoswarms. For instance, spherical building blocks consisting of aligned magnetic nanoparticle chains and microgel shells were developed to form a micronanoswarm [190]. Under rotating magnetic fields, the micronanoswarm can be accurately controlled to move toward a blood clot in an artificial vasculature (Figure 1.12a), and thrombolytic drugs can be released using magnetic hyperthermia (MH). Wang *et al.* also developed nanoparticle swarms containing microbubbles that were able to move toward thrombi through magnetic guidance [191]. As shown in Figure 1.12b, the proposed swarm for thrombolysis was effective in reducing the thrombus area compared to the control groups. The blood clots shrank, and the dark areas became shallow, further indicating the

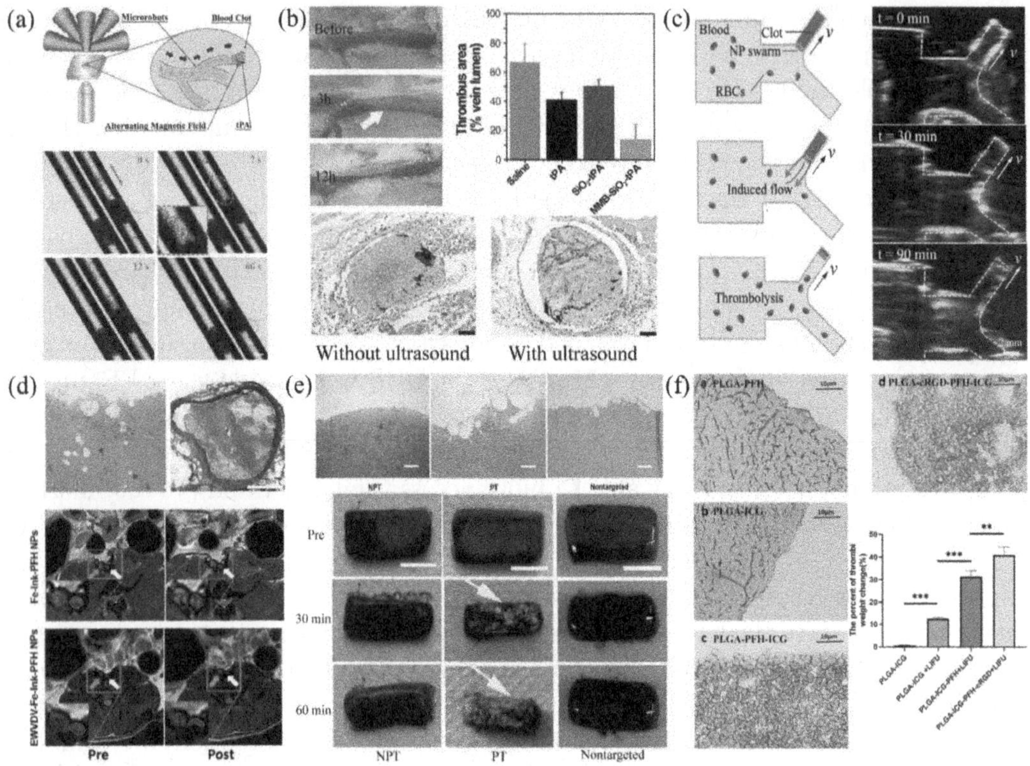

Figure 1.12 Thrombolysis using micronanoswarms. (a) Movement of swarms toward blood clots in artificial vasculature. Reproduced with permission from reference [190]. (b) Thrombolytic results with tPA-loaded swarms and ultrasound. Reproduced with permission from reference [191]. (c) Illustration and experiments of thrombolysis using magnetic field-controlled nanoparticle swarms. Reproduced with permission from reference [192]. (d) Thrombolysis results using PFH phase transition. Reproduced with permission from reference [193]. (e) Thrombolytic effects based on PFH phase transition with targeting capability. Reproduced with permission from reference [194]. (f) Thrombolysis via PFH phase transition. Reproduced with permission from reference [195].

effectiveness of the swarm for thrombolysis. The release of thrombolytic drugs can also be triggered using US, which enhances the drug penetration into clots. Another magnetic nanoparticle swarm with tPA for thrombolysis was also developed under US imaging [192]. The microswarm can be accurately controlled to move along both the short and long axis under magnetic fields. Additionally, the locomotion of the swarm induces fluid convection and enhances shear stress in the high viscous fluid, thereby improving thrombolysis efficiency (Figure 1.12c).

Thrombolysis can also be achieved through the use of perfluorohexane (PFH) phase transition under low-intensity focused US irradiation, which can cause cavitation effect and sonoporation to achieve thrombus destruction. Xu *et al.* developed a nanoparticle swarm loaded with the EWVDV peptide for thrombus targeting and treatment based on this mechanism [193]. *In vitro* experiments have shown that the thrombus can be penetrated, and *in vivo* experiments have demonstrated that the thrombi can be dissolved using the proposed swarm (Figure 1.12d). Other nanoparticle swarms with targeting capabilities have also been developed for thrombolysis [194, 195]. By applying low-intensity focused US, the vaporization of PFH was triggered, and the treatment effect was improved due to the targeting property of the swarm (Figure 1.12e). Additionally, another nanoparticle swarm with the ability to bind to clots was investigated, and the thrombi were surrounded and banded by the swarm. The proposed swarm's thrombi-dissolving capability was validated by comparing the change in thrombi weight in various groups (Figure 1.12f).

Thrombolytic drugs are often fixed onto micronanoswarms for active targeting delivery to reduce their side effects. However, the active agents for thrombolysis may remain inside the body, so their potential cytotoxicity must be further evaluated systematically. Additionally, the safety of PFH phase transition needs to be studied, including potential tissue damage that may occur.

1.5 SUMMARY AND OUTLOOK

Over the last ten years, significant advancements have been achieved in the field of microrobotic swarms and their applications in robotic delivery. Our review focuses on the recent progress made in swarm formation, navigation, localization, and their utilization in imaging-guided targeted delivery. Although considerable efforts have been dedicated to achieving controllable delivery within living organisms, several limitations persist, and further advancements are necessary to effectively control microrobotic swarms for targeted delivery purposes. In this context, we outline the research opportunities and challenges ahead, and we are optimistic that potential solutions are within reach.

(1) Swarm Control *In Vivo*: 3-D Navigation, Long-Range Delivery, and Environmental Adaptability. When it comes to swarm control, it is essential to recognize that the control logic differs from that of single-robot control or multi-robot operation. The control algorithm for swarms demands greater consideration of factors such as access rate, the interaction between swarms and their environments, and even feedback from a statistical perspective [199]. (1) One of the challenges in swarm control is achieving 3D navigation. Most existing collective micro-/nanorobots operate in a 2D space near a substrate or boundary, limiting their capabilities for complex 3D delivery tasks. To enable 3D navigation, it is necessary to address factors such as compensating for gravity and buoyancy forces and developing a robust control algorithm capable of processing multi-dimensional feedback. Additionally, the boundaries of the environment must be reconsidered to facilitate the control process. One potential solution is to employ a 2D swarm formation followed by 3D navigation, which requires a reevaluation of the constraints imposed by boundaries and the controllability of the swarm [55, 200]. (2) Long-range delivery. The integration of swarm control with established techniques, including catheter intervention, holds potential for application. However, the long-range navigation of swarms presents time-consuming obstacles and also impacts the efficiency of accessing building blocks (*e.g.*, magnetic nanoparticles, mobile microorganisms). An assemblage of micro-/nano-objects has the capability to be loaded into the tip of a catheter and subsequently released prior to reaching a challenging anatomical location. This approach enables the swarm to navigate through the narrowed lumen and reach the desired destination. Additionally, by incorporating mini-camera/sensors, the catheter can serve as a valuable imaging device for monitoring the environment in real-time and providing haptic feedback [201]. The convergence of assisted tool navigation and robotic swarms presents a notable avenue for research exploration. 3) Environmental adaptability. The flexible and adjustable morphology of assembled swarm patterns makes them well-suited for utilization in restricted and ever-changing environments. Their exceptional adaptability necessitates rapid responsiveness to external actuation energy, the ability to reconfigure their shape, and consistent control over pattern formation. Achieving this level of swarm intelligence requires the seamless integration of control systems, simultaneous localization, and real-time environment registration to ensure effective operation. Furthermore, a microrobotic swarm necessitates efficient locomotion through complex media (*e.g.*, blood, mucus) and needs to permeate biological barriers during navigation (*e.g.*, mucosal barrier, blood-brain barrier) [202, 203, 204]. Investigating control strategies that address both the penetration of biological barriers and the maintenance of swarm functionality is crucial.

(2) Integration of Microrobotic Swarm, Controller Unit, and Imaging Modality. The integration of a swarm controller unit with *in vivo* imaging techniques is an essential challenge for performing delivery tasks within living organisms. While various imaging techniques can be employed to localize a microswarm within opaque tissues or organs, there are still challenges in integrating imaging and control systems, as well as selecting the appropriate imaging method based on factors such as the navigation location, actuation method, materials of the building blocks, and the specific delivery task [205]. Optical-based imaging, for example, is not well-suited for deep-tissue navigation. Conversely, US imaging can penetrate deep tissues but faces difficulties in achieving sufficient imaging contrast in gas-filled body parts, such as the lungs. In the case of magnetically controlled microrobotic swarms, the formation of patterns and the ability to navigate with multiple degrees of freedom (multi-DoF) are influenced by the strength and bandwidth of the field generator, which can be electromagnetic coils or systems based on permanent magnets [206]. Consequently, integrating these controller units with MRI systems is not feasible, as it can interfere with the magnetic resonance imaging process. The trade-off between imaging and control systems, as well as the development of a swarm control scheme that can be integrated with existing imaging systems, presents a significant challenge. Research attention should be directed toward the integration of navigation and imaging for swarms using the same energy source. The recent proposal of actuating small-scale robots using MRI gradient coils demonstrates the potential of an integrated control and imaging system [207]. In order to achieve an imaging-integrated swarm control scheme, machine learning techniques can be utilized to analyze image feedback and simultaneously enable adaptable swarm control [208]. The control scheme can establish a correlation between the collective behavior of microrobotic swarms and the characteristics of biological environments, facilitating the mapping of physical boundaries and the identification of navigation strategies in complex conditions. One approach is to employ deep neural networks to analyze medical image feedback and track the swarms, subsequently implementing swarm transformation control to adapt to confined environments.

(3) Microrobotic Swarm for Clinical Applications. Recent research endeavors have primarily concentrated on integrating robotic swarms with established techniques, such as closed-loop control systems and medical imaging systems, to conduct preliminary trials at the preclinical level. However, several important considerations must be addressed before the application of microrobotic swarms in clinical settings, particularly in imaging-guided therapy. Firstly, substantial efforts should be devoted to the integration of various systems, encompassing hardware, software, and autonomous control. Existing techniques, including catheters and endoscopes, can be incorporated to assist in delivery and therapy procedures [209, 210]. To enable real-time control of microswarms within living organisms and monitor therapy procedures, it is necessary to develop user interfaces that integrate microrobotic control and feedback processing systems. Autonomous control offers advantages in terms of high manipulation efficiency and relieving medical practitioners from tedious and repetitive tasks. However, the level of autonomy required must be carefully considered, as fully automated systems can entail complex coding efforts and potentially give rise to safety concerns. Secondly, addressing safety concerns is crucial for conducting targeted therapy using microrobotic swarms. These concerns encompass determining the appropriate effective dose of delivery (pharmacokinetics), ensuring the reliability of integrated systems, and ensuring the swarms can effectively permeate biological barriers encountered during therapy procedures [211, 212]. Before designing therapeutic procedures, it is crucial to evaluate the biocompatibility and potential toxicity of microrobotic swarms. Recent studies have highlighted the biocompatibility and biomedical applications of hydrogels, including hydrogel micro/nanoparticles and hydrogel-based micro/nanostructures [213, 214]. These hydrogel-based agents can serve as building blocks to reduce the toxicity of microrobotic swarms. Additionally, the use of bio-hybrid agents, such as particles enclosed within the plasma membrane of human platelets, cell membrane-coated micro/nanorobots, and bio-hybrid microrobots, can enhance the biocompatibility of the swarm [215, 216, 217]. Indeed, the specific application site of microrobotic swarms plays a significant role in determining the acceptable toxicity levels. For instance, in the case of delivering microrobotic swarms within the gastrointestinal (GI) tract of living mice, histological evaluation of the swarm's toxicity may be conducted on various regions such as the stomach, duodenum, jejunum, distal colon, and ileum. This evaluation aims to investigate the biocompatibility and safety of the swarm for oral administration [218, 219]. Comprehensive toxicity evaluation from various perspectives, including materials, dosage, and size of building blocks, may be necessary for swarms in endovascular delivery applications. To test the feasibility of the proposed scheme, it is imperative to conduct *ex vivo* trials and animal tests, necessitating collaboration between roboticists, material specialists, and medical practitioners. Thirdly, identifying a compelling application that aids medical doctors and collaborators in evaluating the procedures involving microrobotic swarms is crucial. Accumulating experiences through such applications can generate greater interest among medical practitioners regarding the use of microrobotic swarms in targeted diagnosis and therapy. The ultimate goal for the application of actively-delivered microrobotic swarms is imaging-guided therapy. However, currently, the proof-of-concept and *in vivo* studies of swarming microrobots in imaging-guided therapy are still limited. Medical imaging systems have yet to be extensively involved in targeted therapy tasks, while imaging-integrated swarm control approaches primarily focus on swarm localization and navigation. Research opportunities exist in bridging the gap between targeted therapy/delivery and imaging-guided swarm control for clinical applications.

Bibliography

[1] Carl Anderson, Guy Theraulaz, and J-L Deneubourg. Self-assemblages in insect societies. *Insectes Sociaux*, 49(2):99–110, 2002.

[2] Tamás Vicsek and Anna Zafeiris. Collective motion. *Physics Reports*, 517(3-4):71–140, 2012.

[3] Jens Elgeti, Roland G Winkler, and Gerhard Gompper. Physics of microswimmers—single particle motion and collective behavior: A review. *Reports on Progress in Physics*, 78(5):056601, 2015.

[4] Orit Peleg, Jacob M Peters, Mary K Salcedo, and Lakshminarayanan Mahadevan. Collective mechanical adaptation of honeybee swarms. *Nature Physics*, 14(12):1193–1198, 2018.

[5] Nathan J Mlot, Craig A Tovey, and David L Hu. Fire ants self-assemble into waterproof rafts to survive floods. *Proceedings of the National Academy of Sciences*, 108(19):7669–7673, 2011.

[6] Christian Peeters and Stéphane De Greef. Predation on large millipedes and self-assembling chains in leptogenys ants from cambodia. *Insectes Sociaux*, 62(4):471–477, 2015.

[7] Michael Rubenstein, Alejandro Cornejo, and Radhika Nagpal. Programmable self-assembly in a thousand-robot swarm. *Science*, 345(6198):795–799, 2014.

[8] Shuguang Li, Richa Batra, David Brown, Hyun-Dong Chang, Nikhil Ranganathan, Chuck Hoberman, Daniela Rus, and Hod Lipson. Particle robotics based on statistical mechanics of loosely coupled components. *Nature*, 567(7748):361–365, 2019.

[9] Metin Sitti and Diederik S Wiersma. Pros and cons: Magnetic *versus* optical microrobots. *Advanced Materials*, 32(20):1906766, 2020.

[10] Yoonho Kim, Hyunwoo Yuk, Ruike Zhao, Shawn A Chester, and Xuanhe Zhao. Printing ferromagnetic domains for untethered fast-transforming soft materials. *Nature*, 558(7709):274–279, 2018.

[11] Antoine Barbot, Haijie Tan, Maura Power, Florent Seichepine, and Guang-Zhong Yang. Floating magnetic microrobots for fiber functionalization. *Science Robotics*, 4(34):eax8336, 2019.

[12] Xiang-Zhong Chen, Bumjin Jang, Daniel Ahmed, Chengzhi Hu, Carmela De Marco, Marcus Hoop, Fajer Mushtaq, Bradley J Nelson, and Salvador Pané. Small-scale machines driven by external power sources. *Advanced Materials*, 30(15):1705061, 2018.

[13] Lidong Yang, Qianqian Wang, and Li Zhang. Model-free trajectory tracking control of two-particle magnetic microrobot. *IEEE Transactions on Nanotechnology*, 17(4):697–700, 2018.

[14] Lei Kong, Carmen C Mayorga-Martinez, Jianguo Guan, and Martin Pumera. Photocatalytic micromotors activated by uv to visible light for environmental remediation, micropumps, reversible assembly, transportation, and biomimicry. *Small*, 16(27):1903179, 2020.

[15] Berta Esteban-Fernández de Ávila, Miguel Angel Lopez-Ramirez, Rodolfo Mundaca-Uribe, Xiaoli Wei, Doris E Ramírez-Herrera, Emil Karshalev, Bryan Nguyen, Ronnie H Fang, Liangfang Zhang, and Joseph Wang. Multicompartment tubular micromotors toward enhanced localized active delivery. *Advanced Materials*, 32(25):2000091, 2020.

[16] Emil Karshalev, Berta Esteban-Fernández de Ávila, Mara Beltrán-Gastélum, Pavimol Angsantikul, Songsong Tang, Rodolfo Mundaca-Uribe, Fangyu Zhang, Jing Zhao, Liangfang Zhang, and Joseph Wang. Micromotor pills as a dynamic oral delivery platform. *ACS Nano*, 12(8):8397–8405, 2018.

[17] Dandan Xu, Yong Wang, Chunyan Liang, Yongqiang You, Samuel Sanchez, and Xing Ma. Self-propelled micro/nanomotors for on-demand biomedical cargo transportation. *Small*, 16(27):1902464, 2020.

[18] Xiankun Lin, Zhiguang Wu, Yingjie Wu, Mingjun Xuan, and Qiang He. Self-propelled micro-/nanomotors based on controlled assembled architectures. *Advanced Materials*, 28(6):1060–1072, 2016.

[19] Yunus Alapan, Oncay Yasa, Oliver Schauer, Joshua Giltinan, Ahmet F Tabak, Victor Sourjik, and Metin Sitti. Soft erythrocyte-based bacterial microswimmers for cargo delivery. *Science Robotics*, 3(17):eaar4423, 2018.

[20] Klaas Bente, Agnese Codutti, Felix Bachmann, and Damien Faivre. Biohybrid and bioinspired magnetic microswimmers. *Small*, 14(29):1704374, 2018.

[21] Leonardo Ricotti, Barry Trimmer, Adam W Feinberg, Ritu Raman, Kevin K Parker, Rashid Bashir, Metin Sitti, Sylvain Martel, Paolo Dario, and Arianna Menciassi. Biohybrid actuators for robotics: A review of devices actuated by living cells. *Science Robotics*, 2(12):eaaq0495, 2017.

[22] Mariana Medina-Sánchez, Lukas Schwarz, Anne K Meyer, Franziska Hebenstreit, and Oliver G Schmidt. Cellular cargo delivery: Toward assisted fertilization by sperm-carrying micromotors. *Nano Letters*, 16(1):555–561, 2016.

[23] Metin Sitti. Miniature soft robots – road to the clinic. *Nature Reviews Materials*, 3(6):74–75, 2018.

[24] Rachel D Field, Priya N Anandakumaran, and Samuel K Sia. Soft medical microrobots: Design components and system integration. *Applied Physics Reviews*, 6(4):041305, 2019.

[25] Juanfeng Ou, Kun Liu, Jiamiao Jiang, Daniela A Wilson, Lu Liu, Fei Wang, Shuanghu Wang, Yingfeng Tu, and Fei Peng. Micro-/nanomotors toward biomedical applications: The recent progress in biocompatibility. *Small*, 16(27):1906184, 2020.

[26] Chuanrui Chen, Emil Karshalev, Jianguo Guan, and Joseph Wang. Magnesium-based micromotors: Water-powered propulsion, multifunctionality, and biomedical and environmental applications. *Small*, 14(23):1704252, 2018.

[27] Bradley J Nelson, Ioannis K Kaliakatsos, and Jake J Abbott. Microrobots for minimally invasive medicine. *Annual Review of Biomedical Engineering*, 12:55–85, 2010.

[28] Metin Sitti, Hakan Ceylan, Wenqi Hu, Joshua Giltinan, Mehmet Turan, Sehyuk Yim, and Eric Diller. Biomedical applications of untethered mobile milli/microrobots. *Proceedings of the IEEE*, 103(2):205–224, 2015.

[29] Lidong Yang, Yabin Zhang, Qianqian Wang, Kai-Fung Chan, and Li Zhang. Automated control of magnetic spore-based microrobot using fluorescence imaging for targeted delivery with cellular resolution. *IEEE Transactions on Automation Science and Engineering*, 17(1):490–501, 2020.

[30] Junyang Li, Xiaojian Li, Tao Luo, Ran Wang, Chichi Liu, Shuxun Chen, Dongfang Li, Jianbo Yue, Shuk-han Cheng, and D Sun. Development of a magnetic microrobot for carrying and delivering targeted cells. *Science Robotics*, 3(19):eaat8829, 2018.

[31] Jinxing Li, Berta Esteban-Fernandez de Avila, Wei Gao, Liangfang Zhang, and Joseph Wang. Micro/nanorobots for biomedicine: Delivery, surgery, sensing, and detoxification. *Science Robotics*, 2(4):eaam6431, 2017.

[32] Berta Esteban-Fernández de Ávila, Miguel Angel Lopez-Ramirez, Daniela F Báez, Adrian Jodra, Virendra V Singh, Kevin Kaufmann, and Joseph Wang. Aptamer-modified graphene-based catalytic micromotors: Off-on fluorescent detection of ricin. *ACS Sensors*, 1(3):217–221, 2016.

[33] Águeda Molinero-Fernández, Adrián Jodra, María Moreno-Guzmán, Miguel Ángel López, and Alberto Escarpa. Magnetic reduced graphene oxide/nickel/platinum nanoparticles micromotors for mycotoxin analysis. *Chemistry–A European Journal*, 24(28):7172–7176, 2018.

[34] Lidong Yang, Yabin Zhang, Qianqian Wang, and Li Zhang. An automated microrobotic platform for rapid detection of *C. diff* toxins. *IEEE Transactions on Biomedical Engineering*, 67(5):1517–1527, 2020.

[35] Yabin Zhang, Ke Yuan, and Li Zhang. Micro/nanomachines: From functionalization to sensing and removal. *Advanced Materials Technologies*, 4(4):1800636, 2019.

[36] Edward B Steager, Mahmut Selman Sakar, Ceridwen Magee, Monroe Kennedy, Anthony Cowley, and Vijay Kumar. Automated biomanipulation of single cells using magnetic microrobots. *The International Journal of Robotics Research*, 32(3):346–359, 2013.

[37] Claudio Pacchierotti, Federico Ongaro, Frank Van den Brink, Changkyu Yoon, Domenico Prattichizzo, David H Gracias, and Sarthak Misra. Steering and control of miniaturized untethered soft magnetic grippers with haptic assistance. *IEEE Transactions on Automation Science and Engineering*, 15(1):290–306, 2017.

[38] Wuming Jing, Sagar Chowdhury, Maria Guix, Jianxiong Wang, Ze An, Benjamin V Johnson, and David J Cappelleri. A microforce-sensing mobile microrobot for automated micromanipulation tasks. *IEEE Transactions on Automation Science and Engineering*, 16(2):518–530, 2018.

[39] Michael P Kummer, Jake J Abbott, Bradley E Kratochvil, Ruedi Borer, Ali Sengul, and Bradley J Nelson. Octomag: An electromagnetic system for 5-dof wireless micromanipulation. *IEEE Transactions on Robotics*, 26(6):1006–1017, 2010.

[40] Christos Bergeles and Guang-Zhong Yang. From passive tool holders to microsurgeons: Safer, smaller, smarter surgical robots. *IEEE Transactions on Biomedical Engineering*, 61(5):1565–1576, 2013.

[41] Arthur W Mahoney and Jake J Abbott. Five-degree-of-freedom manipulation of an untethered magnetic device in fluid using a single permanent magnet with application in stomach capsule endoscopy. *The International Journal of Robotics Research*, 35(1-3):129–147, 2016.

[42] Jake J Abbott, Eric Diller, and Andrew J Petruska. Magnetic methods in robotics. *Annual Review of Control, Robotics, and Autonomous Systems*, 3:57–90, 2020.

[43] U Kei Cheang, Kyoungwoo Lee, Anak Agung Julius, and Min Jun Kim. Multiple-robot drug delivery strategy through coordinated teams of microswimmers. *Applied Physics Letters*, 105(8):083705, 2014.

[44] B Shapiro, S Kulkarni, Alek Nacev, Azeem Sarwar, D Preciado, and Didier A Depireux. Shaping magnetic fields to direct therapy to ears and eyes. *Annual Review of Biomedical Engineering*, 16:455–481, 2014.

[45] Helena Massana-Cid, Fanlong Meng, Daiki Matsunaga, Ramin Golestanian, and Pietro Tierno. Tunable self-healing of magnetically propelling colloidal carpets. *Nature Communications*, 10:2444, 2019.

[46] Berk Yigit, Yunus Alapan, and Metin Sitti. Cohesive self-organization of mobile microrobotic swarms. *Soft Matter*, 16(8):1996–2004, 2020.

[47] Dongdong Jin, Jiangfan Yu, Ke Yuan, and Li Zhang. Mimicking the structure and function of ant bridges in a reconfigurable microswarm for electronic applications. *ACS Nano*, 13(5):5999–6007, 2019.

[48] Jiangfan Yu, Lidong Yang, and Li Zhang. Pattern generation and motion control of a vortex-like paramagnetic nanoparticle swarm. *The International Journal of Robotics Research*, 37(8):912–930, 2018.

[49] Peter J Vach, Debora Walker, Peer Fischer, Peter Fratzl, and Damien Faivre. Pattern formation and collective effects in populations of magnetic microswimmers. *Journal of Physics D: Applied Physics*, 50(11):11LT03, 2017.

[50] Alexey Snezhko and Igor S Aranson. Magnetic manipulation of self-assembled colloidal asters. *Nature Materials*, 10(9):698–703, 2011.

[51] Zhiguang Wu, Jonas Troll, Hyeon-Ho Jeong, Qiang Wei, Marius Stang, Focke Ziemssen, Zegao Wang, Mingdong Dong, Sven Schnichels, Tian Qiu, and Peer Fischer. A swarm of slippery micropropellers penetrates the vitreous body of the eye. *Science Advances*, 4(11):eaat4388, 2018.

[52] Xiaopu Wang, Chengzhi Hu, Lukas Schurz, Carmela De Marco, Xiangzhong Chen, Salvador Pané, and Bradley J Nelson. Surface-chemistry-mediated control of individual magnetic helical microswimmers in a swarm. *ACS Nano*, 12(6):6210–6217, 2018.

[53] Rui Cheng, Weijie Huang, Lijie Huang, Bo Yang, Leidong Mao, Kunlin Jin, Qichuan ZhuGe, and Yiping Zhao. Acceleration of tissue plasminogen activator-mediated thrombolysis by magnetically powered nanomotors. *ACS Nano*, 8(8):7746–7754, 2014.

[54] A Nacev, IN Weinberg, PY Stepanov, S Kupfer, LO Mair, MG Urdaneta, M Shimoji, ST Fricke, and B Shapiro. Dynamic inversion enables external magnets to concentrate ferromagnetic rods to a central target. *Nano Letters*, 15(1):359–364, 2015.

[55] Daniel Ahmed, Thierry Baasch, Nicolas Blondel, Nino Läubli, Jürg Dual, and Bradley J Nelson. Neutrophil-inspired propulsion in a combined acoustic and magnetic field. *Nature Communications*, 8:770, 2017.

[56] Stefano Giovanazzi, Axel Görlitz, and Tilman Pfau. Tuning the dipolar interaction in quantum gases. *Physical Review Letters*, 89(13):130401, 2002.

[57] Pietro Tierno, Steffen Schreiber, Walter Zimmermann, and Thomas M Fischer. Shape discrimination with hexapole-dipole interactions in magic angle spinning colloidal magnetic resonance. *Journal of the American Chemical Society*, 131(15):5366–5367, 2009.

[58] Jiangfan Yu, Ben Wang, Xingzhou Du, Qianqian Wang, and Li Zhang. Ultra-extensible ribbon-like magnetic microswarm. *Nature Communications*, 9:3260, 2018.

[59] C Wilhelm, J Browaeys, A Ponton, and J-C Bacri. Rotational magnetic particles microrheology: The maxwellian case. *Physical Review E*, 67(1):011504, 2003.

[60] Sheldon Green. *Fluid Vortices*. Springer: Dordrecht, Netherlands, 1995.

[61] Sebastian Jaeger, Holger Stark, and Sabine HL Klapp. Dynamics of cluster formation in driven magnetic colloids dispersed on a monolayer. *Journal of Physics: Condensed Matter*, 25(19):195104, 2013.

[62] Jing Yan, Sung Chul Bae, and Steve Granick. Rotating crystals of magnetic janus colloids. *Soft Matter*, 11(1):147–153, 2015.

[63] Koohee Han, Gašper Kokot, Shibananda Das, Roland G Winkler, Gerhard Gompper, and Alexey Snezhko. Reconfigurable structure and tunable transport in synchronized active spinner materials. *Science Advances*, 6(12):eaaz8535, 2020.

[64] Gašper Kokot, Andrey Sokolov, and Alexey Snezhko. Guided self-assembly and control of vortices in ensembles of active magnetic rollers. *Langmuir*, 36(25):6957–6962, 2020.

[65] Qianqian Wang, Lidong Yang, Ben Wang, Edwin Yu, Jiangfan Yu, and Li Zhang. Collective behavior of reconfigurable magnetic droplets *via* dynamic self-assembly. *ACS Applied Materials & Interfaces*, 11(1):1630–1637, 2018.

[66] M Belkin, A Snezhko, IS Aranson, and W-K Kwok. Driven magnetic particles on a fluid surface: Pattern assisted surface flows. *Physical Review Letters*, 99(15):158301, 2007.

[67] Eric Lauga and Thomas R Powers. The hydrodynamics of swimming microorganisms. *Reports on Progress in Physics*, 72(9):096601, 2009.

[68] Li Zhang, Tristan Petit, Yang Lu, Bradley E Kratochvil, Kathrin E Peyer, Ryan Pei, Jun Lou, and Bradley J Nelson. Controlled propulsion and cargo transport of rotating nickel nanowires near a patterned solid surface. *ACS Nano*, 4(10):6228–6234, 2010.

[69] A Snezhko, M Belkin, IS Aranson, and W-K Kwok. Self-assembled magnetic surface swimmers. *Physical Review Letters*, 102(11):118103, 2009.

[70] Soichiro Tottori, Li Zhang, Kathrin E Peyer, and Bradley J Nelson. Assembly, disassembly, and anomalous propulsion of microscopic helices. *Nano Letters*, 13(9):4263–4268, 2013.

[71] Michael Ibele, Thomas E Mallouk, and Ayusman Sen. Schooling behavior of light-powered autonomous micromotors in water. *Angewandte Chemie International Edition*, 48(18):3308–3312, 2009.

[72] Ivo Buttinoni, Julian Bialké, Felix Kümmel, Hartmut Löwen, Clemens Bechinger, and Thomas Speck. Dynamical clustering and phase separation in suspensions of self-propelled colloidal particles. *Physical Review Letters*, 110(23):238301, 2013.

[73] Yiying Hong, Misael Diaz, Ubaldo M Córdova-Figueroa, and Ayusman Sen. Light-driven titanium-dioxide-based reversible microfireworks and micromotor/micropump systems. *Advanced Functional Materials*, 20(10):1568–1576, 2010.

[74] Sergi Hernàndez-Navarro, Pietro Tierno, Joan Anton Farrera, Jordi Ignés-Mullol, and Francesc Sagués. Reconfigurable swarms of nematic colloids controlled by photoactivated surface patterns. *Angewandte Chemie International Edition*, 53(40):10696–10700, 2014.

[75] Fangzhi Mou, Jianhua Zhang, Zhen Wu, Sinan Du, Zexin Zhang, Leilei Xu, and Jianguo Guan. Phototactic flocking of photochemical micromotors. *iScience*, 19:415–424, 2019.

[76] Zhuoyi Deng, Fangzhi Mou, Shaowen Tang, Leilei Xu, Ming Luo, and Jianguo Guan. Swarming and collective migration of micromotors under near infrared light. *Applied Materials Today*, 13:45–53, 2018.

[77] Xiong Liang, Fangzhi Mou, Zhen Huang, Jianhua Zhang, Ming You, Leilei Xu, Ming Luo, and Jianguo Guan. Hierarchical microswarms with leader-follower-like structures: Electrohydrodynamic self-organization and multimode collective photoresponses. *Advanced Functional Materials*, 30(16):1908602, 2020.

[78] Wei Wang, Wentao Duan, Suzanne Ahmed, Thomas E Mallouk, and Ayusman Sen. Small power: Autonomous nano- and micromotors propelled by self-generated gradients. *Nano Today*, 8(5):531–554, 2013.

[79] Xiaoran Wu, Xiang Xue, Jinghang Wang, and Hewen Liu. Phototropic aggregation and light guided long-distance collective transport of colloidal particles. *Langmuir*, 36(24):6819–6827, 2020.

[80] Chuanrui Chen, Fangzhi Mou, Leilei Xu, Shaofei Wang, Jianguo Guan, Zunpeng Feng, Quanwei Wang, Lei Kong, Wei Li, Joseph Wang, and Qingjie Zhang. Light-steered isotropic semiconductor micromotors. *Advanced Materials*, 29(3):1603374, 2017.

[81] Wei Wang, Wentao Duan, Zexin Zhang, Mei Sun, Ayusman Sen, and Thomas E Mallouk. A tale of two forces: Simultaneous chemical and acoustic propulsion of bimetallic micromotors. *Chemical Communications*, 51(6):1020–1023, 2015.

[82] Tailin Xu, Fernando Soto, Wei Gao, Renfeng Dong, Victor Garcia-Gradilla, Ernesto Magaña, Xueji Zhang, and Joseph Wang. Reversible swarming and separation of self-propelled chemically powered nanomotors under acoustic fields. *Journal of the American Chemical Society*, 137(6):2163–2166, 2015.

[83] Zesheng Li, Hongyue Zhang, Daolin Wang, Changyong Gao, Mengmeng Sun, Zhiguang Wu, and Qiang He. Reconfigurable assembly of active liquid metal colloidal cluster. *Angewandte Chemie*, 132(45):20056–20060, 2020.

[84] K Jagajjanani Rao, Fei Li, Long Meng, Hairong Zheng, Feiyan Cai, and Wei Wang. A force to be reckoned with: A review of synthetic microswimmers powered by ultrasound. *Small*, 11(24):2836–2846, 2015.

[85] Tailin Xu, Li-Ping Xu, and Xueji Zhang. Ultrasound propulsion of micro-/nanomotors. *Applied Materials Today*, 9:493–503, 2017.

[86] James Friend and Leslie Y Yeo. Microscale acoustofluidics: Microfluidics driven *via* acoustics and ultrasonics. *Reviews of Modern Physics*, 83(2):647–704, 2011.

[87] Xiaoyun Ding, Sz-Chin Steven Lin, Brian Kiraly, Hongjun Yue, Sixing Li, I-Kao Chiang, Jinjie Shi, Stephen J Benkovic, and Tony Jun Huang. On-chip manipulation of single microparticles, cells, and organisms using surface acoustic waves. *Proceedings of the National Academy of Sciences*, 109(28):11105–11109, 2012.

[88] Henrik Bruus. Acoustofluidics 7: The acoustic radiation force on small particles. *Lab on a Chip*, 12(6):1014–1021, 2012.

[89] Alexander A Doinikov. Acoustic radiation interparticle forces in a compressible fluid. *Journal of Fluid Mechanics*, 444:1–21, 2001.

[90] Steven M Woodside, Bruce D Bowen, and James M Piret. Measurement of ultrasonic forces for particle-liquid separations. *AIChE Journal*, 43(7):1727–1736, 1997.

[91] Jing Yan, Ming Han, Jie Zhang, Cong Xu, Erik Luijten, and Steve Granick. Reconfiguring active particles by electrostatic imbalance. *Nature Materials*, 15(10):1095–1099, 2016.

[92] Fuduo Ma, Sijia Wang, David T Wu, and Ning Wu. Electric-field-induced assembly and propulsion of chiral colloidal clusters. *Proceedings of the National Academy of Sciences*, 112(20):6307–6312, 2015.

[93] Antoine Bricard, Jean-Baptiste Caussin, Nicolas Desreumaux, Olivier Dauchot, and Denis Bartolo. Emergence of macroscopic directed motion in populations of motile colloids. *Nature*, 503(7474):95–98, 2013.

[94] Sumit Gangwal, Olivier J Cayre, Martin Z Bazant, and Orlin D Velev. Induced-charge electrophoresis of metallodielectric particles. *Physical Review Letters*, 100(5):058302, 2008.

[95] Daiki Nishiguchi and Masaki Sano. Mesoscopic turbulence and local order in janus particles self-propelling under an ac electric field. *Physical Review E*, 92(5):052309, 2015.

[96] Qianqian Wang, Jiangfan Yu, Ke Yuan, Lidong Yang, Dongdong Jin, and Li Zhang. Disassembly and spreading of magnetic nanoparticle clusters on uneven surfaces. *Applied Materials Today*, 18:1004189, 2020.

[97] Syun-Ru Yeh, Michael Seul, and Boris I Shraiman. Assembly of ordered colloidal aggregrates by electric-field-induced fluid flow. *Nature*, 386(6620):57–59, 1997.

[98] WD Ristenpart, Ilhan A Aksay, and DA Saville. Electrohydrodynamic flow around a colloidal particle near an electrode with an oscillating potential. *Journal of Fluid Mechanics*, 575:83–109, 2007.

[99] Jinxing Li, Tianlong Li, Tailin Xu, Melek Kiristi, Wenjuan Liu, Zhiguang Wu, and Joseph Wang. Magneto-acoustic hybrid nanomotor. *Nano Letters*, 15(7):4814–4821, 2015.

[100] Songsong Tang, Fangyu Zhang, Jing Zhao, Wael Talaat, Fernando Soto, Emil Karshalev, Chuanrui Chen, Zhihan Hu, Xiaolong Lu, Jinxing Li, Zhihua Lin, Haifeng Dong, Xueji Zhang, Amir Nourhani, and Joseph Wang. Structure-dependent optical modulation of propulsion and collective behavior of acoustic/light-driven hybrid microbowls. *Advanced Functional Materials*, 29(23):1809003, 2019.

[101] Jeremie Palacci, Stefano Sacanna, Asher Preska Steinberg, David J Pine, and Paul M Chaikin. Living crystals of light-activated colloidal surfers. *Science*, 339(6122):936–940, 2013.

[102] Suzanne Ahmed, Dillon T Gentekos, Craig A Fink, and Thomas E Mallouk. Self-assembly of nanorod motors into geometrically regular multimers and their propulsion by ultrasound. *ACS Nano*, 8(11):11053–11060, 2014.

[103] Zhihua Lin, Tieyan Si, Zhiguang Wu, Changyong Gao, Xiankun Lin, and Qiang He. Light-activated active colloid ribbons. *Angewandte Chemie International Edition*, 56(43):13517–13520, 2017.

[104] Murat Kaynak, Adem Ozcelik, Amir Nourhani, Paul E Lammert, Vincent H Crespi, and Tony Jun Huang. Acoustic actuation of bioinspired microswimmers. *Lab on a Chip*, 17(3):395–400, 2017.

[105] Jizhai Cui, Tian-Yun Huang, Zhaochu Luo, Paolo Testa, Hongri Gu, Xiang-Zhong Chen, Bradley J Nelson, and Laura J Heyderman. Nanomagnetic encoding of shape-morphing micromachines. *Nature*, 575:164–168, 2019.

[106] Hui Xie, Mengmeng Sun, Xinjian Fan, Zhihua Lin, Weinan Chen, Lei Wang, Lixin Dong, and Qiang He. Reconfigurable magnetic microrobot swarm: Multimode transformation, locomotion, and manipulation. *Science Robotics*, 4(28):eaav8006, 2019.

[107] Xiaoguang Dong and Metin Sitti. Controlling two-dimensional collective formation and cooperative behavior of magnetic microrobot swarms. *The International Journal of Robotics Research*, 39(5):617–638, 2020.

[108] C. K. Schmidt, M. Medina-Sanchez, R. J. Edmondson, and O. G. Schmidt. Engineering Microrobots for Targeted Cancer Therapies from a Medical Perspective. *Nature Communications*, 11(1):5618, 2020.

[109] J Yu, D Jin, and L Zhang. Mobile paramagnetic nanoparticle-based vortex for targeted cargo delivery in fluid. In *Proceedings of the IEEE International Conference on Robotics and Automation*, pages 6594–6599. IEEE, 2017.

[110] H Xie, X Fan, M Sun, Z Lin, Q He, and L Sun. Programmable generation and motion control of a snakelike magnetic microrobot swarm. *IEEE-ASME Transactions on Mechatronics*, 24(2):902–912, 2019.

[111] F Xiong, S Huang, and N Gu. Magnetic nanoparticles: Recent developments in drug delivery system. *Drug Development and Industrial Pharmacy*, 44(5):697–706, 2018.

[112] J Lu, J Wang, and D Ling. Surface engineering of nanoparticles for targeted delivery to hepatocellular carcinoma. *Small*, 14(43):1702037, 2018.

[113] J Yu and L Zhang. Reconfigurable colloidal microrobotic swarm for targeted delivery. In *Proceedings of the International Conference on Ubiquitous Robots*, pages 615–616. IEEE, 2019.

[114] Wenxing Song, Munitta Muthana, Joy Mukherjee, Robert J Falconer, Catherine A Biggs, and Xiubo Zhao. Magnetic-silk core–shell nanoparticles as potential carriers for targeted delivery of curcumin into human breast cancer cells. *ACS Biomaterials Science & Engineering*, 3(6):1027–1038, 2017.

[115] W Song, X Su, DA Gregory, W Li, Z Cai, and X Zhao. Magnetic alginate/chitosan nanoparticles for targeted delivery of curcumin into human breast cancer cells. *Nanomaterials*, 8(11):907, 2018.

[116] K Dukenbayev, IV Korolkov, DI Tishkevich, AL Kozlovskiy, SV Trukhanov, YG Gorin, EE Shumskaya, EY Kaniukov, DA Vinnik, MV Zdorovets, M Anisovich, AV Trukhanov, D Tosi, and C Molardi. Fe3o4 nanoparticles for complex targeted delivery and boron neutron capture therapy. *Nanomaterials*, 9(4):494, 2019.

[117] Byung-Wook Park, Jiang Zhuang, Oncay Yasa, and Metin Sitti. Multifunctional bacteria-driven microswimmers for targeted active drug delivery. *ACS Nano*, 11(9):8910–8923, 2017.

[118] Dominic De Lanauze, Ouajdi Felfoul, Jean-Philippe Turcot, Mahmood Mohammadi, and Sylvain Martel. Three-dimensional remote aggregation and steering of magnetotactic bacteria microrobots for drug delivery applications. *The International Journal of Robotics Research*, 33(3):359–374, 2014.

[119] Abdulaziz M Aldayel, Hannah L O'Mary, Solange A Valdes, Xu Li, Sachin G Thakkar, Bahar E Mustafa, and Zhengrong Cui. Lipid nanoparticles with minimum burst release of tnf-α sirna show strong activity against rheumatoid arthritis unresponsive to methotrexate. *Journal of Controlled Release*, 283:280–289, 2018.

[120] Ania Servant, Famin Qiu, Mariarosa Mazza, Kostas Kostarelos, and Bradley J Nelson. Controlled *in Vivo* swimming of a swarm of bacteria-like microrobotic flagella. *Advanced Materials*, 27(19):2981–2988, 2015.

[121] Ouajdi Felfoul, Mahmood Mohammadi, Samira Taherkhani, Dominic De Lanauze, Yong Zhong Xu, Dumitru Loghin, Sherief Essa, Sylwia Jancik, Daniel Houle, Michel Lafleur, Louis Gaboury, Maryam Tabrizian, Neila Kaou1, Michael Atkin, Té Vuong, Gerald Batist, Nicole Beauchemin, Danuta Radzioch, and Sylvain Martel. Magneto-aerotactic bacteria deliver drug-containing nanoliposomes to tumour hypoxic regions. *Nature Nanotechnology*, 11:941–947, 2016.

[122] ZK Ghezeli, M Hekmati, and H Veisi. Synthesis of imatinib-loaded chitosan-modified magnetic nanoparticles as an anti-cancer agent for ph responsive targeted drug delivery. *Applied Organometallic Chemistry*, 33(10):e4833, 2019.

[123] Zeinab Hosseinidoust, Babak Mostaghaci, Oncay Yasa, Byung-Wook Park, Ajay Vikram Singh, and Metin Sitti. Bioengineered and biohybrid bacteria-based systems for drug delivery. *Advanced Drug Delivery Reviews*, 106:27–44, 2016.

[124] Dumitru Loghin, Charles Tremblay, and Sylvain Martel. Improved three-dimensional remote aggregations of magnetotactic bacteria for tumor targeting. In *2016 International Conference on Manipulation, Automation and Robotics at Small Scales (MARSS)*, pages 1–6. IEEE, 2016.

[125] Rika Wright Carlsen, Matthew R Edwards, Jiang Zhuang, Cecile Pacoret, and Metin Sitti. Magnetic steering control of multi-cellular bio-hybrid microswimmers. *Lab on a Chip*, 14(19):3850–3859, 2014.

[126] Juan Jiang, Shi-jin Yang, Jian-cheng Wang, Li-juan Yang, Zhen-zhong Xu, Ting Yang, Xiao-yan Liu, and Qiang Zhang. Sequential treatment of drug-resistant tumors with rgd-modified liposomes containing sirna or doxorubicin. *European Journal of Pharmaceutics and Biopharmaceutics*, 76(2):170–178, 2010.

[127] Xiaju Cheng, Rui Sun, Ling Yin, Zhifang Chai, Haibin Shi, and Mingyuan Gao. Light-triggered assembly of gold nanoparticles for photothermal therapy and photoacoustic imaging of tumors in vivo. *Advanced Materials*, 29(6):1604894, 2017.

[128] Elizabeth Higbee-Dempsey, Ahmad Amirshaghaghi, Matthew J Case, Joann Miller, Theresa M Busch, and Andrew Tsourkas. Indocyanine green–coated gold nanoclusters for photoacoustic imaging and photothermal therapy. *Advanced Therapeutics*, 2(9):1900088, 2019.

[129] Sun-Hwa Seo, Bo-Mi Kim, Ara Joe, Hyo-Won Han, Xiaoyuan Chen, Zhen Cheng, and Eue-Soon Jang. Nir-light-induced surface-enhanced raman scattering for detection and photothermal/photodynamic therapy of cancer cells using methylene blue-embedded gold nanorod@ sio2 nanocomposites. *Biomaterials*, 35(10):3309–3318, 2014.

[130] Lu Wang, Yuanyuan Yuan, Shudong Lin, Jinsheng Huang, Jian Dai, Qing Jiang, Du Cheng, and Xintao Shuai. Photothermo-chemotherapy of cancer employing drug leakage-free gold nanoshells. *Biomaterials*, 78:40–49, 2016.

[131] Jibin Song, Feng Wang, Xiangyu Yang, Bo Ning, Mary G Harp, Stephen H Culp, Song Hu, Peng Huang, Liming Nie, Jingyi Chen, et al. Gold nanoparticle coated carbon nanotube ring with enhanced raman scattering and photothermal conversion property for theranostic applications. *Journal of the American Chemical Society*, 138(22):7005–7015, 2016.

[132] Shuyan Yang, Defan Yao, Yanshu Wang, Weitao Yang, Bingbo Zhang, and Dengbin Wang. Enzyme-triggered self-assembly of gold nanoparticles for enhanced retention effects and photothermal therapy of prostate cancer. *Chemical Communications*, 54(70):9841–9844, 2018.

[133] Xiaoqing Ren, Rui Zheng, Xiaoling Fang, Xiaofei Wang, Xiaoyan Zhang, Wuli Yang, and Xianyi Sha. Red blood cell membrane camouflaged magnetic nanoclusters for imaging-guided photothermal therapy. *Biomaterials*, 92:13–24, 2016.

[134] Nardine S. Abadeer and Catherine J. Murphy. Recent progress in cancer thermal therapy using gold nanoparticles. *Journal of Physical Chemistry C*, 120(9): 2016.

[135] Yang Liu, Bridget M Crawford, and Tuan Vo-Dinh. Gold nanoparticles-mediated photothermal therapy and immunotherapy. *Immunotherapy*, 10(13):1175–1188, 2018. PMID: 30236026.

[136] Yang Liu, Jeffrey R Ashton, Everett J Moding, Hsiangkuo Yuan, Janna K Register, Andrew M Fales, Jaeyeon Choi, Melodi J Whitley, Xiaoguang Zhao, Yi Qi, et al. A plasmonic gold nanostar theranostic probe for in vivo tumor imaging and photothermal therapy. *Theranostics*, 5(9):946, 2015.

[137] Feng Hu, Yan Zhang, Guangcun Chen, Chunyan Li, and Qiangbin Wang. Double-walled au nanocage/sio2 nanorattles: integrating sers imaging, drug delivery and photothermal therapy. *Small*, 11(8):985–993, 2015.

[138] Ke Jiang, David A Smith, and Anatoliy Pinchuk. Size-dependent photothermal conversion efficiencies of plasmonically heated gold nanoparticles. *The Journal of Physical Chemistry C*, 117(51):27073–27080, 2013.

[139] Sanghak Park, Woo Jin Lee, Sungmin Park, Doowon Choi, Sungjee Kim, and Nokyoung Park. Reversibly ph-responsive gold nanoparticles and their applications for photothermal cancer therapy. *Scientific Reports*, 9(1):1–9, 2019.

[140] Ruili Zhang, Linlin Wang, Xiaofei Wang, Qian Jia, Zhuang Chen, Zuo Yang, Renchuan Ji, Jie Tian, and Zhongliang Wang. Acid-induced in vivo assembly of gold nanoparticles for enhanced photoacoustic imaging-guided photothermal therapy of tumors. *Advanced Healthcare Materials*, 9(14):2000394, 2020.

[141] Yu Yang, Jingjing Liu, Chao Liang, Liangzhu Feng, Tingting Fu, Ziliang Dong, Yu Chao, Yonggang Li, Guang Lu, Meiwan Chen, et al. Nanoscale metal–organic particles with rapid clearance for magnetic resonance imaging-guided photothermal therapy. *ACS Nano*, 10(2):2774–2781, 2016.

[142] Sungyun Kim, Song Yi Lee, and Hyun-Jong Cho. Berberine and zinc oxide-based nanoparticles for the chemo-photothermal therapy of lung adenocarcinoma. *Biochemical and Biophysical Research Communications*, 501(3):765–770, 2018.

[143] Sudip Mondal, Panchanathan Manivasagan, Subramaniyan Bharathiraja, Madhappan Santha Moorthy, Van Tu Nguyen, Hye Hyun Kim, Seung Yun Nam, Kang Dae Lee, and Junghwan Oh. Hydroxyapatite coated iron oxide nanoparticles: a promising nanomaterial for magnetic hyperthermia cancer treatment. *Nanomaterials*, 7(12):426, 2017.

[144] Bianca P Meneses-Brassea, Edgar A Borrego, Dawn S Blazer, Mohamed F Sanad, Shirin Pourmiri, Denisse A Gutierrez, Armando Varela-Ramirez, George C Hadjipanayis, and Ahmed A El-Gendy. Ni-cu nanoparticles and their feasibility for magnetic hyperthermia. *Nanomaterials*, 10(10):1988, 2020.

[145] LH Nguyen, VTK Oanh, PH Nam, DH Doan, NX Truong, NX Ca, PT Phong, LV Hong, and TD Lam. Increase of magnetic hyperthermia efficiency due to optimal size of particles: Theoretical and experimental results. *Journal of Nanoparticle Research*, 22:1–16, 2020.

[146] Eirini Myrovali, N Maniotis, Antonios Makridis, Anastasia Terzopoulou, Vitalis Ntomprougkidis, K Simeonidis, D Sakellari, Orestis Kalogirou, Theodoros Samaras, Ruslan Salikhov, et al. Arrangement at the nanoscale: Effect on magnetic particle hyperthermia. *Scientific Reports*, 6(1):37934, 2016.

[147] Ben Wang, Kai Fung Chan, Jiangfan Yu, Qianqian Wang, Lidong Yang, Philip Wai Yan Chiu, and Li Zhang. Reconfigurable swarms of ferromagnetic colloids for enhanced local hyperthermia. *Advanced Functional Materials*, 28(25):1705701, 2018.

[148] Sangmin Jeon, Bum Chul Park, Seungho Lim, Hong Yeol Yoon, Yoo Sang Jeon, Byung-Soo Kim, Young Keun Kim, and Kwangmeyung Kim. Heat-generating iron oxide multigranule nanoclusters for enhancing hyperthermic efficacy in tumor treatment. *ACS Applied Materials & Interfaces*, 12(30):33483–33491, 2020.

[149] Qianling Lu, Xinyu Dai, Peng Zhang, Xiao Tan, Yuejiao Zhong, Cheng Yao, Mei Song, Guili Song, Zhenghai Zhang, Gang Peng, et al. Fe3o4@ au composite magnetic nanoparticles modified with cetuximab for targeted magneto-photothermal therapy of glioma cells. *International Journal of Nanomedicine*, 13:2491, 2018.

[150] Janani Sadhasivam and Abimanyu Sugumaran. Magnetic nanocarriers: Emerging tool for the effective targeted treatment of lung cancer. *Journal of Drug Delivery Science and Technology*, 55:101493, 2020.

[151] Hassan A Albarqi, Leon H Wong, Canan Schumann, Fahad Y Sabei, Tetiana Korzun, Xiaoning Li, Mikkel N Hansen, Pallavi Dhagat, Abraham S Moses, Olena Taratula, et al. Biocompatible nanoclusters with high heating efficiency for systemically delivered magnetic hyperthermia. *ACS Nano*, 13(6):6383–6395, 2019.

[152] Pradip Das, Miriam Colombo, and Davide Prosperi. Recent advances in magnetic fluid hyperthermia for cancer therapy. *Colloids and Surfaces B: Biointerfaces*, 174:42–55, 2019.

[153] Ziba Hedayatnasab, Faisal Abnisa, and Wan Mohd Ashri Wan Daud. Review on magnetic nanoparticles for magnetic nanofluid hyperthermia application. *Materials & Design*, 123:174–196, 2017.

[154] Yundong Tang, Rodolfo CC Flesch, Tao Jin, Yueming Gao, and Minhua He. Effect of nanoparticle shape on therapeutic temperature distribution during magnetic hyperthermia. *Journal of Physics D: Applied Physics*, 54(16):165401, 2021.

[155] Ali F Abu-Bakr and Andrey Yu Zubarev. On the theory of magnetic hyperthermia: clusterization of nanoparticles. *Philosophical Transactions of the Royal Society A*, 378(2171):20190251, 2020.

[156] Cristina Blanco-Andujar, Aurelie Walter, Geoffrey Cotin, Catalina Bordeianu, Damien Mertz, Delphine Felder-Flesch, and Sylvie Begin-Colin. Design of iron oxide-based nanoparticles for mri and magnetic hyperthermia. *Nanomedicine*, 11(14):1889–1910, 2016.

[157] AF Abu-Bakr and A Yu Zubarev. Hyperthermia in a system of interacting ferromagnetic particles under rotating magnetic field. *Journal of Magnetism and Magnetic Materials*, 477:404–407, 2019.

[158] Saeid Ebrahimisadr, Bagher Aslibeiki, and Reza Asadi. Magnetic hyperthermia properties of iron oxide nanoparticles: The effect of concentration. *Physica C: Superconductivity and Its Applications*, 549:119–121, 2018.

[159] Ihab M Obaidat, Venkatesha Narayanaswamy, Sulaiman Alaabed, Sangaraju Sambasivam, and Chandu VV Muralee Gopi. Principles of magnetic hyperthermia: a focus on using multifunctional hybrid magnetic nanoparticles. *Magnetochemistry*, 5(4):67, 2019.

[160] Xiaoli Liu, Yifan Zhang, Yanyun Wang, Wenjing Zhu, Galong Li, Xiaowei Ma, Yihan Zhang, Shizhu Chen, Shivani Tiwari, Kejian Shi, et al. Comprehensive understanding of magnetic hyperthermia for improving antitumor therapeutic efficacy. *Theranostics*, 10(8):3793, 2020.

[161] Jaber Keyvan Rad, Zeinab Alinejad, Samideh Khoei, and Ali Reza Mahdavian. Controlled release and photothermal behavior of multipurpose nanocomposite particles containing encapsulated gold-decorated magnetite and 5-fu in poly (lactide-co-glycolide). *ACS Biomaterials Science & Engineering*, 5(9):4425–4434, 2019.

[162] Xianxian, Yao, Xingxing, Niu, Kexin, Ma, Ping, Huang, Julia, Grothe. Graphene quantum dots-capped magnetic mesoporous silica nanoparticles as a multifunctional platform for controlled drug delivery, magnetic hyperthermia, and photothermal therapy. *Small*, 13(2), 2017.

[163] Xiaohui Yan, Qi Zhou, Melissa Vincent, Yan Deng, Jiangfan Yu, Jianbin Xu, Tiantian Xu, Tao Tang, Liming Bian, Yi-Xiang Wang, Kostas Kostarelos, and Li Zhang. Multifunctional biohybrid magnetite microrobots for imaging-guided therapy. *Science Robotics*, 2(12):eaaq1155, 2017.

[164] Xian Wang, Tiancong Wang, Guanqiao Shan, Junhui Law, Changsheng Dai, Zhuoran Zhang, and Yu Sun. Robotic control of a magnetic swarm for on-demand intracellular measurement. In *2020 IEEE International Conference on Robotics and Automation (ICRA)*, pages 11385–11391. IEEE, 2020.

[165] Sylvain Martel, Ouajdi Felfoul, Jean-Baptiste Mathieu, Arnaud Chanu, Samer Tamaz, Mahmood Mohammadi, Martin Mankiewicz, and Nasr Tabatabaei. Mri-based medical nanorobotic platform for the control of magnetic nanoparticles and flagellated bacteria for target interventions in human capillaries. *The International Journal of Robotics Research*, 28(9):1169–1182, 2009.

[166] Qianqian Wang, Kai Fung Chan, Kathrin Schweizer, Xingzhou Du, Dongdong Jin, Simon Chun Ho Yu, Bradley J Nelson, and Li Zhang. Ultrasound doppler-guided real-time navigation of a magnetic microswarm for active endovascular delivery. *Science Advances*, 7(9):eabe5914, 2021.

[167] Chen Shen, Xiaoxiong Wang, Zhixing Zheng, Chuang Gao, Xin Chen, Shiguang Zhao, and Zhifei Dai. Doxorubicin and indocyanine green loaded superparamagnetic iron oxide nanoparticles with pegylated phospholipid coating for magnetic

resonance with fluorescence imaging and chemotherapy of glioma. *International Journal of Nanomedicine*, 14:101, 2019.

[168] Qi Xia, Zikang Chen, Yuping Zhou, and Ruiyuan Liu. Near-infrared organic fluorescent nanoparticles for long-term monitoring and photodynamic therapy of cancer. *Nanotheranostics*, 3(2):156, 2019.

[169] Yongfeng Zhao, Bo Pang, Hannah Luehmann, Lisa Detering, Xuan Yang, Deborah Sultan, Scott Harpstrite, Vijay Sharma, Cathy S Cutler, Younan Xia, et al. Gold nanoparticles doped with 199au atoms and their use for targeted cancer imaging by spect. *Advanced Healthcare Materials*, 5(8):928–935, 2016.

[170] Zhen Fan, Leming Sun, Yujian Huang, Yongzhong Wang, and Mingjun Zhang. Bioinspired fluorescent dipeptide nanoparticles for targeted cancer cell imaging and real-time monitoring of drug release. *Nature Nanotechnology*, 11(4):388–394, 2016.

[171] Qian Chen, Xiaodong Liu, Jianfeng Zeng, Zhenping Cheng, and Zhuang Liu. Albumin-nir dye self-assembled nanoparticles for photoacoustic ph imaging and ph-responsive photothermal therapy effective for large tumors. *Biomaterials*, 98:23–30, 2016.

[172] Shuai Yue, Xiaoting Sun, Ning Wang, Yaning Wang, Yue Wang, Zhangrun Xu, Mingli Chen, and Jianhua Wang. Sers–fluorescence dual-mode ph-sensing method based on janus microparticles. *ACS Applied Materials & Interfaces*, 9(45):39699–39707, 2017.

[173] Yuan-Yuan Huang, Ye Tian, Xiao-Qin Liu, Zhongwei Niu, Qing-Zheng Yang, Vaidhyanathan Ramamurthy, Chen-Ho Tung, Yu-Zhe Chen, and Li-Zhu Wu. Luminescent supramolecular polymer nanoparticles for ratiometric hypoxia sensing, imaging and therapy. *Materials Chemistry Frontiers*, 2(10):1893–1899, 2018.

[174] Manos Gkikas, Thomas Peponis, Tomaz Mesar, Celestine Hong, Reginald K Avery, Emmanuel Roussakis, Hyung-Jin Yoo, Anushri Parakh, Manuel Patino, Dushyant V Sahani, et al. Systemically administered hemostatic nanoparticles for identification and treatment of internal bleeding. *ACS Biomaterials Science & Engineering*, 5(5):2563–2576, 2019.

[175] Hao Zhang, Tingting Wang, Weibao Qiu, Yaobao Han, Qiao Sun, Jianfeng Zeng, Fei Yan, Hairong Zheng, Zhen Li, and Mingyuan Gao. Monitoring the opening and recovery of the blood–brain barrier with noninvasive molecular imaging by biodegradable ultrasmall cu2–x se nanoparticles. *Nano Letters*, 18(8):4985–4992, 2018.

[176] Jiangfan Yu, Qianqian Wang, Mengzhi Li, Chao Liu, Lidai Wang, Tiantian Xu, and Li Zhang. Characterizing nanoparticle swarms with tuneable concentrations for enhanced imaging contrast. *IEEE Robotics and Automation Letters*, 4(3):2942–2949, 2019.

[177] Ben Wang, Kostas Kostarelos, Bradley J Nelson, and Li Zhang. Trends in micro-/nanorobotics: materials development, actuation, localization, and system integration for biomedical applications. *Advanced Materials*, 33(4):2002047, 2021.

[178] Guanying Chen, Indrajit Roy, Chunhui Yang, and Paras N Prasad. Nanochemistry and nanomedicine for nanoparticle-based diagnostics and therapy. *Chemical Reviews*, 116(5):2826–2885, 2016.

[179] Zhenghuan Zhao, Zijian Zhou, Jianfeng Bao, Zhenyu Wang, Juan Hu, Xiaoqin Chi, Kaiyuan Ni, Ruifang Wang, Xiaoyuan Chen, Zhong Chen, et al. Octapod iron oxide nanoparticles as high-performance t 2 contrast agents for magnetic resonance imaging. *Nature Communications*, 4(1):2266, 2013.

[180] Qianqian Wang, Lidong Yang, Jiangfan Yu, Philip Wai Yan Chiu, Yong-Ping Zheng, and Li Zhang. Real-time magnetic navigation of a rotating colloidal microswarm under ultrasound guidance. *IEEE Transactions on Biomedical Engineering*, 67(12):3403–3412, 2020.

[181] Oana Hosu, Mihaela Tertis, and Cecilia Cristea. Implication of magnetic nanoparticles in cancer detection, screening and treatment. *Magnetochemistry*, 5(4):55, 2019.

[182] Huige Zhou, Xiaoyang Hou, Ying Liu, Tianming Zhao, Qiuyu Shang, Jinglong Tang, Jing Liu, Yuqing Wang, Qiuchi Wu, Zehao Luo, et al. Superstable magnetic nanoparticles in conjugation with near-infrared dye as a multimodal theranostic platform. *ACS Applied Materials & Interfaces*, 8(7):4424–4433, 2016.

[183] Nathalie M Pinkerton, Marian E Gindy, Victoria L Calero-DdelC, Theodore Wolfson, Robert F Pagels, Derek Adler, Dayuan Gao, Shike Li, Ruobing Wang, Margot Zevon, et al. Single-step assembly of multimodal imaging nanocarriers: Mri and long-wavelength fluorescence imaging. *Advanced Healthcare Materials*, 4(9):1376–1385, 2015.

[184] Ziliang Dong, Liangzhu Feng, Wenwen Zhu, Xiaoqi Sun, Min Gao, He Zhao, Yu Chao, and Zhuang Liu. Caco3 nanoparticles as an ultra-sensitive tumor-ph-responsive nanoplatform enabling real-time drug release monitoring and cancer combination therapy. *Biomaterials*, 110:60–70, 2016.

[185] Michael Schäferling. Nanoparticle-based luminescent probes for intracellular sensing and imaging of ph. *Wiley Interdisciplinary Reviews: Nanomedicine and Nanobiotechnology*, 8(3):378–413, 2016.

[186] Amani L Lee, Clifford T Gee, Bradley P Weegman, Samuel A Einstein, Adam R Juelfs, Hattie L Ring, Katie R Hurley, Sam M Egger, Garrett Swindlehurst, Michael Garwood, et al. Oxygen sensing with perfluorocarbon-loaded ultraporous mesostructured silica nanoparticles. *ACS Nano*, 11(6):5623–5632, 2017.

[187] Naga VS Vallabani, Sanjay Singh, and Ajay S Karakoti. Magnetic nanoparticles: current trends and future aspects in diagnostics and nanomedicine. *Current Drug Metabolism*, 20(6):457–472, 2019.

[188] Gaurav Pandey, Rashmi Chaudhari, Bhavana Joshi, Sandeep Choudhary, Jaspreet Kaur, and Abhijeet Joshi. Fluorescent biocompatible platinum-porphyrin–doped polymeric hybrid particles for oxygen and glucose biosensing. *Scientific Reports*, 9(1):1–12, 2019.

[189] Ayesha Chaudhary, Michael J McShane, and Rohit Srivastava. Glucose response of dissolved-core alginate microspheres: towards a continuous glucose biosensor. *Analyst*, 135(10):2620–2628, 2010.

[190] Meihua Xie, Wei Zhang, Chengying Fan, Chu Wu, Qishuai Feng, Jiaojiao Wu, Yingze Li, Rui Gao, Zhenguang Li, Qigang Wang, et al. Bioinspired soft microrobots with precise magneto-collective control for microvascular thrombolysis. *Advanced Materials*, 32(26):2000366, 2020.

[191] Siyu Wang, Xixi Guo, Weijun Xiu, Yang Liu, Lili Ren, Huaxin Xiao, Fang Yang, Yu Gao, Chenjie Xu, and Lianhui Wang. Accelerating thrombolysis using a precision and clot-penetrating drug delivery strategy by nanoparticle-shelled microbubbles. *Science Advances*, 6(31):eaaz8204, 2020.

[192] Qianqian Wang, Ben Wang, Jiangfan Yu, Kathrin Schweizer, B. J. Nelson, and Li Zhang. Reconfigurable magnetic microswarm for thrombolysis under ultrasound imaging. In *IEEE International Conference on Robotics and Automation*, pages 10285–10291. IEEE, 2020.

[193] Jie Xu, Jun Zhou, Yixin Zhong, Yu Zhang, Jia Liu, Yuli Chen, Liming Deng, Danli Sheng, Zhigang Wang, Haitao Ran, et al. Phase transition nanoparticles as multimodality contrast agents for the detection of thrombi and for targeting thrombolysis: in vitro and in vivo experiments. *ACS Applied Materials & Interfaces*, 9(49):42525–42535, 2017.

[194] Yixin Zhong, Yu Zhang, Jie Xu, Jun Zhou, Jia Liu, Man Ye, Liang Zhang, Bin Qiao, Zhi-gang Wang, Hai-tao Ran, et al. Low-intensity focused ultrasound-responsive phase-transitional nanoparticles for thrombolysis without vascular damage: a synergistic nonpharmaceutical strategy. *ACS Nano*, 13(3):3387–3403, 2019.

[195] Sheng Bai, Jintang Liao, Bo Zhang, Min Zhao, Baiyang You, Pan Li, Haitao Ran, Zhigang Wang, Ruizheng Shi, and Guogang Zhang. Multimodal and multifunctional nanoparticles with platelet targeting ability and phase transition efficiency for the molecular imaging and thrombolysis of coronary microthrombi. *Biomaterials Science*, 8(18):5047–5060, 2020.

[196] Ting Huang, Ni Li, and Jianqing Gao. Recent strategies on targeted delivery of thrombolytics. *Asian Journal of Pharmaceutical Sciences*, 14(3):233–247, 2019.

[197] Alyssa M Flores, Jianqin Ye, Kai-Uwe Jarr, Niloufar Hosseini-Nassab, Bryan R Smith, and Nicholas J Leeper. Nanoparticle therapy for vascular diseases. *Arteriosclerosis, Thrombosis, and Vascular Biology*, 39(4):635–646, 2019.

[198] Yunn-Hwa Ma, Chih-Hsin Liu, Yueh Liang, Jyh-Ping Chen, and Tony Wu. Targeted delivery of plasminogen activators for thrombolytic therapy: An integrative evaluation. *Molecules*, 24(18):3407, 2019.

[199] Lidong Yang, Jiangfan Yu, and Li Zhang. Statistics-based automated control for a swarm of paramagnetic nanoparticles in 2-d space. *IEEE Transactions on Robotics*, 36(1):254–270, 2020.

[200] Fengtong Ji, Dongdong Jin, Ben Wang, and Li Zhang. Light-driven hovering of a magnetic microswarm in fluid. *ACS Nano*, 14(6):6990–6998, 2020.

[201] Yoonho Kim, German A Parada, Shengduo Liu, and Xuanhe Zhao. Ferromagnetic soft continuum robots. *Science Robotics*, 4(33):eaax7329, 2019.

[202] Zhiguang Wu, Ye Chen, Daniel Mukasa, On Shun Pak, and Wei Gao. Medical micro/nanorobots in complex media. *Chemical Society Reviews*, 49:8088–8112, 2020.

[203] Hakan Ceylan, Immihan C Yasa, Ugur Kilic, Wenqi Hu, and Metin Sitti. Translational prospects of untethered medical microrobots. *Progress in Biomedical Engineering*, 1(1):012002, 2019.

[204] Dongdong Jin and Li Zhang. Microrobotics-embodied intelligence weaves a better future. *Nature Machine Intelligence*, 2(11):663–664, 2020.

[205] Guido T van Moolenbroek, Tania Patiño, Jordi Llop, and Samuel Sánchez. Engineering intelligent nanosystems for enhanced medical imaging. *Advanced Intelligent Systems*, 2(10):2000087, 2020.

[206] Lidong Yang and Li Zhang. Motion control in magnetic microrobotics: From individual and multiple to swarm. *Annual Review of Control, Robotics, and Autonomous Systems*, 4:1–26, 2021.

[207] Onder Erin, Hunter B Gilbert, Ahmet Fatih Tabak, and Metin Sitti. Elevation and azimuth rotational actuation of an untethered millirobot by mri gradient coils. *IEEE Transactions on Robotics*, 35(6):1323–1337, 2019.

[208] Frank Cichos, Kristian Gustavsson, Bernhard Mehlig, and Giovanni Volpe. Machine learning for active matter. *Nature Machine Intelligence*, 2(2):94–103, 2020.

[209] James W Martin, Bruno Scaglioni, Joseph C Norton, Venkataraman Subramanian, Alberto Arezzo, Keith L Obstein, and Pietro Valdastri. Enabling the future of colonoscopy with intelligent and autonomous magnetic manipulation. *Nature Machine Intelligence*, 2:595–606, 2020.

[210] Guillaume Lapouge, Philippe Poignet, and Jocelyne Troccaz. Towards 3d ultrasound guided needle steering tobust to uncertainties, noise and tissue heterogeneity. *IEEE Transactions on Biomedical Engineering*, page DOI: 10.1109/TBME.2020.3022619, 2020.

[211] Changyong Gao, Yong Wang, Zihan Ye, Zhihua Lin, Xing Ma, and Qiang He. Biomedical micro-/nanomotors: From overcoming biological barriers to *in Vivo* imaging. *Advanced Materials*, page DOI: 10.1002/adma.202000512, 2020.

[212] Ben Wang, K Kostarelos, Bradley J Nelson, and Li Zhang. Trends in micro-/nano-robotics: Materials development, actuation, localization, and system integration for biomedical applications. *Advanced Materials*, page DOI: 10.1002/adma.202002047, 2020.

[213] Kun Xue, Xiaoyuan Wang, Pei Wern Yong, David James Young, Yun-Long Wu, Zibiao Li, and Xian Jun Loh. Hydrogels as emerging materials for translational biomedicine. *Advanced Therapeutics*, 2(1):1800088, 2019.

[214] Mohammad Hosein Ayoubi-Joshaghani, Khaled Seidi, Mehdi Azizi, Mehdi Jaymand, Tahereh Javaheri, Rana Jahanban-Esfahlan, and Michael R Hamblin. Potential applications of advanced nano/hydrogels in biomedicine: Static, dynamic, multi-stage, and bioinspired. *Advanced Functional Materials*, 30(45):2004098, 2020.

[215] Jia Zhuang, Hua Gong, Jiarong Zhou, Qiangzhe Zhang, Weiwei Gao, Ronnie H Fang, and Liangfang Zhang. Targeted gene silencing *in Vivo* by platelet membrane-coated metal-organic framework nanoparticles. *Science Advances*, 6(13):eaaz6108, 2020.

[216] Berta Esteban-Fernández de Ávila, Weiwei Gao, Emil Karshalev, Liangfang Zhang, and Joseph Wang. Cell-like micromotors. *Accounts of Chemical Research*, 51(9):1901–1910, 2018.

[217] Lukas Schwarz, Mariana Medina-Sánchez, and Oliver G Schmidt. Hybrid biomicromotors. *Applied Physics Reviews*, 4(3):031301, 2017.

[218] Jinxing Li, Soracha Thamphiwatana, Wenjuan Liu, Berta Esteban-Fernández de Ávila, Pavimol Angsantikul, Elodie Sandraz, Jianxing Wang, Tailin Xu, Fernando Soto, Valentin Ramez, Xiaolei Wang, Weiwei Gao, Liangfang Zhang, and Joseph Wang. Enteric micromotor can selectively position and spontaneously propel in the gastrointestinal tract. *ACS Nano*, 10(10):9536–9542, 2016.

[219] Zhiguang Wu, Lei Li, Yiran Yang, Peng Hu, Yang Li, So-Yoon Yang, Lihong V Wang, and Wei Gao. A microrobotic system guided by photoacoustic computed tomography for targeted navigation in intestines *in Vivo*. *Science Robotics*, 4(32):eaax0613, 2019.

II

Collective Control

CHAPTER 2

Disassembly and Spreading of Collective Nanoparticle Chains for Microrobotic Delivery

2.1 INTRODUCTION

Microrobots actuated by external energy sources (magnetic field [1, 2, 3, 4, 5], electric field [6], and light [7, 8, 9, 10]) have shown promising applications, such as biosensing [11] and minimally invasive surgery [12]. Indeed, microrobots can serve as fluidic tweezers [13, 14] or grippers [15], enabling micromanipulation of cells and proteins. However, real-time tracking of individual microrobots remains a challenging task, primarily due to their small size. Additionally, the limited interaction between an individual microrobot and its cargo can result in reduced efficiency when performing manipulation tasks. These challenges need to be addressed to enhance the tracking capabilities and improve the interaction between microrobots and their manipulated objects for more efficient and precise micromanipulation. Collective behaviors are prevalent in the biological realm, where groups of individuals come together to engage in cooperative tasks [16, 17]. In the face of environmental stimuli, a cohesive swarm has the ability to migrate, assemble, or disassemble. Utilizing swarming intelligence, it becomes feasible to create a collective of artificial microrobots capable of undertaking tasks that would be unattainable for a solitary agent [18, 19, 20, 21]. The application of a swarm shows advantages compared with an individual microrobot. The relatively high area density of swarming microrobots contributes to enhancing the contrast of medical imaging [22, 23, 24] and manipulate a large amount of cargo in one batch [25].

The utilization of a swarm offers notable advantages when compared to an individual microrobot. The relatively dense arrangement of swarming microrobots [22, 23, 24] enhances the contrast of medical imaging. Additionally, swarms have the capability to manipulate a significant quantity of cargo simultaneously allowing for efficient

DOI: 10.1201/9781032665788-2

batch processing [25]. The implementation of a magnetic field is widely recognized as an effective method to induce interactions among magnetic entities, utilizing various external energy sources. In contrast, interactions with nonmagnetic media [26, 27] are generally considered negligible. Various swarm have been proposed such as magnetic asters [28], rings [29, 30], carpets [31], and rollers [32], using time-dependent magnetic fields. By controlling the applied magnetic field, it is possible to adjust these energy-dissipative structures and enable them to perform micromanipulation tasks on interfaces or flat surfaces. This tunability allows for precise manipulation and control over the structures' actions. The utilization of swarms demonstrates the broad application of active colloidal suspensions as fundamental building blocks. This is primarily attributed to their rapid response, as well as their diverse and controllable interactions in response to external stimuli [33, 34, 35, 36]. Among them, magnetite nanoparticles are considered as promising candidates because they are able to be functionalized [37, 38], and have applied to medical imaging [39, 40] and biosensing [41]. Indeed, magnetite nanoparticles have a natural tendency to cluster, particularly when exposed to magnetic fields. This clustering phenomenon leads to a decrease in the surface-to-volume ratio, which consequently reduces the efficiency of surface reactions and diminishes the reproducibility of magnetic nanoparticle-based procedures, including magnetic hyperthermia[42]. The application of magnetic dipole-dipole repulsion has been employed as a method to disassemble micrometer-sized particles on a flat surface [43]. When subjected to a time-dependent magnetic field, aggregated microparticles can be effectively separated into individual components. However, this technique cannot be employed for nanoparticle-based processes, particularly on irregular surfaces. For the reason of the small size [44, 45],the repulsive forces generated between magnetic nanoparticles are insufficient to disperse the clusters. In practical applications, biological tissues and organs often possess micrometer-scale or even millimeter-scale structures, which deviate from a flat surface [46]. As a result, nanoparticle clusters have a tendency to become trapped in the recessed regions of an uneven surface, complicating the disassembly and spreading process. Therefore, additional research is required to explore effective methods for disassembling nanoparticle clusters on uneven surfaces.

In this chapter, we propose the use of a dynamic magnetic field to achieve reversible disassembly of paramagnetic nanoparticle chains. This process allows for controlled distribution of smaller chain segments, while simultaneously reducing the likelihood of recombination by increasing the distances between the disassembled parts. The lengths of the chains can be adjusted, enabling control over their velocity within confined environments, such as bifurcated microvasculature, ensuring controllable motion. Moreover, due to the reversible nature of the assembly/disassembly process, paramagnetic nanoparticles have the potential to alter their clustering form as required, exhibiting behavior akin to a swarm-like entity. The controllable disassembly process comprises two essential elements: (1) the spreading of the chains using repulsive magnetic dipole-dipole forces, and (2) the fragmentation behavior of the paramagnetic particle chains. The dynamic magnetic fields are characterized, and individual models are developed to describe the behaviors of the particle chains. To estimate the length distribution, an analytical model is developed, which demonstrates good agreement with the experimental results. Furthermore, the induced tumbling motion of the nanoparticle chains enables their spread on patterned surfaces when subjected to a rotating magnetic field. The study also demonstrates the disassembly and spreading of nanoparticle clusters on an uneven surface, specifically the bladder of a swine organ. The disassembled nanoparticles can be readily reassembled using a magnetic needle. The reversible process can be monitored using ultrasound imaging, and the resulting dynamic ultrasound contrast is also applicable for eliminating noise signals.

2.2 MATHEMATICAL MODELING AND SIMULATION

Various research groups have proposed different techniques to disrupt chains composed of micro- or nanoparticles. One effective method involves the use of rotating magnetic fields, which can break long particle chains into several smaller segments. However, a challenge arises as these particles tend to attract one another, leading to the formation of longer chains once again due to magnetic attractive forces. Consequently, achieving both the dispersion and fragmentation of magnetic nanoparticle chains are crucial factors in the disassembly process.

2.2.1 Spreading

To facilitate the spreading of nanoparticle chains, it is necessary to apply forces that prompt the chains to move in different directions. In order to meet this requirement, magnetically induced repulsive forces are employed between the paramagnetic nanoparticle chains. These forces work to push the chains apart, allowing for their dispersion and preventing them from rejoining into longer chains.

Here, we assume that an external uniform magnetic field perpendicular to the substrate (*i.e.*, X-Y plane in Figure 2.1a) is applied, which can align the particle chains to Z-axis due to magnetic torques. The chains will be repelled from each other due to the induced repulsive interaction forces. The schematic drawing of the forces exerted on the ith chain are shown in Figure 2.1a. The red arrows indicate the magnetic forces, while the blue arrow indicates the resultant force of friction and hydrodynamic drags. In order to depict the spreading process, the original status of the chains is shown at t_1 and the final status is shown at t_2 . The chains will encounter friction and drags as they moving outwardly, resulting a force balance of each chain

$$M_a \frac{\mathrm{d}^2\mathbf{r}_i(t)}{\mathrm{d}t^2} = \mathbf{F}_i^m + \mathbf{F}_i^d + \mathbf{F}_i^f \tag{2.1}$$

where M_a and $\mathbf{r}_i(t)$ are the mass and the location of the ith chain at the moment t, respectively.

The magnetic force ($\mathbf{F}(\mathbf{P}) \in \mathbb{R}^{3\times1}$) acting on a magnetic dipole can be described as

$$\mathbf{F}(\mathbf{P}) = \nabla\left(\mathbf{m}_c(\mathbf{P}) \cdot \mathbf{B}(\mathbf{P})\right) \tag{2.2}$$

where $\mathbf{m}_c(\mathbf{P}) \in \mathbb{R}^{3\times1}$ and $\mathbf{B}(\mathbf{P}) \in \mathbb{R}^{3\times1}$ are the induced magnetic dipole moment of the chains and the magnetic field at the point $\mathbf{P} \in \mathbb{R}^{3\times1}$, respectively.

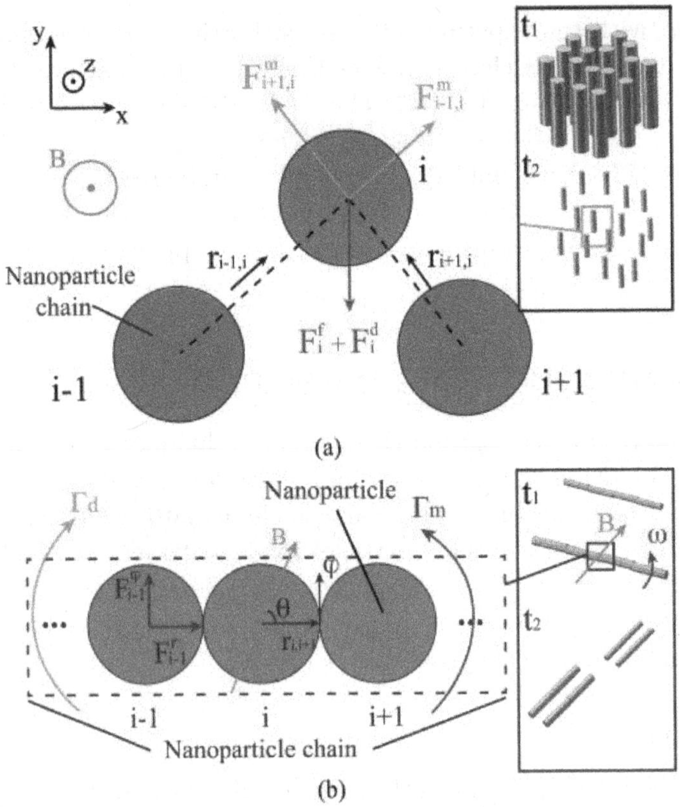

Figure 2.1 Two important elements in disassembly: (a) spreading and (b) fragmentation. (a) Top view of the chains. The forces exerted on the ith chain by the $(i-1)$th and $(i+1)$th chains. $\mathbf{r}_{i+1,i}$ is the unit vector pointing from the centers of the $(i+1)$th chain to the ith chain. The $(i+1)$th chain exerts its magnetic interaction force $\mathbf{F}^m_{i+1,i}$ on the ith chain. Simultaneously, the ith chain encounters a hydrodynamic drag force of $\mathbf{F}^d_i$ and a friction force of $\mathbf{F}^f_i$. (b) Schematic depiction of a part of a paramagnetic nanoparticle chain with a phase lag of θ, which is the angle between the direction of the external magnetic field B and the long axis of the chain $\hat{\mathbf{r}}_{i,i+1}$. φ represents the vector perpendicular to $\hat{\mathbf{r}}_{i,i+1}$. Γ_m and Γ_d indicate the magnetic torque and fluidic drag encountered by the rotating chains. The magnetic interaction forces exerted on the $(i-1)$th particle, which are perpendicular and parallel to the long axis of the chain, are indicated by F^{φ}_{i-1} and F^{r}_{i-1}, respectively.

$$\mathbf{B}(\mathbf{P}) = \sum_{i=1}^{n} \tilde{\mathbf{B}}_i(\mathbf{P}) I_i = \tilde{\mathbf{B}}(\mathbf{P})\mathbf{I} \tag{2.3}$$

where n is the number of the electromagnetic coils, $\tilde{\mathbf{B}}_i(\mathbf{P}) \in \mathbb{R}^{3\times 1}$ is a matrix depends on the measuring position in the working space of the magnetic system, and $\mathbf{I} \in \mathbb{R}^{3\times 1}$ is a vector of the applied current in each coil.

In this part, the chains are regarded as uniform cylinders with the same size and magnetic dipole moment. Therefore, the magnetic dipole moment of each chain can be described as

$$\mathbf{m}_c(\mathbf{P}) = V_p \chi_p \frac{\mathbf{B}(\mathbf{P})}{\mu_0} = a_c^2 l \pi \chi_p \frac{\mathbf{B}(\mathbf{P})}{\mu_0} \tag{2.4}$$

where V_p is the volume of the chain, and χ_p is the effective magnetic susceptibility constant of the nanoparticles. The cylinder has a length of l and a radius of the cross section of a_c , and the permeability of the free space is μ_0. The expression of the magnetic chain–chain force $\mathbf{F}_i^m$ exerted on the ith chain by the rest $N-1$ chains can be expressed as

$$\mathbf{F}_i^m = \frac{3\mu_0}{4\pi} \sum_{\substack{j=1 \\ i\neq j}}^{N} \frac{m_{ci} m_{cj}}{r_{ij}^4} \left[\left(1 - 5\left(\hat{\mathbf{m}} \cdot \hat{\mathbf{r}}_{ij}\right)^2\right) \hat{\mathbf{r}}_{ij} + 2\left(\hat{\mathbf{m}} \cdot \hat{\mathbf{r}}_{ij}\right) \hat{\mathbf{m}} \right] \tag{2.5}$$

where m_{ci} and m_{cj} are the strengths of the magnetic dipole moments of the ith and jth chains, and $\hat{\mathbf{r}}_{ij}$ is the unit vector between the centers of the corresponding two chains, which has a distance of r_{ij}. A unit vector of the magnetic field is indicated as $\hat{\mathbf{m}}$.

In the experiments conducted, the nanoparticle chains are spread within the same plane, with the magnetic field vector $\hat{\mathbf{m}}$ positioned orthogonally to the substrate, while the vector $\hat{\mathbf{r}}_{ij}$ is parallel to the substrate. As a result, the dot product terms become zero, eliminating their contribution. This causes the magnetic interaction force $\mathbf{F}_i^m$ to point outwardly, resulting in the repulsion of the ith chain from the adjacent chains. It is important to note that magnetic dipole-dipole interactions not only generate strong attractive or repulsive forces between the chains but also have the potential to modify the material's magnetization. However, in this chapter, the model disregards the alteration of magnetic dipoles induced by neighboring particles, as their influence is considered negligible.

As the chains disperse under the influence of dipole forces, they experience hydrodynamic drag opposing their motion. In this particular study, the Reynolds number is approximately 0.006. Within this range, the hydrodynamic drag encountered by a chain can be mathematically represented [47]

$$\mathbf{F}_i^d = 3\pi\eta d_e \left(w_{\parallel} f_{E\parallel} + w_{\perp} f_{E\perp}\right) \tag{2.6}$$

$$d_e = d_{\perp} E^{1/3} = d_{\parallel} E^{-2/3} \tag{2.7}$$

where η and d_e are the dynamic viscosity of water and the effective diameter of the chain, respectively. The chain has relative velocity components of $w_{\parallel}$ and $w_{\perp}$, being parallel and perpendicular to the long axis of the chain. $E = \frac{d_{\parallel}}{d_{\perp}}$ is the aspect ratio, and the Stokes correction factors are expressed as $f_{E_{\parallel}} = (4/5 + E/5)E^{-1/3}$ and $f_{E_{\perp}} = (3/5 + E/5)E^{-1/3}$, respectively ($1 < E < 6$). The chains have parallel and normal diameters of $d_{\parallel}$ and $d_{\perp}$, respectively.

Based on the estimation, the drag $\mathbf{F}_i^d \approx 2.1 \times 10^{-11}$ N ($E = 2.2$, $\eta = 8 \times 10^{-4}$ N $\cdot$ s/m^2, $w_{\perp} = 3.1 \times 10^{-5}$ m/s, $w_{\parallel} = 0$, $d_{\parallel} = 1.335 \times 10^{-4}$ m, and $d_{\perp} = 3 \times 10^{-5}$ m). The estimated value of the magnetic dipole force has been made as $\mathbf{F}_i^m \approx 2.49 \times 10^{-8}$ N

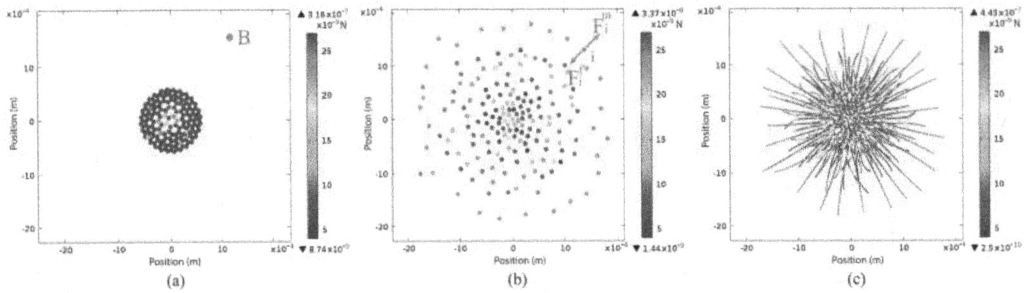

Figure 2.2 Simulation results using COMSOL: (a) Original status of the gathered particles and (b) status at t = 70 s. Each spot represents a magnetic nanoparticle chain, and the colors of the spots indicate the magnitudes of the forces exerted on the chains. The resultant magnetic force F_i^m and the friction F_i^f are labeled with the red arrows, and at this moment the ith particle reaches a force balance. (c) Trajectories of all particles, and the color change represents the change of the force strengths. The friction F_i^f is set to 1.1×10^{-8} N.

(r_{ij} = 100 µm), which is estimated in the situation of existing two chains. Comparing to it, the drag forces are negligible.

The estimation of the friction is difficult due to the complexity of the contact conditions between the chains and the substrate. In fact, the mass of each chain is estimated to be 2×10^{-9} kg, the magnetic interaction force is estimated to be 2.49×10^{-8} N, and the average velocity during spreading is approximately 3.1×10^{-5} m/s. Therefore, the accelerating period is calculated to be extremely short. Meanwhile, because the inertial forces can be neglected in this case, the moving velocity is regarded as a constant during the spreading process, and the friction forces are counterbalanced by the magnetic forces. The friction should be in the same order of magnitude as the magnetic forces, and smaller than the magnetic force generated at the beginning of the spreading. For an approximate estimation, the friction encountered in the microscale can be expressed as $F_f = \tau A_e$. [48], where τ is the shear strength between the chains and the silicon substrate, and A_e is the effective contact area.

In this simulation, the particles are initially confined within a circular area with a radius of 600 µm, as illustrated in Figure 2.2a. The colors assigned to the particles represent their real-time force conditions. At t = 70 s (Figure 2.2b), the spreading of the particles becomes evident, with the outer particles experiencing weaker forces compared to the inner ones. The change in interaction forces is depicted in Figure 2.2c. The simulation employs key parameters listed in Table 2.1. As the distances between the particle chains increase, the magnetic repulsive forces diminish, making it more challenging to overcome friction. Consequently, the velocities of the particles decrease, as illustrated in Figure 2.3. Each curve in Figure 2.3 exhibits a decreasing slope over time, with some curves reaching a plateau before 70 s (for instance, the curve for 8 mT levels out at 60 s and 6 mT at 40 s).

TABLE 2.1 Key parameters used in the simulation

Parameter	Value
Origin position	mesh based
Refinement factor	1
Area of release [mm^2]	3.6×10^{-7}
a [m]	3×10^{-5}
l [m]	1.34×10^{-4}
χ_p	0.95
μ_0 [$V \cdot s/(A \cdot m)$]	1.257×10^{-6}
B [T]	0.01

2.2.2 Fragmentation

To disrupt a magnetic nanoparticle chain, rotating magnetic fields can be employed. The behavior of chain disassembly is estimated using a model that considers a single uniform particle chain. The chain consists of (2N + 1) beads with a radius of a, with the middle bead located at the origin of the coordinate system, and the remaining particles labeled from -N to N. Since the particles are paramagnetic, their magnetizations are assumed to always align parallel to the external magnetic field. The application of the rotating magnetic fields induces dipolar magnetic interactions and torques on the chain, as the long axes of the chains are not parallel to the individual particle dipole moments. Consequently, this leads to the rotation of the chains.

Figure 2.1b provides a schematic representation of the fragmentation process. The blue and yellow arrows in the figure represent the actuating magnetic torque and the drag torque experienced by the chain, respectively. The magnetic forces acting on

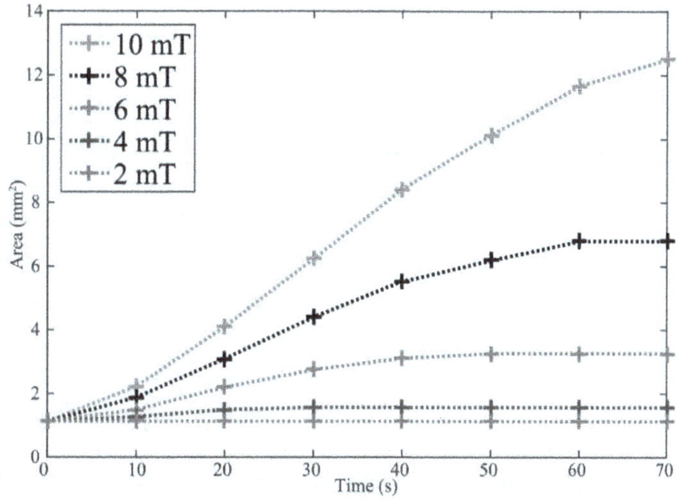

Figure 2.3 Simulation results showing the relationship between the spreading area and the time.

the ith particle, while considering the interaction forces between particles, can be expressed as follows:

$$\mathbf{F}_i = F_i^{\varphi}\mathbf{u}_{\varphi} + F_i^{r}\mathbf{u}_r \tag{2.8}$$

$$F_i^r = \frac{3\mu_0 m^2}{4\pi}\left(1 - 3\cos^2\theta\right)\left[\sum_{j=-N}^{i-1}\frac{1}{r_{ij}^4} - \sum_{j=i+1}^{N}\frac{1}{r_{ij}^4}\right] \tag{2.9}$$

$$F_i^{\varphi} = \frac{3\mu_0 m^2}{4\pi}\sum_{\substack{j=-N\\ j\neq i}}^{N}\frac{2\sin(\theta)\left(\hat{\mathbf{m}}\cdot\hat{\mathbf{r}}_{ij}\right)}{r_{ij}^4} \tag{2.10}$$

where F_i^{φ} and F_i^r are the magnitudes of the forces exerted along $\mathbf{u}_{\varphi}$ and $\mathbf{u}_r$, which are perpendicular to and along the axis of the chain, respectively. $\mathbf{u}_r$ always points to the Nth particle [49]. The phase lag is represented as θ, which is the angle between the magnetic field $\mathbf{B}$ and the vector $\hat{\mathbf{r}}_{i,i+1}$. The magnetic dipole moment of each paramagnetic nanoparticle is m. The centers of the ith particle and the jth particle have a distance of r_{ij}, and the unit vector pointing from the ith particle to the jth particle is $\hat{\mathbf{r}}_{ij}$. Consider the ith particle ($-N < i < 0$), when the chain rotates stably, the direction of the resultant magnetic force exerted on the ith particle points to the Nth particle. The fragmentation process at the ith particle will take place when $\mathbf{F}_i^r$ becomes repulsive, which means the resultant force points to the $-N$th particle. Thus, F_i^r is a negative value to satisfy Eq. (2.8). Moreover, due to the value of $\sum_{j=-N}^{i-1} 1/r_{ij}^{14} - \sum_{j=i+1}^{N} 1/r_{ij}^{14}$ being negative ($-N < i < 0$), the unstable range of the chain is $|\cos\theta| < \sqrt{1/3}$, and the critical value for θ is 54.7°, beyond which the chain will not be stable.

When a chain rotates with a constant angular speed ω, a balance between the magnetic torque Γ_m and the hydrodynamic drag torque Γ_d due to the viscosity of the fluid is reached. If ω increases to the edge of breaking, the fragmentation of the chain will occur. The total torque about the center Γ_m of the chain is obtained by summing up all the torques exerted by the neighboring particle pairs, to be

$$\Gamma_m = 2\sum_{i=1}^{N}\left(F_i^{\varphi} r_i\right) = \frac{3\mu_0 m^2}{4\pi}\sin(2\theta)\sum_{i=1}^{N}\left(2r_i\sum_{\substack{j=-N\\ i\neq j}}^{N}\frac{1}{r_{ij}^4}\right) \tag{2.11}$$

where r_i is the distance between the ith particle and the center of the chain. If only the particle-particle interactions from the nearest neighbor are taken into consideration, the magnetic torque on the chain can be simplified to be [50]

$$\Gamma_m = \frac{3\mu_0 m^2}{4\pi}\sin(2\theta)4aN\frac{1}{(2a)^4} = \frac{3\mu_0 m^2 N}{16\pi a^3}\sin(2\theta) \tag{2.12}$$

where a is the radius of each particle. Meanwhile, the opposing viscous drag is estimated with the shape factor reported by Wilhelm *et al.* [51] as

$$\Gamma_d = \frac{64\pi a^3}{3}\frac{N^3}{\left(\ln(N) + \frac{1.2}{N}\right)}\eta\omega \tag{2.13}$$

where ω is the angular velocity of the rotating chains. Therefore, a modified Mason Number R_T [52], *i.e.*, a parameter to estimate the stability of a rotating particle chain, can be obtained, by dividing the viscous drag torque Γ_d by the driven magnetic torque Γ_m, as

$$R_T = 64\frac{\mu_0 \eta \omega}{\chi_p^2 B^2}\frac{N^2}{\left(\ln(N) + \frac{1.2}{N}\right)}. \tag{2.14}$$

If $R_T < 1$, the magnetic torque is stronger than the viscous drag torque, and the chain keeps stable. Just prior to chain fragmentation, the viscous torque equals to the magnetic torque exerted on the chain, so $R_T = 1$ and the chain rotates following the magnetic field. But, if R_T grows beyond unity, chain fragmentation occurs.

2.2.3 Disassembly

Rotating magnetic fields are widely used to break a particle chain into shorter pieces, and the chains will be broken and reformed regularly following the fields. To realize the on-demand disassembly, fragmentation is one of the requirements, and simultaneously, the reassembly of the chains has to be avoided. We have developed a dynamic magnetic field of combining fragmentation and spreading to realize the disassembly of nanoparticle chains in a controllable manner. Figures 2.4a and 2.4b show the 3D and 2D depictions of the applied dynamic magnetic fields. (1) A tumbling field, rotating perpendicularly to the substrate, and (2) the phase-changing motion: The plane that the field tumbling in keeps shifting with an angle of θ and a frequency of f are simultaneously applied.

The schematic disassembly process is shown in Figure 2.4a. P_1 represents the plane in which the tumbling field initially rotates, and it changes to P_2 with one step. The nanoparticle chain is represented as the black dot chains in Figure 2.4a. At stage I, the particle chain undergoes tumbling motion in P_1, from S_1 to S_2. Then, the plane of the tumbling motion changes from P_1 to P_2, and the chain follows the shifting between phases, as shown in stage II. This stage is referred to as the phase-changing motion, and the chain rotates from S_2 to S_3 (from P_2 to P_3). Once the phase-changing motion is complete, the chain begins tumbling in P_2, from S_3 to S_4, as depicted in stage III. During the disassembly process, the tumbling magnetic field generates chain-chain interaction forces that repel each other outwardly. Since the chains tumble on or near the substrate side-by-side, the likelihood of assembly is greatly reduced. To facilitate disassembly, the frequency of the tumbling field should be kept low enough (*e.g.*, 1 Hz) to allow sufficient time for the interaction forces to increase the chain-chain distances. Additionally, the translational locomotion of all the particle chains due to the tumbling motion should be limited to an acceptable range. Furthermore, the phase-changing motion is employed for effective disassembly of nanoparticle chains. In order to achieve this, the frequency of the phase-changing motion should be set relatively high (*e.g.*, 10–20 Hz).

According to Eqs. (2.9) and (2.14), the fragmentation behavior and length distribution of the disassembled chains are directly influenced by the phase lag. Hence,

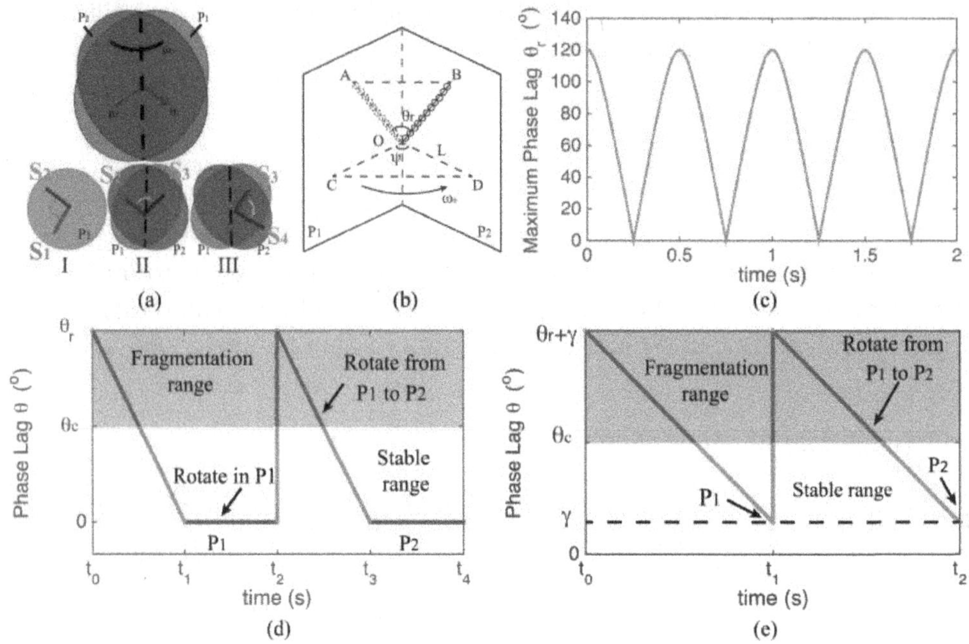

Figure 2.4 (a) and (b) Schematic depictions of the magnetic field proposed for the disassembly of paramagnetic nanoparticle chains. P_1 and P_2 are two phases that the nanoparticle chains rotate in, with n_1 and n_2 as their normal directions, respectively. $S1$–$S4$ are the four steps of a chain, with a length of L, in a disassembly cycle. ψ and θ_r are the angles between two phases and the chain rotates, respectively. The phase-changing signal has an angular velocity of ω_θ. (c) Change of the maximum phase lag θ_r with time. (d) and (e) Phase lags in SPLM and DPLM. In (d) and (e), θ_c and γ are the critical value of the fragmentation threshold and the minimum value of the phase lag, respectively. In the blue region, the chains are unstable and fragmentations can occur, and the white part is the stable region for the chains.

it is crucial to examine the phase lag in order to develop various models based on the rotation speed of the chains (ω_α) and the average rotation speed of the phase-changing signal (ω_θ). By investigating the phase lag, different models can be devised to better understand and predict the dynamics of the disassembly process.

(1) Maximum Value of Phase Lag: In order to determine the maximum value of the phase lag, the influence of the tumbling motion is considered. The phase-changing order is controlled by preprogrammed sequences implemented using a control PC. Since the phase-changing order follows a step order, the low-frequency tumbling motion occurring between two phases can be disregarded. As a result, the angle between the chain and the intersection of two phases remains constant between consecutive phases. The expression for the actual angle of rotation undergone by the chain can be derived as depicted in Figure 2.4b. Hence, the angle between the chain and the intersection of two phases remains constant throughout consecutive phases. The formula for calculating the actual angle of rotation of the chain can be derived as depicted in Figure 2.4b

$$\sin\frac{\theta_r - \phi_0}{2} = \frac{\sqrt{2}}{2}\sqrt{1-\cos\psi}\cos(2\pi f t) \tag{2.15}$$

where θ_r is the angle between the two chains, which is also the maximum phase lag of the chains in this case, and ϕ_0 is the origin phase of the chain. If $\phi_0 = 0$, the chains lie down on the substrate, and they are vertical to the subsection of the two phases. The rotating frequency of the tumbling motion is represented by f, and t is the time. If ψ is set to be 120° and f is 1 Hz, the maximum phase lag θ_r can be depicted using MATLAB as shown in Figure 2.4c.

(2) Static-Phase-Lag Model ($\omega_\alpha > \omega_\theta$): When the average angular velocity of the input phase-changing order, ω_θ, is slower than the angular velocity of the rotating chains ω_α, a static-phase-lag model (SPLM) is established to estimate the fragmentation behavior in this scenario. In the SPLM, after the rotating field transitions to a new phase, it remains stationary for a certain period known as the phase-stop-period (PSP), before transitioning to the next phase. The phase lag of the chains under this model is illustrated in Figure 2.4d. The SPLM allows for the prediction and analysis of the fragmentation behavior under these specific conditions where the average angular velocity of the phase-changing order is slower than that of the rotating chains.

Herein, we define the average angular velocity of the input phase-changing signal ω_θ and the experimental angular velocity of the rotating chain ω_α as

$$\omega_\theta = \frac{\psi}{T_{\text{PSPO}}} \tag{2.16}$$

$$\omega_\alpha = \frac{\theta_r}{T_r} \tag{2.17}$$

where ψ is the angle between two phases, and T_{PSPO} is the duration of the PSP in the predefined program (the length of the duration is the same as $t_2 - t_0$ in Figure 2.4d, which is the period between the phase-changing signals. T_r is the duration of the chains shifting from one phase to another (*i.e.*, $t_1 - t_0$ in Figure 2.4d). The slope of the red curve indicates the process of the chains rotating from phase 1 to phase 2. Since the Reynolds number in the experiment is small enough, the inertial torque can be neglected [53]. Therefore, the torques applied to the chains are balanced, and we can assume that the phase lag decreases at a constant rate. As $\omega_\alpha > \omega_\theta$, the chains will reach the new phase before the end of PSP, and the phase lag from t_1 to t_2 remains zero (the frequency of the tumbling motion is low enough, and the corresponding phase lag can be neglected), represented by the blue line in the figure. In the green part of the figure, the disassembly of the chains is very likely to occur, while the white part represents a stable range for the chain. In this case, increasing the frequency of the phase-changing signal has no influence on the disassembly results of the chains until this frequency reaches a critical value (the angular velocity of the chains), which will lead to another model.

(3) Dynamic-Phase-Lag Model ($\omega_\alpha = \omega_\theta$): When the frequency of the input phase-changing signal increases, until there are no stops for the chains in any phases (*i.e.*, $T_{\text{PSPO}} = T_r = t_1 - t_0$ in Figure 2.4e), the dynamic-phase-lag model (DPLM) can express the phase lags, as shown in Figure 2.4e. The chains will not stop, and therefore, a minimum phase lag of γ always exists in the motion cycle. In this velocity range, the frequency of the phase-changing motion will greatly affect the disassembly results. Because the maximum value θ_r keeps changing sinusoidally, the phase lag of these two cases does not change linearly.

2.2.4 Assembly

There are various techniques available for assembling the scattered fragments. One approach involves using a permanent magnet tip to collect chains of magnetic particles through the magnetic field gradient. However, as the distance from the tip increases, the magnetic gradient significantly decreases. Therefore, it is necessary to explore a more efficient method. To disrupt the chain-like aggregation, a rotating magnetic field can be employed. This not only breaks the chains but also generates fluidic vortices as the chains rotate. These vortices, produced by the fragmented pieces, exert a strong fluidic interaction on other fragments. By selecting an appropriate frequency, the fluidic microvortices can attract smaller rotating pieces, facilitating the formation of larger clusters. Ultimately, this process allows for the successful reassembly of most of the fragments.

2.3 MAGNETIC ACTUATION SETUP AND NANOPARTICLES

2.3.1 Hardware for Magnetic Actuation

The experimental studies were carried out using a three-axis Helmholtz electromagnetic coils setup, as depicted in Figure 2.5. The maximum strength of the magnetic field was 10 mT, with a minimum step size of 0.1 mT. Control signals were generated using a Sensoray 826 card, and the current was amplified to produce magnetic fields in the working space. The magnetic fields required for disassembling the chains were generated based on the sequence proposed in the modeling part, as shown in Figures 2.4a and 2.4b. The order of the dynamic field was determined by the control PC. Through this numerically controlled setup, various parameters such as the frequency of tumbling motion, phase-changing frequency, strength, and original phase of the magnetic field could be pre-defined through programming. The magnetic actuation experiments were conducted in an open tank filled with deionized water. A silicon wafer was used as the substrate for the disassembly process, with its polished surface enhancing the imaging contrast during observation.

2.3.2 Synthesis of Paramagnetic Nanoparticles

The synthesis of magnetite paramagnetic nanoparticles was previously described in reference [54]. In this method, $FeCl_3 \cdot 6H_2O$ (1.35 g, 5 mmol) was dissolved in ethylene glycol (40 mL) to obtain a clear solution. Next, NaAc (3.6 g) and polyethylene glycol

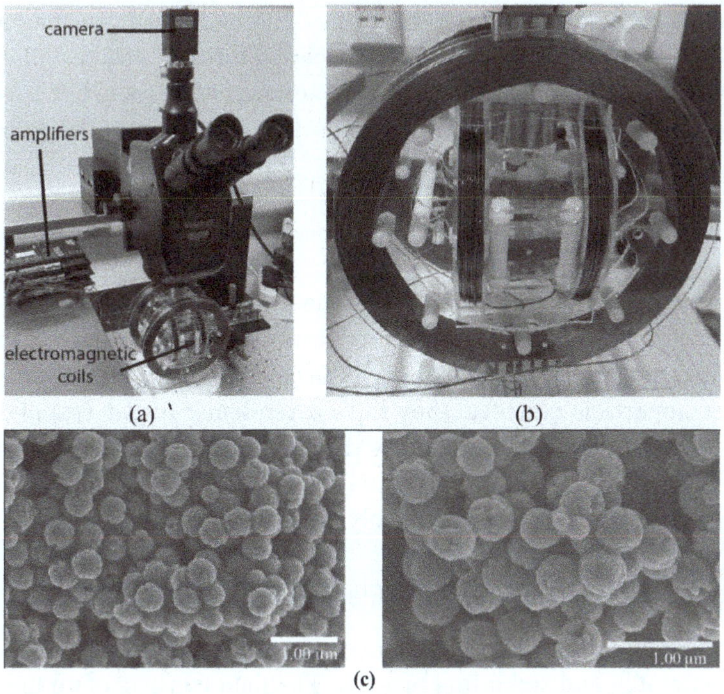

Figure 2.5 (a) and (b) Set of three-axis Helmholtz electromagnetic coils are used for generating the dynamic magnetic fields. A PointGrey camera is for recording the experiments and three Maxon motor controllers are served as the amplifiers. (c) SEM micrographs showing the magnetic nanoparticle aggregations.

(1.0 g) were added to the solution. The mixture was vigorously stirred for 30 minutes and then transferred to a Teflon stainless-steel autoclave with a capacity of 50 mL. The autoclave was sealed and heated to 200 °C, maintaining this temperature for 8–72 hours. After cooling to room temperature, the resulting black product was identified as magnetite nanoparticles. The nanoparticles were washed multiple times with ethanol and dried at 60 °C for 6 hours. SEM images depicting the nanoparticles are shown in Figure 2.5c. Based on these images, the average particle diameter was calculated to be approximately 500 nm, a value that will be used for modeling and estimating the disassembly performance in the subsequent analysis.

2.3.3 Gathering of Paramagnetic Nanoparticles

To begin the experiment, a single drop of nanoparticle suspension measuring 6 μL was added to the tank. The particles were initially gathered by placing a permanent magnet beneath the tank. To enhance the gathering process, the magnet was slightly moved within a small region. Subsequently, the particle clusters were transferred to the workspace of the electromagnetic coils for further manipulation. Initially, an in-plane oscillating magnetic field with a strength of 10 mT was applied. The magnetic field oscillated at an angle of 40°. As a result of the magnetic interactions, the particles were attracted to each other, leading to the formation of large clusters characterized by spindle-shaped aggregations. The high-strength magnetic fields ensured a strong combination among the particles. Moreover, the oscillating magnetic fields induced the motion of the aggregations across a wide sector-shaped area, allowing the remaining microparticles to be drawn toward the main body of the particle cluster.

2.4 CHALLENGE AND DISCUSSION

The analysis mentioned above is based on the assumption of a smooth plane. However, in practical applications, biological tissues and organs often possess microscale or even millimeter-scale structures on their surfaces, making them non-planar. When it comes to nanoparticle clusters, they have a tendency to get trapped in the lower regions of uneven surfaces, which makes disassembly and spreading more challenging. Consequently, a more intricate actuating field is necessary to facilitate chain fragmentation while preventing reassembly simultaneously.

2.4.1 Design of the Dynamic Magnetic Field (DMF)

A dynamic magnetic field (DMF) has been designed (Figure 2.6a) to perform the proposed disassembly and spreading process. The field consists of an in-plane rotating magnetic field (B_{xy}) and an out-of-plane oscillating magnetic field (B_z), and the resultant field could be generated by a three-axis Helmholtz coil system. The out-of-plane oscillating component is expressed as

$$\mathbf{B}_z = B\cos\theta_m \cdot \sin(2\pi f_z t)\hat{\mathbf{z}} \tag{2.18}$$

where B is the maximum field strength, θ_m is the minimal precession angle, and f_z is the vertical oscillating frequency. Two sinusoidal fields with a 90° phase difference combine into the in-plane rotating component, as

$$\mathbf{B}_{xy} = \mathbf{B}_x + \mathbf{B}_y = B\sin\theta_m \cdot [\sin(2\pi f_{xy} t)\hat{\mathbf{x}} + \cos(2\pi f_{xy} t)\hat{\mathbf{y}}] \tag{2.19}$$

where f_{xy} is the in-plane rotating frequency. During actuation, the time-dependent precession angle $\theta(t)$ is changing between θ_m and $\pi - \theta_m$. The magnetic field strength $B(t)$ reaches maximum value B when $\theta(t) = \theta_m$ and $\pi - \theta_m$, and minimal value $B_{min} = B\sin\theta_m$ when $\theta(t) = 90°$. Figure 2.6b shows the visualization of the superposition of the dynamic field over a cycle. The lower in-plane rotating frequency (1 Hz) and higher out-of-plane oscillating frequency (10 Hz) shape the field trajectory like a lotus flower.

The actuation and disassembly process of a particle chain near a substrate is schematically demonstrated in Figure 2.6c. We assume the effect of the boundary to the drag force is negligible, and the viscous drag coefficient remains constant along the chain. First, the magnetic attraction between nanoparticles leads to the formation of nanoparticle chains (stage I). In this stage, the angular velocity of chain is close to zero and meanwhile, the magnetic field reaches the maximum value. Therefore, a stable particle chain is yielded when the magnetic torque reaches the maximum value and viscous drag is negligible. To induce fragmentation of chains, we decrease

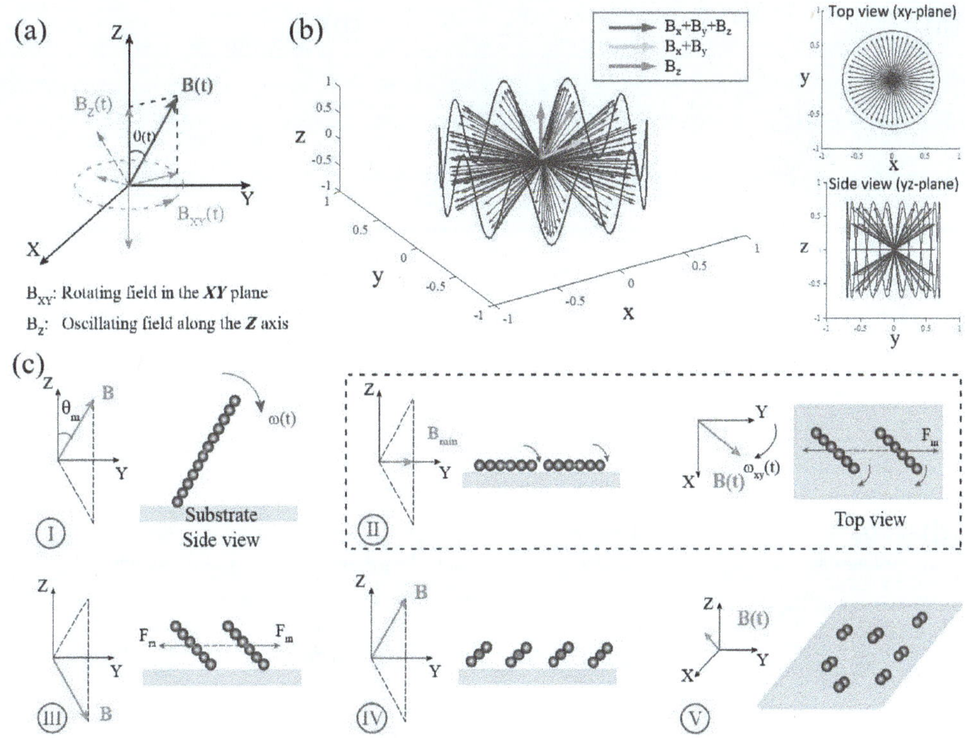

Figure 2.6 (a) Schematic demonstration of the DMF, B_{xy} and B_z refer to the in-plane rotating field and out-of-plane oscillating field, respectively. $\theta(t)$ is the time-dependent precession angle. (b) Visualization of the superposition field, including an in-plane rotating field ($B_x + B_y$) and an out-of-plane oscillating field (B_z). The top and side view illustrate the rotating and oscillating components of the field, respectively. (c) Schematic demonstration of the proposed disassembly and spreading process actuated by the DMF. $\omega(t)$ refers to the angular velocity of nanoparticle chains, F_m refers to the magnetic repulsive forces between chains.

the field strength and simultaneously increase the angular velocity of the field as illustrated in stage II. When $\theta_m = 90°$, angular velocity reaches the maximum value while $B(t) = B_{min}$, resulting in an increase of viscous drag and fragmentation of chain consequently. In this stage, a magnetic repulsive force (F_m) between chains is induced due to the simultaneous rotation of chains in the XY plane. The repulsive force is maximized in stage III (maximum field strength), where the distances between chains are further enlarged and reduces the chance of reassembly. Repeating the process of I-III yields shorter nanoparticle chains and increases the coverage area of nanoparticles (stage IV). Finally, a number of shorter chains is obtained from the disassembly of the initial nanoparticles chain and gradually spreading to a larger area (stage V).

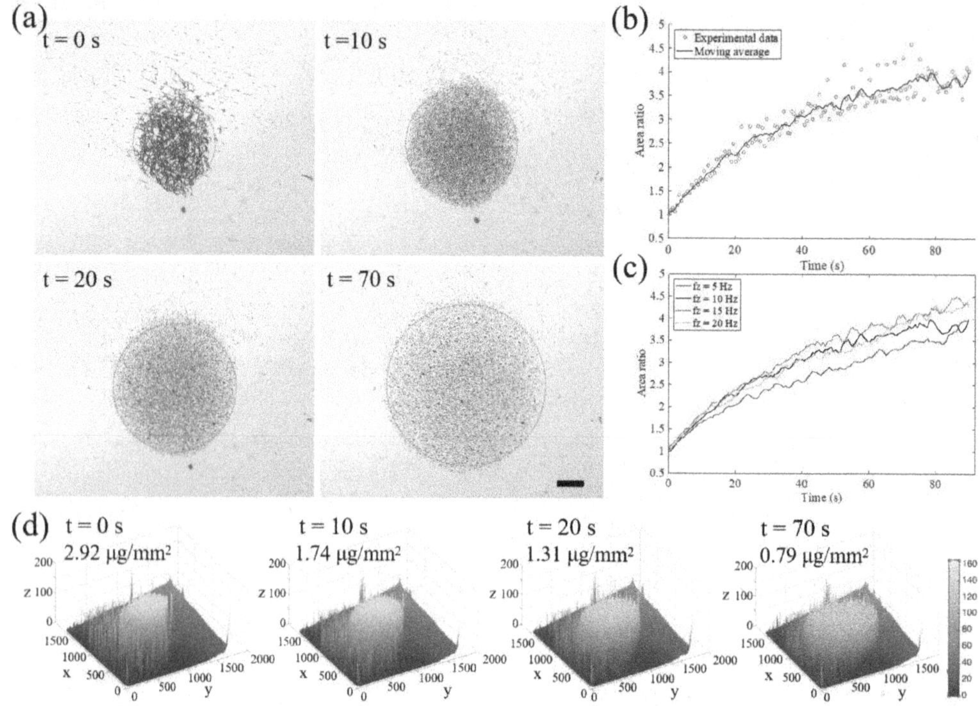

Figure 2.7 (a) Disassembly and spreading process of Fe_3O_4 nanoparticles. The coverage area is tracked and included in the blue circles. Applied field parameters are $B = 8$ Hz, $\theta_m = 30°$, f_{xy}= 3 Hz and $f_z = 10$ Hz. (b) Changing of the coverage area during actuation. Dots are the tracking results from experiments. Curve refers to the moving average over a sliding window with a length of 4 (average value of four neighboring data). (c) The changes of coverage area actuated by DMF with four different out-of-plane oscillating frequencies (f_z). Curves are the moving average of the tracking results over a sliding window with a length of 4. (d) Changing of area density of nanoparticles during the actuation from (A). Scale bar is 500 μm.

2.4.2 Validation of the Disassembly and Spreading Strategy on a Flat Surface

Experiments of the disassembly of Fe_3O_4 clusters are shown in Figure 2.7a. Add 3 μL of Fe_3O_4 nanoparticle suspension (2 mg/mL) into the tank, which is filled with 1.5 wt.% polyvinylpyrrolidone (PVP) aqueous solution with a silicon wafer as the substrate. Based on SEM images, the average diameter of nanoparticles is 300 nm (JEOL system model JSM-7800F). Using PVP aqueous solution, set up a low Reynolds number environment ($\sim 1 \times 10^{-3}$). First, through a rotating magnetic field with field gradient toward the center of the tank to gather these nanoparticles. During actuation, the coverage area of nanoparticles is tracked by a designed LabVIEW program in real time. Above 90% of the nanoparticles are contained in the tracking area (blue circles in Figure 2.7a). Figures 2.7b and 2.7c show changes of the coverage area during actuation and the coverage area of nanoparticles increases to 450% of the initial area. As mentioned above, magnetic chain-chain repulsion results in spreading of the nanoparticles. Therefore, in spreading process of the nanoparticles, oscillating frequencies of the external field have little effect (Figure 2.7c). Moreover, the area density of nanoparticles declines from 2.92 μg/mL to 0.79 μg/mL in this process as correspondingly shown in Figure 2.7d, indicating the nanoparticles clusters disassemble and obtain a larger coverage area.

In order to better understand the mechanism of disassembly and spreading process, an analytical model is established based on the counterbalance relationship between magnetic torque and drag torque a particle chain experienced. Based on our analysis, the disassembly process is caused by the out-of-plane oscillating field, and the in-plane rotating field is used to prevent the reassembly of the disassembled short chains. Therefore, to simplify the first-step analysis, we only consider the out-of-plane field (Figure 2.8a). For a nanoparticle chain of N particles, the driven magnetic torque can be expressed as [55]

$$\Gamma_m = \frac{3\mu_0 m^2(t)(N-1)}{4\pi(2R)^3}\sin(2\alpha) \tag{2.20}$$

where μ_0 is the magnetic permeability for free space and R is the particle radius. $m(t) = V_p\chi_p B(t)/\mu_o$ is the induced dipole moment of a particle, where $V_p = \frac{4}{3}\pi R^3$ is the volume of the nanoparticle and χ_p is the effective magnetic susceptibility.

$$L = 2NR. \tag{2.21}$$

In the disassembly process of chains, when the velocity reaches the maximum value (stage II, Figure 2.6c), nanoparticle chains have the most possibility to fragmentate. Figure 2.8b shows the maximum angular velocity is 108.8 rad/s, which becomes 111.6 rad/s with the consideration of a 3 Hz in-plane rotation ($\sim$ 0.7% increases). α refers to the phase lag between the long axis of the chain and the applied field (vertical oscillating field). The drag torque of a nanoparticle chain considering the shape factor is expressed as [56]

$$\Gamma_d = \frac{8\pi R^3}{3}\frac{N^3}{\ln(\frac{N}{2}) + \frac{2.4}{N}}\eta\omega(t) \tag{2.22}$$

where η is the viscosity of the surrounding fluid and $\omega(t)$ is the angular velocity of the chain in the YZ plane. According to the definition, the modified Mason number in our case can be expressed as [57]

$$R_T = 16\frac{\mu_0\eta\omega(t)}{\chi_p^2 B^2(t)}\frac{N^3}{(N-1)(\ln(\frac{N}{2}) + \frac{2.4}{N})}. \tag{2.23}$$

The field strength $B(t)$ and angular velocity $\omega(t)$ are both time-dependent parameters and need further derived. The field strength is defined by the oscillating angle as $B(t) = B\cos\varphi(t)$, shown in Figure 2.8a, and the angular velocity $\omega(t)$ can be obtained from the derivative of the oscillating angle. The changes of $B(t)$ and $\omega(t)$ with time are plotted in Figure 2.8b. When $\varphi(t) = 0$, $\omega(t)$ reaches the maximum velocity and the drag torque reaches the maximum value as we discussed in Eq. (2.22). When $R_T = 1$, there is a critical case, where the drag torque equals the maximum

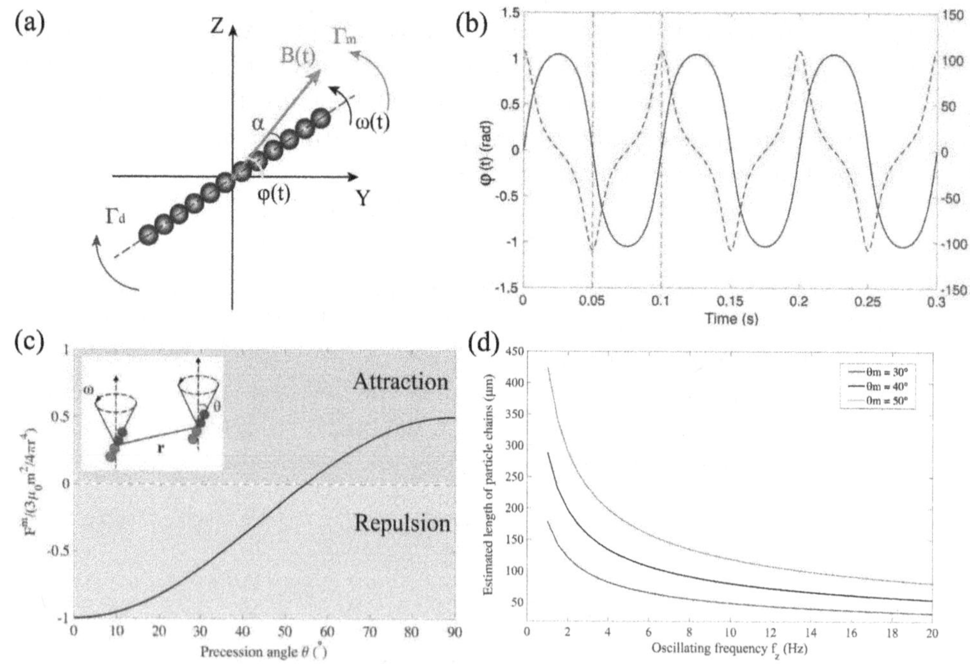

Figure 2.8 (a) Schematic of a nanoparticle chain actuated by the DMF in the YZ plane. $\varphi(t)$ refers to the oscillating angle between the long axis of the chain and the XY plane, α refers to the phase lag, and $\omega(t)$ is the angular velocity. Γ_m and Γ_d are magnetic torque and drag torque, respectively. (b) Changing of the oscillating angle $\varphi(t)$ (black line) and the angular velocity $\omega(t)$ (blue dashed line). Red dashed lines indicate the maximum angular velocity. Applied field parameters are $\theta_m = 30°$ and $f_z = 10$ Hz. (c) Relationship of magnetic interaction between chains over a cycle and applied precession angles. (d) Estimated lengths of particle chains (L) versus input oscillating frequency under θ_m of 30°, 40° and 50°.

driven magnetic torque. Therefore, the number (N) of nanoparticles of chain can be solved providing $R_T = 1$, and the length of nanoparticle chain is calculated by Higher input oscillating frequency will further reduce the importance of the in-plane component. Therefore, the in-plane rotation component is neglected to simplify analysis. The fragmentation of a nanoparticle chain and chain-chain interaction both act on the disassembly process. To prevent reassembly, we could try to avoid the magnetic attraction between chains or limit it in a negligible range. Over a cycle, the mean magnetic interaction between magnetic chains can be expressed as [58]

$$F_m = -\frac{3\mu_0 m^2}{4\pi r^4}\left(\frac{3\cos^2\theta - 1}{2}\right) \tag{2.24}$$

where r is the center distance between chains. Eq. (2.24) indicates that the precession angle can determine the magnetic interaction (attraction or repulsion). Figure 2.8c shows the relationship between the input precession angle and the sign of net interaction, if $54.7° < \theta < 90°$ the interaction is attractive while it is repulsive if $0° < \theta < 54.7°$. The dipolar interaction vanished at a particular angle of 54.7°. Based on Eqs. (2.20)–(2.23), numerical solutions of lengths can be calculated on MATLAB. The relationship between the length of chains and oscillating frequency at three minimal precession angles is shown in Figure 2.8d. In the case of actuation with a relatively high f_z and a small θ_m, it is easier to obtain relatively shorter chains indicated by the results.

Based on the analysis, it is capable of improving the disassembly process by increasing the exerted viscous drag. An approach through applying the DMF with a higher out-of-plane oscillating frequency (f_z) to increase the angular velocity of nanoparticle chains. The experimental results actuated by the DMF with four different f_z are shown in Figure 2.9a. To quantitatively investigate the length distributions of disassembled nanoparticle chains (Figure 2.9b), we designed and utilized a MATLAB image processing algorithm. Nanoparticle chains have a chance to overlap, applying a static magnetic field with a pitch angle of 60° to the XY plane at the final stage of each process to avoid that. Length-based data are calculated on the ground of the sum of lengths within a range (*e.g.*, 40–50 μm) divided by the total lengths of all nanoparticle chains. Nanoparticles stuck on the substrate are the main formative factor of noise signals. Therefore, the length-based calculation can effectively decrease the disturbance of the noise signals. The data shows the peak range of lengths (marked with dashed ellipse in Figure 2.9b) decreases with the increase of the out-of-plane oscillating frequency f_z. The peak range is 80–100 μm when f_z is 4 Hz, and it further decreases to 50–70 μm and 30–50 μm when the f_z increases to 10 Hz and 20 Hz, respectively. In comparison to the length distribution when f_z = 4 Hz, lengths of nanoparticle chains shorter than 100 μm increase around 30% in the case of 20 Hz, and even becomes 116.5% by summing the total percentage of lengths shorter than 50 μm. The results indicate that increasing the oscillating frequency can improve the disassembly process and have good agreement with the analysis in Figure 2.8d.

Based on our analytical model, the disassembly and spreading process can be tuned by adjusting the input minimal precession angle. The results of the actuation with four different θ_m and the length distribution of nanoparticle chains are shown in Figures 2.9c and 2.9d, respectively. The percentage of lengths in the 30–100 μm accounts for over 60% of the total when $\theta_m = 40°$, and it schematically decreases to 13.2% ($\theta_m = 70°$) with a larger θ_m. However, in the case of 70°, more particle chains are reassembled to clusters and the chains shorter than 200 μm account for less than 30%. By contrast, this percentage with $\theta_m = 40°$ increases to around three times (~86.3%). The nanoparticle clusters experimentally show that it is hard to be disassembled with higher input θ_m, and when $\theta_m = 70°$ many clusters can be clearly observed. Analyze results from these experiments in three aspects. First, the repulsion between particle chains (Eq. (2.24)) is decreased by the increased precession angles, providing a higher possibility for the reassembly of the chains. Here, we use the $\theta_m = 30°$-case for an example, where the change range of precession angle is 30° to 150°. The net magnetic chain-chain interaction is attraction when $54.7° < \theta(t) < 125.3°$, and repulsion when $30° < \theta(t) < 54.7°$ and $125.3° < \theta(t) < 150°$. The angular velocity of chain varies with time, and the time with a different stage of interaction can be calculated. The time of chains subjected

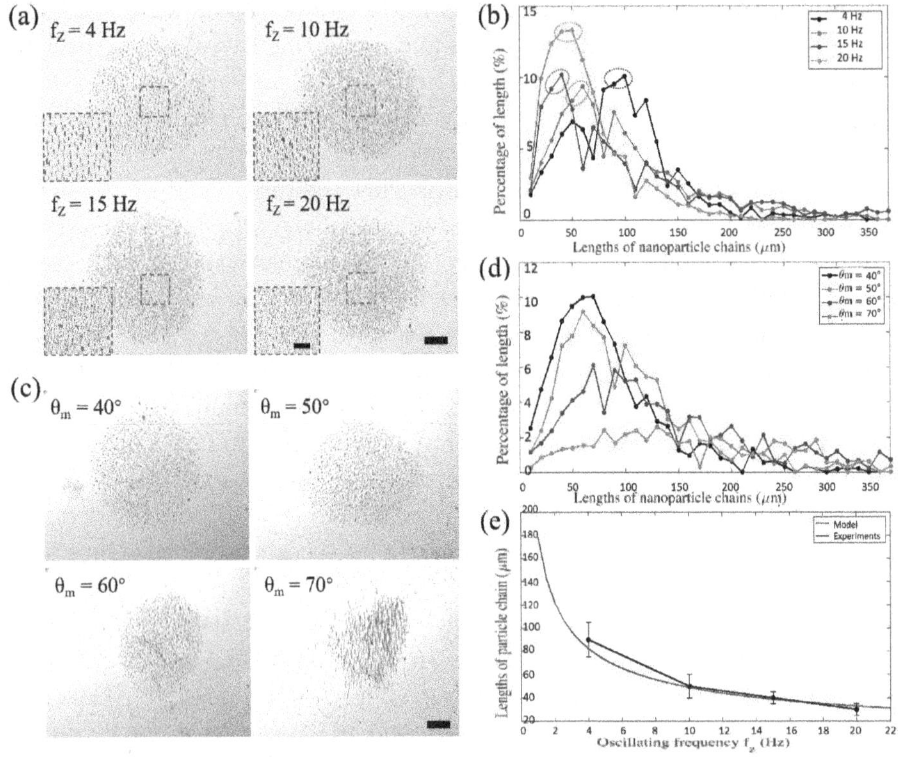

Figure 2.9 (a) Experimental results after a 60 s disassembly process at four different out-of-plane frequencies (f_z). The applied field parameters are $B = 8$ mT, $f_{xy} =$ 3 Hz, and $\theta_m = 30°$. Scale bar is 600 μm. Inset are the enlarged view of partial areas marked with dashed rectangles. Scale bar is 200 μm. (b) Distribution of chain lengths after the disassembly with input f_z of 4 Hz, 10 Hz, 15 Hz, and 20 Hz. The peak ranges are correspondingly pointed out by dashed ellipses. Data are obtained from images of (a). (c) Experimental results after a 60 s disassembly process at four different minimal precession angles (θ_m). The applied field parameters are $B = 8$ mT, $f_{xy} = 3$ Hz, and $f_z = 10$ Hz. Scale bar is 600 μm. (d) Distribution of chain lengths after the disassembly with input θ_m of 40°, 50°, 60°, and 70°. Data are obtained from images of (c). (e) Comparison of particle chain lengths between experimental results and the analytical model when θ_m of 30°. Error bars denote the standard deviation from three trials.

to repulsion accounts for 73.2% of a cycle, *i.e.*, around 2.73 times the time of attraction. Spreading of nanoparticle chains is governed by the exerted magnetic force from neighboring chains and drag from the substrate. Due to the time-dependence of the chain-chain interaction, we analyze the effective interaction between chains by using the integral of magnetic interaction in a time slot ($\int F_m(t)dt$) as the criterion. The repulsion is four times stronger than attraction, we learn from calculated results, indicating that the interaction between chains is dominated by the magnetic repulsion.

However, the dominant interaction is attraction in the $\theta_m = 70°$-case. Although the drag by the substrate can counteract part of the attraction between chains, clusters still exist. Second, the change range of precession angles is narrowed down and the maximum angular velocity is decreased with larger θ_m. The insufficient drag torque cannot break the stabilization of relatively long chains. Third, the precession angle defines the magnetic strength, and the minimal magnetic field is increased with θ_m ($B_{min} = B \sin \theta_m$). Mason number (Eq. (2.23)) is decreased by the increased magnetic torque, reducing the chance for triggering fragmentation of chains. Our modeling results indicate that we could obtain more effective results with a smaller input θ_m in the case of the same input f_z, which has a good agreement with our experimental results. However, there is a limitation in defining the θ_m. If the driven magnetic torque falls below a critical value, nanoparticle chains will reach the step-out frequency [59]. Once actuating over the step-out frequency, the asynchronous chains with stops and backward motions will diminish the drag torque. In the following experiments, the θ_m is set as 30°.

A comparison of chain length between experiments and the model is plotted in Figure 2.9e. We use the peak range (marked in Figure 2.9b) to represent the experimental results. The difference between the results from experiments and analytical model is mainly caused by the following two reasons. First, the interaction between nanoparticle chains. Mason number is originally applied to examine the stability of an individual nanoparticle chain. During experiment, the interaction among multiple chains affects the stability of a chain. The lengths of chains at input $f_z = 4$ Hz–15 Hz are higher than the estimation value from the analytical model (Figure 2.9e), indicating that the chains in experiments are more stable than that in the model. Therefore, a higher f_z is acquired to obtain the desired length of chains. Second, the simplicity of the analytical model. For the estimation of chain lengths, we only consider the effect of the out-of-plane oscillating field. The phase lag α between the chain and the applied field in the XY plane is not taken into consideration, which may cause a minor effect on the chain lengths. However, the good agreement between the experimental results and the model indicates the feasibility of our proposed analytical model.

2.4.3 Validation of the Disassembly and Spreading Strategy on Patterned Surfaces

In order to further expand the application of the proposed strategy, we perform the disassembly and spreading process on a patterned surface. We bound two Kapton foils on the substrate at a certain distance as shown in Figure 2.10, which have a varied thickness from 25 μm to 150 μm. Add nanoparticle clusters into the depression formed by the substrate and foil steps. Under a 60 s continuous actuation, disassembled chains gradually cross the 25 μm high steps and spread to a larger area. We then use steps of 100 μm height to repeat the experiment. As shown in Figure 2.10b, all the disassembled chains cannot cross the higher steps under the same actuation. Over half of the nanoparticle chains are shorter than 80 μm as shown in Figure 2.9b, and they are hard to cross the steps of 100 μm height (t = 60 s, Figure 2.10b). In reality, because of being subjected the stronger repulsive forces, the relatively longer chains

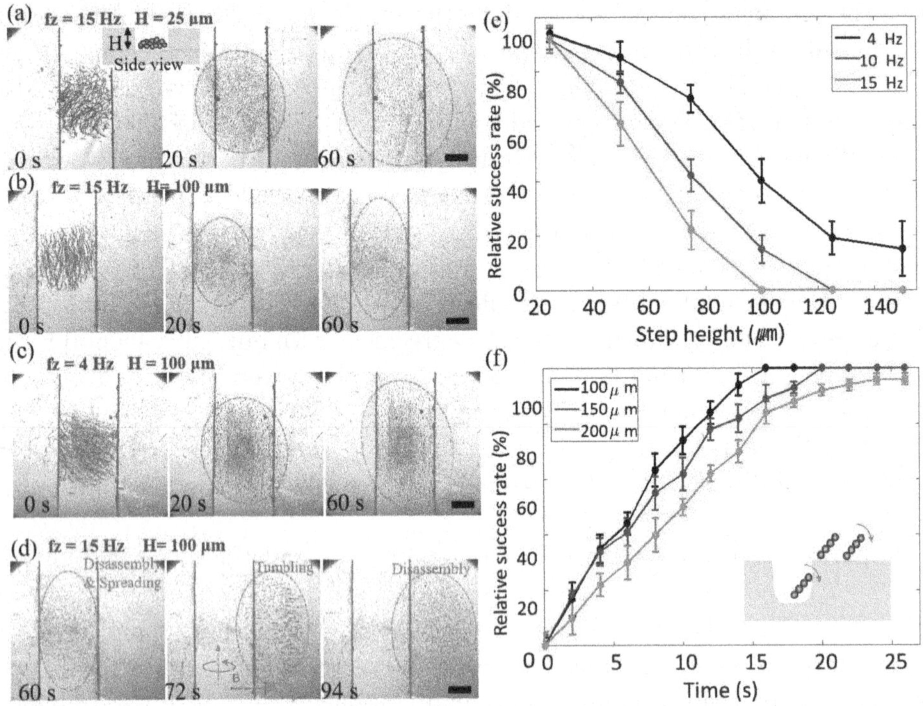

Figure 2.10 Disassembly and spreading process on patterned surfaces. (a) Conducting the process on a patterned surface with the step height (H) of 25 μm. Blue circles indicate the coverage area of nanoparticles, and yellow areas refer to the coverage area above the steps. Field parameters: $B = 8$ mT, $f_z = 15$ Hz, $\theta_m = 30°$. (b) Conducting the process with H of 100 μm and f_z of 15 Hz. (c) Conducting the process with H of 100 μm and f_z of 4 Hz. (d) Nanoparticles are actuated by the DMF and the following rotating field. The tumbling field has a frequency of 1 Hz (72 s). (e) Relative success rate versus step height actuated by the DMF with f_z of 4 Hz, 10 Hz, and 15 Hz. (f) Changes of relative success rate under the actuation of a rotating field with H of 100 μm, 150 μm, and 200 μm. Error bars are standard deviations from three trials. All scale bars are 800 μm.

can cross the steps. Tuning the input f_z to 4 Hz to obtain better cross-step ability. We get longer chains and part of the chains are able to cross the 100 μm steps (Figure 2.10c). The coverage area of chains in Figures 2.10a–c exhibits ellipse-like shapes differ from the circular area in Figure 2.7a, because steps hinder the spreading of chains. Therefore, the anisotropic boundary condition affects the final shape of the coverage area. Alternatively, we could exert an out-of-plane rotating field with the rotating axis parallel to the XY plane to actuate the stuck nanoparticles in Figure 2.10b. Under the applied rotating field, nanoparticle chains move toward the right side by tumbling motion (t = 72 s, Figure 2.10d) because of the friction asymmetry caused by the boundary [60]. These nanoparticles are able to cross the steps gradually even the step heights are higher than the length of the chains. We can change the frequency and yaw angle of the external field to tune the velocity and actuation direction of nanoparticle chains, respectively. It is beneficial for these chains to cross the steps and the realization of the disassembly process (t = 94 s). The relative success rate is used as the criterion to evaluate the expansion ability of nanoparticles by using only the DMF (Figure 2.10e). The rate is defined as the coverage area above the steps (yellow areas in Figures 2.10a and 2.10c) divided by the area in the control group that performed on a flat substrate. The area from the control group is calculated by subtracting the area in the depression in Figure 2.10 from the total coverage area. The success rates reach higher than 50% with step heights smaller than or equal to 50 μm. The rate increases with a lower f_z due to the longer disassembled chains. With an input f_z of 4 Hz, approximately 20% of chains are able to cross the 125 μm step. In the case of different step heights, the success rates of nanoparticles crossing steps as shown in Figure 2.10f. Use an input f_z = 15 Hz to disassemble the clusters and then change to a 1 Hz rotating field to actuate them (similar to Figures 2.10b and 2.10d). Tumbling motion is an effective approach on patterned surfaces. Above 90% of nanoparticle chains are capable of crossing a 200 μm step in 25 s, indicating the drag asymmetry at the two ends of the chain can overcome its own gravity [61].

2.4.4 *Ex Vivo* Validation on the Surface of Bladder with Ultrasound Imaging Guidance

Figures 2.11 and 2.12 shows *ex vivo* experiments, which demonstrate the application of proposed disassembly and spreading strategy on a surface of a bladder of swine. We fill the bladder with 1.8% aqueous solution of urea and place it at the center of

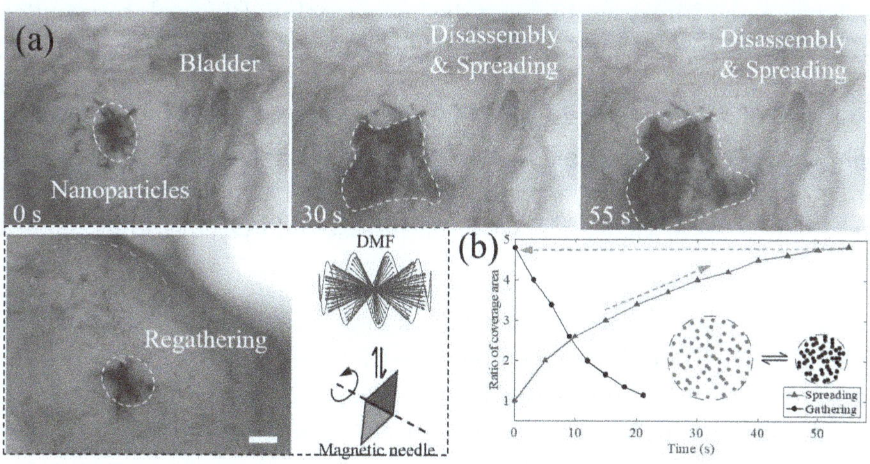

Figure 2.11 Reversible disassembly and regathering of Fe_3O_4 nanoparticles inside a bladder of swine. (a) The coverage area increases gradually under the actuation of the DMF (0–55 s). The disassembled nanoparticles are regathered again using a magnetic needle, where blue polygon indicates the previous coverage area of nanoparticles before the regathering process. Scale bar is 4 mm. (b) Changes of coverage area during spreading and regathering process in comparison with the initial area (t = 0 s in (a)). The regathering process follows the disassembly process as indicated by the red arrows.

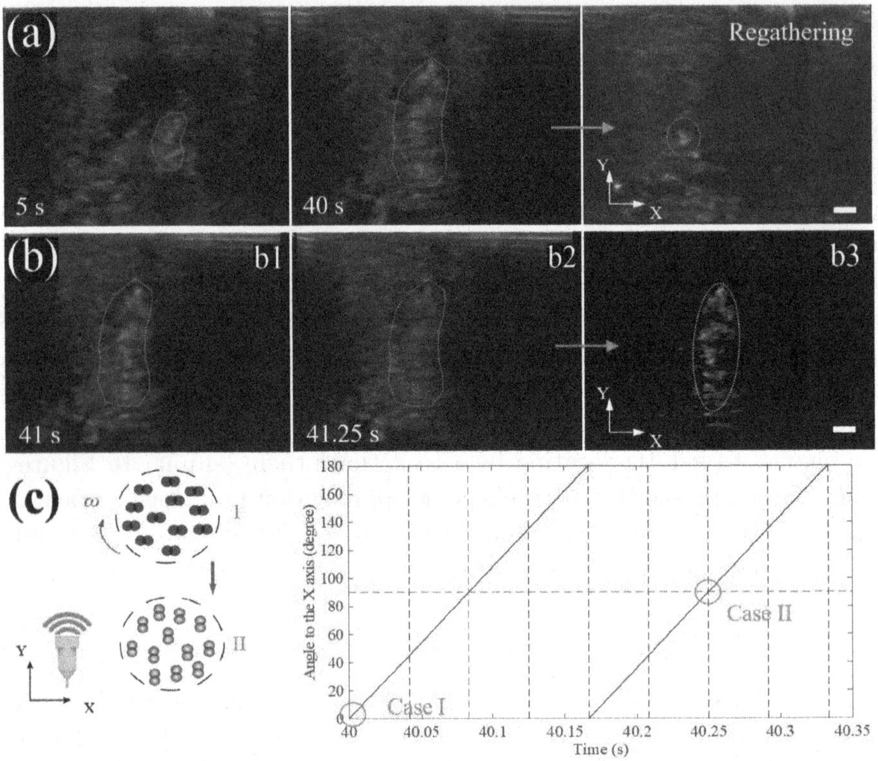

Figure 2.12 Reversible disassembly and regathering of Fe_3O_4 nanoparticles inside a bladder of swine. (a) Ultrasound images during actuation. Blue polygons indicate the area of nanoparticles. Scale bar is 3 mm. (b) Dynamic ultrasound contrast and image processing. (b1) and (b2) refer to the highest and lowest contrast during actuation. (b3) is obtained by subtracting (b2) from (b1) and doubling the pixel intensity. The yellow ellipse represents the fitted edge using image thresholding. Scale bar: 3 mm. (c) Change of angle (blue line) between nanoparticle chain's long axis (projected on XY plane) and X axis. Black dashed lines: ultrasound system frames. Red dashed line: angle of 90°.

the Helmholtz coil system. By using a pipette, we inject nanoparticle suspension into the bladder. Under actuation of the DMF, nanoparticles gradually spread toward lower area density (t = 0–55 s), and the effect of the micrometer-scale irregularity on the inner surface of organ is negligible [62]. These disassembled nanoparticles can be regathered again. We place a magnetic needle of strength 60 mT (measured on the tip of the needle) near the bladder and move it along a circular trajectory to actuate nanoparticles on the surface. Finally, under the effect of the magnetic gradient disassembled nanoparticles are gathered. Figure 2.11b shows changes of the coverage area during the spreading-gathering process. The final coverage area of nanoparticles swells up to 480%, and these nanoparticles can be regathered within 25 s. Additionally, using ultrasound imaging we can monitor this reversible process (Figure 2.12a). During actuation, the applied field controls the orientation of these nanoparticle chains, *i.e.*, the angle between ultrasound wave propagation direction and the particle chains is time-dependent [63]. Therefore, there is a periodical change of ultrasound contrast due to the amount of scattered ultrasound waves changing. As illustrated in Figure 2.12c, the angle between the long axis of chains (the projection in the XY plane) and the X axis changes from 0° to 180° twice in one actuation cycle (blue lines). The nanoparticle chain has an input f_{xy} of 3 Hz and the display frame rate of the ultrasound system is 24 fps, *i.e.*, one acquired frame per 1/24 s as indicated by the dashed black lines. In case I (corresponding to Figure 2.12b1), the projection of the long axis is perpendicular to the wave propagation direction. Therefore, the scattered waves by these chains reach the highest amount, and the best ultrasound contrast in a cycle is exhibited. Unlike case I, in case II (corresponding to Figure 2.12b2), the projection of particle chains is parallel to the wave propagation direction, resulting in a decrease of contrast. The noise signals can be eliminated and nanoparticles are located (b3) by using the processing of image difference (subtract pixels in (b2) from (b1)). By utilizing the periodic contrast, the nanoparticles can be effectively located from noise signals under ultrasound feedback.

2.5 CONCLUSION

We have developed a strategy to actuate the disassembly and spreading of magnetic clusters on an uneven surface using dynamic magnetic fields. Under the actuation of the dynamic magnetic field (DMF), nanoparticle clusters are effectively disassembled into short chains, and the coverage area of nanoparticles is increased simultaneously. The enlarged separation distance between nanoparticle chains also decreases the possibility of reassembly. The length of nanoparticle chains is controlled by regulating the input parameters (f_z, θ_m) and estimated from the torque-balance-based analytical model. Moreover, the nanoparticle chains are able to cross the steps and spread on patterned surfaces due to the induced tumbling motion. The proposed disassembly strategy is experimentally demonstrated that it can be applied on a surface of a bladder of swine, where nanoparticle clusters are disassembled, and the final coverage area of nanoparticles increases by over 480%. In addition, we also demonstrate the regathering of the assembled nanoparticles, making the entire process reversible and controllable. Combining the ultrasound imaging technique and process of image difference, this reversible process of the nanoparticles is tracked in a robust fashion. The proposed disassembly technique provides a new method to tune the coverage area and surface-to-volume ratio and will improve the reproducibility of magnetic nanoparticle-based applications.

Bibliography

[1] Katherine Villa, Ludmila Krejčová, Filip Novotný, Zbynek Heger, Zdeněk Sofer, and Martin Pumera. Cooperative multifunctional self-propelled paramagnetic microrobots with chemical handles for cell manipulation and drug delivery. *Advanced Functional Materials*, 28(43), 2018, Art. no. 1804343.

[2] Debora Walker, Benjamin T Käsdorf, Hyeon-Ho Jeong, Oliver Lieleg, and Peer Fischer. Enzymatically active biomimetic micropropellers for the penetration of

mucin gels. *Science Advances*, 1(11), 2015, Art. no. e1500501.

[3] Wenqi Hu, Guo Zhan Lum, Massimo Mastrangeli, and Metin Sitti. Small-scale soft-bodied robot with multimodal locomotion. *Nature*, 554(7690):81–85, 2018.

[4] Hen-Wei Huang, Mahmut Selman Sakar, Andrew J Petruska, Salvador Pané, and Bradley J Nelson. Soft micromachines with programmable motility and morphology. *Nature Communications*, 7, 2016, Art. no. 12263.

[5] Lidong Yang, Qianqian Wang, and Li Zhang. Model-free trajectory tracking control of two-particle magnetic microrobot. *IEEE Transactions on Nanotechnology*, 17(4):697–700, 2018.

[6] Gabriel Loget and Alexander Kuhn. Electric field-induced chemical locomotion of conducting objects. *Nature Communications*, 2(1), 2011, Art. no. 535.

[7] Amir Masoud Pourrahimi, Katherine Villa, Carmen Lorena Manzanares Palenzuela, Yulong Ying, Zdeněk Sofer, and Martin Pumera. Catalytic and light-driven zno/pt janus nano/micromotors: Switching of motion mechanism via interface roughness and defect tailoring at the nanoscale. *Advanced Functional Materials*, 29(22), 2019, Art. no. 1808678.

[8] Katherine Villa, C Lorena Manzanares Palenzuela, Zdeněk Sofer, Stanislava Matějková, and Martin Pumera. Metal-free visible-light photoactivated c3n4 bubble-propelled tubular micromotors with inherent fluorescence and on/off capabilities. *ACS Nano*, 12(12):12482–12491, 2018.

[9] Chuanrui Chen, Songsong Tang, Hazhir Teymourian, Emil Karshalev, Fangyu Zhang, Jinxing Li, Fangzhi Mou, Yuyan Liang, Jianguo Guan, and Joseph Wang. Chemical/light-powered hybrid micromotors with “on-the-fly” optical brakes. *Angewandte Chemie*, 130(27):8242–8246, 2018.

[10] Baohu Dai, Jizhuang Wang, Ze Xiong, Xiaojun Zhan, Wei Dai, Chien-Cheng Li, Shien-Ping Feng, and Jinyao Tang. Programmable artificial phototactic microswimmer. *Nature Nanotechnology*, 11(12):1087–1092, 2016.

[11] Lidong Yang, Yabin Zhang, Qianqian Wang, Kai-Fung Chan, and Li Zhang. Automated control of magnetic spore-based microrobot using fluorescence imaging for targeted delivery with cellular resolution. *IEEE Transactions on Automation Science and Engineering*, 17(1):490–501, 2020.

[12] Giuseppe Tortora, Tommaso Ranzani, Iris De Falco, Paolo Dario, and Arianna Menciassi. A miniature robot for retraction tasks under vision assistance in minimally invasive surgery. *Robotics*, 3(1):70–82, 2014.

[13] Zhihua Lin, Xinjian Fan, Mengmeng Sun, Changyong Gao, Qiang He, and Hui Xie. Magnetically actuated peanut colloid motors for cell manipulation and patterning. *ACS Nano*, 12(3):2539–2545, 2018.

[14] Qi Zhou, Tristan Petit, Hongsoo Choi, Bradley J Nelson, and Li Zhang. Dumbbell fluidic tweezers for dynamical trapping and selective transport of microobjects. *Advanced Functional Materials*, 27(1), 2017, Art. no. 1604571.

[15] Eric Diller and Metin Sitti. Three-dimensional programmable assembly by untethered magnetic robotic micro-grippers. *Advanced Functional Materials*, 24(28):4397–4404, 2014.

[16] Tamás Vicsek and Anna Zafeiris. Collective motion. *Physics Reports*, 517(3-4):71–140, 2012.

[17] Carl Anderson, Guy Theraulaz, and J-L Deneubourg. Self-assemblages in insect societies. *Insectes Sociaux*, 49(2):99–110, 2002.

[18] Tailin Xu, Fernando Soto, Wei Gao, Renfeng Dong, Victor Garcia-Gradilla, Ernesto Magaña, Xueji Zhang, and Joseph Wang. Reversible swarming and separation of self-propelled chemically powered nanomotors under acoustic fields. *Journal of the American Chemical Society*, 137(6):2163–2166, 2015.

[19] A Snezhko, M Belkin, IS Aranson, and W-K Kwok. Self-assembled magnetic surface swimmers. *Physical Review Letters*, 102(11), 2009, Art. no. 118103.

[20] Jing Yan, Ming Han, Jie Zhang, Cong Xu, Erik Luijten, and Steve Granick. Reconfiguring active particles by electrostatic imbalance. *Nature Materials*, 15(10):1095–1099, 2016.

[21] Helena Massana-Cid, Fanlong Meng, Daiki Matsunaga, Ramin Golestanian, and Pietro Tierno. Tunable self-healing of magnetically propelling colloidal carpets. *Nature Communications*, 10(1), 2019, Art. no. 2444.

[22] Ania Servant, Famin Qiu, Mariarosa Mazza, Kostas Kostarelos, and Bradley J Nelson. Controlled in vivo swimming of a swarm of bacteria-like microrobotic flagella. *Advanced Materials*, 27(19):2981–2988, 2015.

[23] Zhiguang Wu, Jonas Troll, Hyeon-Ho Jeong, Qiang Wei, Marius Stang, Focke Ziemssen, Zegao Wang, Mingdong Dong, Sven Schnichels, Tian Qiu, and Peer Fischer. A swarm of slippery micropropellers penetrates the vitreous body of the eye. *Science Advances*, 4(11), 2018, Art. no. eaat4388.

[24] Salvador Pané, Josep Puigmartí-Luis, Christos Bergeles, Xiang-Zhong Chen, Eva Pellicer, Jordi Sort, Vanda Počepcová, Antoine Ferreira, and Bradley J Nelson. Imaging technologies for biomedical micro- and nanoswimmers. *Advanced Materials Technologies*, 4(4), 2019, Art. no. 1800575.

[25] Jiangfan Yu, Ben Wang, Xingzhou Du, Qianqian Wang, and Li Zhang. Ultra-extensible ribbon-like magnetic microswarm. *Nature Communications*, 9(1), 2018, Art. no. 3260.

[26] Kyle J Solis and James E Martin. Complex magnetic fields breathe life into fluids. *Soft Matter*, 10(45):9136–9142, 2014.

[27] Qianqian Wang, Lidong Yang, Ben Wang, Edwin Yu, Jiangfan Yu, and Li Zhang. Collective behavior of reconfigurable magnetic droplets via dynamic self-assembly. *ACS Applied Materials & Interfaces*, 11(1):1630–1637, 2019.

[28] Alexey Snezhko and Igor S Aranson. Magnetic manipulation of self-assembled colloidal asters. *Nature Materials*, 10(9):698–703, 2011.

[29] Fernando Martinez-Pedrero, Andrejs Cebers, and Pietro Tierno. Dipolar rings of microscopic ellipsoids: Magnetic manipulation and cell entrapment. *Physical Review Applied*, 6(3), 2016, Art. no. 034002.

[30] Randall M Erb, Hui S Son, Bappaditya Samanta, Vincent M Rotello, and Benjamin B Yellen. Magnetic assembly of colloidal superstructures with multipole symmetry. *Nature*, 457(7232):999–1002, 2009.

[31] Fernando Martinez-Pedrero and Pietro Tierno. Magnetic propulsion of self-assembled colloidal carpets: Efficient cargo transport via a conveyor-belt effect. *Physical Review Applied*, 3(5), 2015, Art. no. 051003.

[32] Gašper Kokot and Alexey Snezhko. Manipulation of emergent vortices in swarms of magnetic rollers. *Nature Communications*, 9(1), 2018, Art. no. 2344.

[33] Fan Yang, Fangzhi Mou, Yuzhou Jiang, Ming Luo, Leilei Xu, Huiru Ma, and Jianguo Guan. Flexible guidance of microengines by dynamic topographical pathways in ferrofluids. *ACS Nano*, 12(7):6668–6676, 2018.

[34] Alexey Snezhko. Complex collective dynamics of active torque-driven colloids at interfaces. *Current Opinion in Colloid & Interface Science*, 21:65–75, 2016.

[35] Zhihua Lin, Changyong Gao, Meiling Chen, Xiankun Lin, and Qiang He. Collective motion and dynamic self-assembly of colloid motors. *Current Opinion in Colloid & Interface Science*, 35:51–58, 2018.

[36] Bo Li, Di Zhou, and Yilong Han. Assembly and phase transitions of colloidal crystals. *Nature Reviews Materials*, 1(2), 2016, Art. no. 15011.

[37] Rui Hao, Ruijun Xing, Zhichuan Xu, Yanglong Hou, Song Gao, and Shouheng Sun. Synthesis, functionalization, and biomedical applications of multifunctional magnetic nanoparticles. *Advanced Materials*, 22(25):2729–2742, 2010.

[38] Hongdong Cai, Xiao An, Jun Cui, Jingchao Li, Shihui Wen, Kangan Li, Mingwu Shen, Linfeng Zheng, Guixiang Zhang, and Xiangyang Shi. Facile hydrothermal synthesis and surface functionalization of polyethyleneimine-coated iron oxide nanoparticles for biomedical applications. *ACS Applied Materials & Interfaces*, 5(5):1722–1731, 2013.

[39] Zhi Wei Tay, Prashant Chandrasekharan, Andreina Chiu-Lam, Daniel W Hensley, Rohan Dhavalikar, Xinyi Y Zhou, Elaine Y Yu, Patrick W Goodwill,

Bo Zheng, Carlos Rinaldi, and Steven M. Conolly. Magnetic particle imaging-guided heating in vivo using gradient fields for arbitrary localization of magnetic hyperthermia therapy. *ACS Nano*, 12(4):3699–3713, 2018.

[40] Kyung Hyun Min, Hyun Su Min, Hong Jae Lee, Dong Jin Park, Ji Young Yhee, Kwangmeyung Kim, Ick Chan Kwon, Seo Young Jeong, Oscar F Silvestre, Xiaoyuan Chen, Yu-Shik Hwang, Eun-Cheol Kim, and Sang Cheon Lee. ph-controlled gas-generating mineralized nanoparticles: a theranostic agent for ultrasound imaging and therapy of cancers. *ACS Nano*, 9(1):134–145, 2015.

[41] Emilia S Olson, Jahir Orozco, Zhe Wu, Christopher D Malone, Boemha Yi, Wei Gao, Mohammad Eghtedari, Joseph Wang, and Robert F Mattrey. Toward in vivo detection of hydrogen peroxide with ultrasound molecular imaging. *Biomaterials*, 34(35):8918–8924, 2013.

[42] Ben Wang, Kai Fung Chan, Jiangfan Yu, Qianqian Wang, Lidong Yang, Philip Wai Yan Chiu, and Li Zhang. Reconfigurable swarms of ferromagnetic colloids for enhanced local hyperthermia. *Advanced Functional Materials*, 28(25), 2018, Art. no. 1705701.

[43] Yang Gao, Alexander van Reenen, Martien A Hulsen, Arthur M de Jong, Menno WJ Prins, and Jaap MJ den Toonder. Disaggregation of microparticle clusters by induced magnetic dipole–dipole repulsion near a surface. *Lab on a Chip*, 13(7):1394–1401, 2013.

[44] James E Martin and Alexey Snezhko. Driving self-assembly and emergent dynamics in colloidal suspensions by time-dependent magnetic fields. *Reports on Progress in Physics*, 76(12), 2013, Art. no. 126601.

[45] Jiangfan Yu, Tiantian Xu, Zheyu Lu, Chi Ian Vong, and Li Zhang. On-demand disassembly of paramagnetic nanoparticle chains for microrobotic cargo delivery. *IEEE Transactions on Robotics*, 33(5):1213–1225, 2017.

[46] CM Disney, PD Lee, JA Hoyland, MJ Sherratt, and BK Bay. A review of techniques for visualising soft tissue microstructure deformation and quantifying strain ex vivo. *Journal of Microscopy*, 272(3):165–179, 2018.

[47] E Loth. Drag of non-spherical solid particles of regular and irregular shape. *Powder Technology*, 182(3):342–353, 2008.

[48] Eui-Sung Yoon, R Arvind Singh, Hyun-Jin Oh, and Hosung Kong. The effect of contact area on nano/micro-scale friction. *Wear*, 259(7-12):1424–1431, 2005.

[49] Sonia Melle, Gerald G Fuller, and Miguel A Rubio. Structure and dynamics of magnetorheological fluids in rotating magnetic fields. *Physical Review E*, 61(4):4111, 2000.

[50] Harpreet Singh, Paul E Laibinis, and T Alan Hatton. Rigid, superparamagnetic chains of permanently linked beads coated with magnetic nanoparticles.

synthesis and rotational dynamics under applied magnetic fields. *Langmuir*, 21(24):11500–11509, 2005.

[51] C Wilhelm, Julien Browaeys, A Ponton, and J-C Bacri. Rotational magnetic particles microrheology: the maxwellian case. *Physical Review E*, 67(1):011504, 2003.

[52] Alexander Van Reenen, Arthur M de Jong, Jaap MJ den Toonder, and Menno WJ Prins. Integrated lab-on-chip biosensing systems based on magnetic particle actuation–a comprehensive review. *Lab on a Chip*, 14(12):1966–1986, 2014.

[53] Y Gao, MA Hulsen, TG Kang, and JMJ Den Toonder. Numerical and experimental study of a rotating magnetic particle chain in a viscous fluid. *Physical Review E*, 86(4):041503, 2012.

[54] Hong Deng, Xiaolin Li, Qing Peng, Xun Wang, Jinping Chen, and Yadong Li. Monodisperse magnetic single-crystal ferrite microspheres. *Angewandte Chemie International Edition*, 44(18):2782–2785, 2005.

[55] Ioannis Petousis, Erik Homburg, Roy Derks, and Andreas Dietzel. Transient behaviour of magnetic micro-bead chains rotating in a fluid by external fields. *Lab on a Chip*, 7(12):1746–1751, 2007.

[56] C Wilhelm, J Browaeys, A Ponton, and J-C Bacri. Rotational magnetic particles microrheology: the maxwellian case. *Physical Review E*, 67(1), 2003, Art. no. 011504.

[57] Y Gao, MA Hulsen, TG Kang, and JMJ Den Toonder. Numerical and experimental study of a rotating magnetic particle chain in a viscous fluid. *Physical Review E*, 86(4), 2012, Art. no. 041503.

[58] Stefano Giovanazzi, Axel Görlitz, and Tilman Pfau. Tuning the dipolar interaction in quantum gases. *Physical Review Letters*, 89(13), 2002, Art. no. 130401.

[59] Sonia Melle, Gerald G Fuller, and Miguel A Rubio. Structure and dynamics of magnetorheological fluids in rotating magnetic fields. *Physical Review E*, 61(4):4111–4117, 2000.

[60] Charles E Sing, Lothar Schmid, Matthias F Schneider, Thomas Franke, and Alfredo Alexander-Katz. Controlled surface-induced flows from the motion of self-assembled colloidal walkers. *Proceedings of the National Academy of Sciences*, 107(2):535–540, 2010.

[61] Li Zhang, Tristan Petit, Yang Lu, Bradley E Kratochvil, Kathrin E Peyer, Ryan Pei, Jun Lou, and Bradley J Nelson. Controlled propulsion and cargo transport of rotating nickel nanowires near a patterned solid surface. *ACS Nano*, 4(10):6228–6234, 2010.

[62] Robin Menzel, Markus Böl, and Tobias Siebert. Importance of contraction history on muscle force of porcine urinary bladder smooth muscle. *International Urology and Nephrology*, 49(2):205–214, 2017.

[63] Qianqian Wang, Lidong Yang, Jiangfan Yu, Chi-Ian Vong, Philip Wai Yan Chiu, and Li Zhang. Magnetic navigation of a rotating colloidal swarm using ultrasound images. In *2018 IEEE/RSJ International Conference on Intelligent Robots and Systems*, pages 5380–5385. IEEE, 2018.

CHAPTER 3

Adaptive Pattern and Motion Control of Collective Nanoparticles

3.1 INTRODUCTION

The field of untethered magnetic micro/nanorobots has garnered significant attention for its vast potential in biomedical applications [1, 2, 3, 4]. Researchers have explored different types of microrobots, including helical-shaped microswimmers [5], soft microrobots [6], spore-based microrobots [7], and even bacteria [8, 9, 10]. However, due to their small sizes and volumes, individual microrobots have limitations in terms of their loading capacity for drugs or materials. Additionally, real-time *in vivo* imaging of a single microrobotic agent poses significant challenges [11]. To address these limitations, microrobotic swarms consisting of a high concentration of nanoagents and controllable patterns have emerged as promising alternatives [12, 13, 14, 15, 16, 17]. Taking inspiration from swarm behaviors observed in nature, researchers have reported various types of swarm behaviors at the micro/nanoscale, which can be broadly classified into two categories: equilibrium and active (maintained out of thermodynamic equilibrium) [18]. Equilibrium periodic collectives are formed through self-assembly, but once formed, the connections between individual agents remain mostly fixed [19, 20, 21, 22, 23, 24].

On the other hand, dynamic swarm behaviors are typically triggered by highly dynamic external fields that provide continuous energy input, enabling the swarm to perform navigated locomotion as a collective entity [25, 26, 27, 28]. The formation of dynamic swarms can be induced by fluidic and magnetic interactions. Fluidic interactions, in particular, play a significant role in the generation of collectives [26, 29]. These swarms are primarily formed through interactions exerted by the surrounding fluid, known as fluidic-induced swarms. In contrast, magnetic field-induced swarms are generated through direct interactions between the agents induced by externally applied magnetic fields [27, 30]. The movement of the agents in these swarms is facilitated by magnetic forces, with fluidic interactions playing a minor role in swarm generation and reconfiguration. Previous studies have reported the generation and

 DOI: 10.1201/9781032665788-3

navigated motion of vortex-like paramagnetic nanoparticle swarms (VPNS) [29]. By adjusting the actuation parameters, these swarms can undergo pattern reconfiguration to adapt to complex and tortuous environments, such as narrow channel networks, thereby enabling targeted delivery with high spatial and temporal resolution from a statistical perspective. However, effectively maneuvering these swarms typically requires extensive training of human operators to understand the mechanisms and characteristics involved. It becomes overwhelming for operators to manually control multiple parameters (*e.g.*, aspect ratio, long-axis orientation, and position) of the swarm simultaneously. In this context, the development of automatic control strategies and embodied intelligence for the swarms becomes crucial to make optimized and autonomous decisions for adaptive motion and pattern tuning [31]. While control algorithms for rigid monolithic microrobots have been extensively investigated [32, 33, 34], the control of microrobotic swarms is still a relatively unexplored area. The physical model and governing mechanisms of a microrobotic swarm differ significantly from those of a monolithic microrobot, posing challenges in the development of optimized control methods. Firstly, swarms may consist of thousands or even millions of individual elements, and as a result, control commands may not take immediate effect at the swarm scale, requiring time for most elements to adjust their motion. Additionally, swarms require continuous and stable energy input, and drastic changes in external inputs can alter the agent-agent interactions, potentially disrupting the stability of the swarm pattern.

In this chapter, we introduce the generation of an elliptical swarm composed of paramagnetic nanoparticles with a dynamic-equilibrium structure. This is achieved by applying programmed elliptical magnetic fields. In comparison to previously reported microrobotic swarms, such as fluidic-induced swarms [27] and vortex-like paramagnetic nanoparticle swarms [29], elliptical swarms exhibit higher adaptability to external confined environments and possess greater motion dexterity. The generation mechanisms of the elliptical swarm are analyzed, and the reversible pattern reconfiguration capability is presented. We demonstrate the adaptive navigation of the swarm through a microchannel with varying constrictions, showcasing its ability to maneuver in complex environments. Furthermore, we design a control architecture comprising a feedforward controller and a feedback fuzzy logic controller to automatically adjust the aspect ratio, long-axis orientation, and position of the swarms. To validate the effectiveness and compatibility of the proposed control strategy, we also apply the same control architecture to another type of swarm, namely, a ribbon-like microswarm [27]. The small control errors observed in both cases indicate the efficacy of the proposed strategy for these two types of swarms. Moreover, the control architecture we propose has the potential to facilitate the development of control methods for various types of swarms at small scales.

3.2 GENERATION AND RECONFIGURATION OF AN EPNS

A VPNS can be generated using an in-plane rotating magnetic field. The heterogeneous pattern reconfiguration of the swarm has yet been systematically investigated.

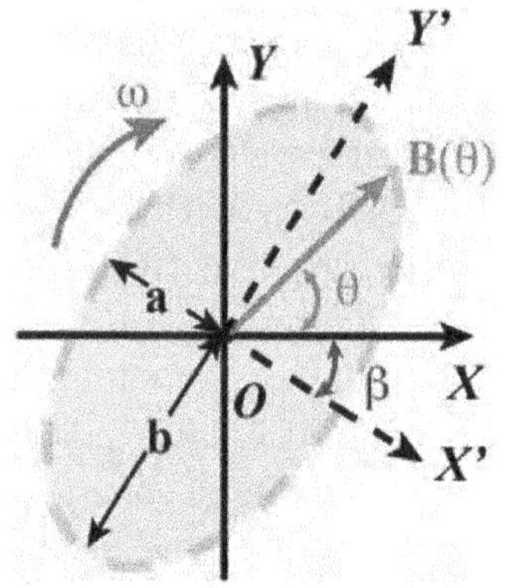

Figure 3.1 Schematic of the elliptical rotating magnetic field. The red arrow indicates the magnetic field at the moment, which has a rotation angle θ with the direction of the long axis. The field strength is $|\mathbf{B}(\theta)|$. The yellow dashed ellipse is the trajectory of $\mathbf{B}(\theta)$, whose short axis is a and long axis is b. The angular velocity of the field is set constant, as ω. The short axis of the ellipse has an angle β with X-axis.

In this work, the elliptical paramagnetic nanoparticle swarm (EPNS) triggered by elliptical rotating magnetic field is achieved and analyzed.

3.2.1 Elliptical Magnetic Field

The schematic of the elliptical magnetic field is demonstrated in Figure 3.1. The parametric equation of the elliptical field is expressed as

$$\mathbf{B}(\theta)_{\mathcal{X}-\mathcal{Y}} = \begin{bmatrix} \cos\beta & -\sin\beta & 0 \\ \sin\beta & \cos\beta & 0 \\ 0 & 0 & 1 \end{bmatrix} \begin{bmatrix} a\cos\theta\cdot\mathbf{x} \\ b\sin\theta\cdot\mathbf{y} \\ 0 \end{bmatrix}_{\mathcal{X}'-\mathcal{Y}'} \tag{3.1}$$

where $\mathbf{B}(\theta)$ is the elliptical magnetic field, β is the angle between $\mathcal{X}$-$\mathcal{Y}$ and $\mathcal{X}'$-$\mathcal{Y}'$ coordinates. The variables are labeled in Figure 3.1. The field ratio $\gamma \in (0,1]$ is defined as

$$\gamma = a/b. \tag{3.2}$$

Therefore, when γ is larger (closer to 1), the difference between the long axis and short axis of the elliptical field is smaller, andvice versa.

Paramagnetic nanoparticles tend to form chain-like structures with the existence of external magnetic fields. Mason number can be expressed as [35]

$$R_T = \Gamma_d/\Gamma_m = 64\frac{\mu_0\eta\omega}{\chi_p^2 B^2(\theta)}\frac{N^2}{\ln(N)+1.2/N} \tag{3.3}$$

where Γ_d is drag torque, Γ_m is the magnetic torque exerted on nanoparticle chains, μ_0 is the permeability of free space, η is fluid viscosity, ω is the angular velocity of the particle chains, χ_p is the effective magnetic susceptibility, $B(\theta)$ is the field strength at θ, and a particle chain consists (2N+1) particles. Based on Eq. (3.3),

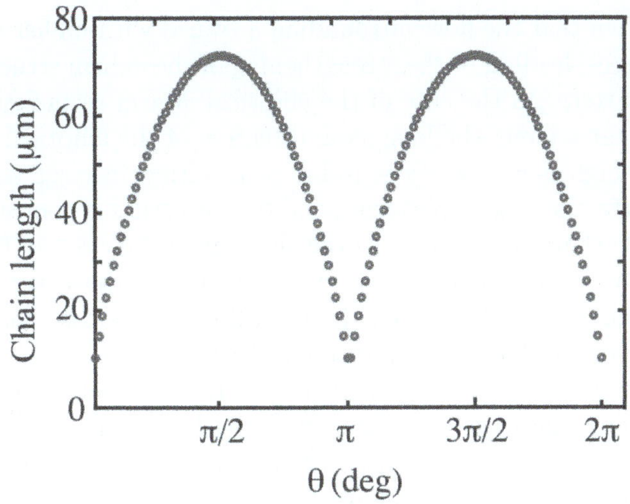

Figure 3.2 Change in the chain length with respect to θ in an elliptical magnetic field. The short-axial direction of the field is set as 0°. In this case, a = 5 mT and b = 10 mT.

the chain lengths are positively related to the applied field strength. Therefore, actuated by the elliptical rotating field, the lengths of particle chains change accordingly (Figure 3.2), which is one of the critical factors for the generation of an EPNS. Based on Eq. (3.1), the field strength (in coordinate $\mathcal{X}'$-$\mathcal{Y}'$) can be expressed as

$$|\mathbf{B}(\theta)_{\mathcal{X}'-\mathcal{Y}'}| = \sqrt{a^2 \cos^2\theta + b^2 \sin^2\theta}. \tag{3.4}$$

The largest and smallest field strengths will be reached when $|\mathbf{B}(\theta)_{\mathcal{X}'-\mathcal{Y}'}|$ points the long axis and short axis of the ellipse, respectively.

3.2.2 Reconfiguration Stage I: Fluidic-Induced

(1) Generation of an EPNS: When a circular swarm just reconfigure into an elliptical shape, reconfiguration stage I dominates. The mechanisms are schematically demonstrated in Figure 3.3a. A vortex-like swarm (VPNS) is first generated using a rotating magnetic field, an elliptical field is then applied to change the length distribution of the particle chains. When the magnetic field vector points along the long axis of the ellipse, the field strength reaches the largest value, which enlarges the agent–agent attractive interactions [35]. At the moment, individual particles and short particle chains will assemble with each other to form long chains, as shown by the blue dashed arrows in Figure 3.3a, Part 1. Because the applied angular velocity is fixed, longer chains can induce flow with higher velocity, as shown

$$\mathbf{U}(\theta) \propto \pi f L(\theta) \tag{3.5}$$

where θ is labeled in Figure 3.1, $\mathbf{U}(\theta)$ represents the flow velocity of the point locates on the swarm contour when the angle is θ, f is the rotating frequency of the field, and $L(\theta)$ is the estimated chain length at the angle of θ. Previous investigations

[29, 36] have shown that the flow surrounding a swarm with higher velocity can exert larger inward forces, leading to the strengthening of the swarm structure and the contraction of its pattern. In the case of the elliptical swarm reconfiguration, when the particle chain rotates along the long-axial direction of the elliptical field, long chains are formed and high flow velocity is induced, resulting in large constraining forces [29]. Consequently, the swarm pattern along this direction is contracted. Conversely, when the particle chains rotate toward the short-axial direction of the elliptical field, the chains tend to disassemble into shorter ones due to the lower field strength, as illustrated in Figure 3.3a, Part 2. The induced flow in this case has a lower velocity, and the inward forces along the short-axial direction of the field are weak as well. Consequently, the swarm pattern along this direction is weakly confined. As a result, the swarm elongates into an elliptical pattern with its long-axial direction perpendicular to that of the applied field. Based on this analysis, it can be concluded that the swarm's behavior during reconfiguration stage I is mainly influenced by fluidic factors. However, further characterization is required to fully understand the fluidic field induced during this process.

(2) Fluidic Field Induced by an EPNS: Herein, we consider an elliptical vortex performing rigid body rotation with a uniform vorticity ξ. The center of the vortex is located at $(x, y) = (0, 0)$. The motion of a tiny part of the fluid, *i.e.*, a fluid particle that can totally represent all characteristics of the fluid at the specific location, in a 2D flow of an incompressible fluid is governed by

$$\dot{x} = \frac{\partial \Psi}{\partial y}, \quad \dot{y} = -\frac{\partial \Psi}{\partial x} \tag{3.6}$$

where Ψ is a stream function and (x, y) is the real-time location of the fluid particle. If an EPNS with an elliptical vortex is considered, the induced stream function is given by

$$\psi_v = -\frac{1}{4}e^{-2\kappa}\cos 2\nu - \frac{1}{2}\kappa \tag{3.7}$$

where (κ, ν) is an elliptic coordinates fixed on the vortex. The transformation from (κ, ν) to Cartesian coordinates (X',Y') reads

$$\begin{cases} X' = p\sinh\kappa\sin\nu \\ Y' = p\cosh\kappa\cos\nu \end{cases} \tag{3.8}$$

where $p^2 = (1-\xi^2)/\xi$. The X' - Y' is fixed on the vortex (Figure 3.1) and rotates with the vortex, which correspond to the minor and major axes, respectively. If no external flow is existed, it can be obtained

$$\dot{\kappa} = \frac{h^2}{2}\left(-\Omega + p^{-2}e^{-2t}\right)\sin 2\nu \tag{3.9}$$

$$\dot{\nu} = \frac{h^2}{2}\left[-\Omega\sinh 2\kappa - p^{-2}\left(e^{-2\kappa\cos 2\nu - 1}\right)\right] \tag{3.10}$$

where $\Omega = r/(r+1)^2$, $h^2 = \left(\cosh^2\kappa - \cosh^2\nu\right)^{-1}$. The equation governs the motion of a fluid particle in the flow.

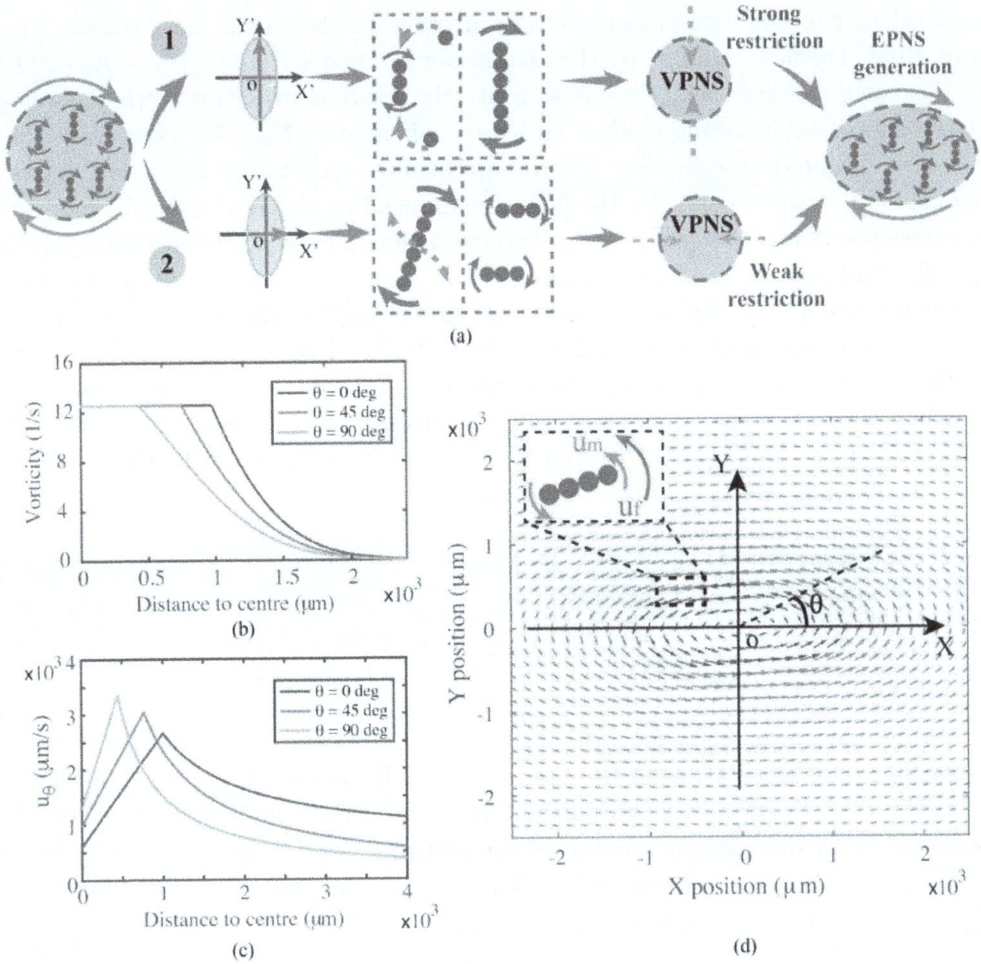

Figure 3.3 (a) Schematic mechanism of the reconfiguration stage I. The grey circles indicate nanoparticles, and the blue regions are the core part of the swarm. The blue and green arrows represent the rotational direction of particle chains and the swarm (the direction of the induced flow), respectively. Thicker arrows indicate larger flow velocity. The green dashed arrows show the assembly/disassembly behaviors of the nanoparticle chains. The orange dashed arrows represent the restriction forces exerted on the swarm. (b) Vorticity distribution with respect to the distance to the swarm center. (c) Tangential velocity distribution of the induced flow with respect to the distance to the swarm center. (d) Clear depiction of u_θ in 2D space. The blue and red arrows indicate the flow velocity inside and outside the vortex core, respectively. The size of the arrows represents the magnitude of the flow velocity. Herein, K_c is set as 1.

Moreover, because the core part of the swarm is assumed as rigid-body rotation, and the core is actuated by external magnetic field, the vorticity will not decay with distance from the swarm center. In fact, the vorticity inside the swarm core keeps constant. Meanwhile, based on the schematic model shown in Figure 3.3a, we need to consider two critical factors in order to model the flow velocity in the core. First, the flow induced by the chains can be modeled as $U_m(\theta) = K_c \cdot \pi f L(\theta)$. In this case, the flow velocity has a positively linear relationship with the velocity of the end of the rotating chains, and the coefficient is K_c. The exact value of K_c can be calibrated case-by-case using experimental calibration data. By deploying nonmagnetic tracing particles, the flow rate induced by the swarm can be monitored. Knowing the flow rate $U_m(\theta)$, the applied frequency f, and the chain lengths $L(\theta)$ in a specific condition, K_c can be calibrated. Herein, in order to give a general introduction about the deduction process, we give a typical example with $K_c = 1$. Second, after the swarm is generated, an overall flow field surrounding the swarm will be formed. Inside the core part, the nanoparticle chains will perform self-rotation due to the magnetic field, and simultaneously, orbiting around the center of the swarm, which validates the existence of the overall background flow. As a result, the vorticity ξ_z and the flow velocity u_θ can be expressed as

$$\xi_z = \frac{\Gamma_0}{\pi ab}(r(\theta) < R(\theta)) \tag{3.11}$$

$$u_\theta = \pi K_c f L(\theta) + \frac{\Gamma_0}{C} \cdot \frac{r(\theta)}{R(\theta)}(r(\theta) < R(\theta)) \tag{3.12}$$

$$C = \pi[3(a+b) - \sqrt{(3a+b)(a+3b)}] \tag{3.13}$$

where Γ_0 is the circulation of the swarm, $r(\theta)$indicates the point (r, θ) in elliptical coordinate (κ, ν), $R(\theta)$ indicates the distance from the center of the swarm to the point (R, θ) locating on the contour of the swarm.

Then ambient flow induced by the swarm is then investigated. The vorticity equation of a vortex can be expressed as

$$\frac{D\vec{\xi}}{Dt} = (\vec{\xi} \cdot \nabla)\vec{u} + \eta \nabla^2 \vec{\xi} \tag{3.14}$$

where D/Dt is Lagrangian derivative, η is the kinetic viscosity of the fluid. Without losing generality, based on Eq. (3.14), we use Lamb–Oseen vortex as a representative example to solve [37], and the results are shown as

$$\xi_z = \frac{\Gamma_0}{4\pi\eta t} \exp\left(\frac{-r(\theta)^2}{4\eta t}\right)(r(\theta) > R(\theta)) \tag{3.15}$$

$$u_\theta = \left(\frac{\Gamma_0}{2\pi r(\theta)}\right)\left[1 - \exp\left(-\frac{r(\theta)^2}{4vt}\right)\right](r(\theta) > R(\theta)) \tag{3.16}$$

where η is the kinetic viscosity of the fluid. By combining Eqs. (3.11)–(3.16), the distribution of the vorticity and the velocity of the induced flow field are obtained, as plotted in Figures 3.3b and 3.3c, respectively. Herein, the swarm ratio, maximum chain length, and applied frequency are defined to be 2200 μm, and 5 Hz, respectively. In the core part of the swarm, the vorticity is uniform, and when $r(\theta) > R(\theta)$, the vorticity decays. The long-axial direction of the swarm is set as 0°. Meanwhile, from the model, the flow velocity along the short axis of the swarm has the largest value

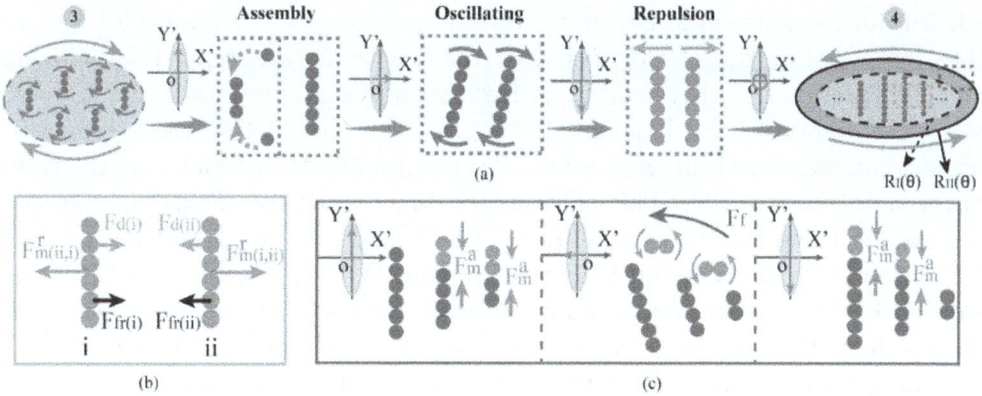

Figure 3.4 (a) Schematic mechanism of the reconfiguration stage II. The blue and green arrows represent the rotational direction of particle chains and the swarm, respectively. The green dashed arrows show the assembly behaviors of the nanoparticle chains. The orange arrows represent the repulsive interactions exerted on the nanoparticles. (b) Schematics of the forces exerted on neighboring nanoparticle chains. The blue and red particles shows the different magnetizations. The red, green, and black arrows indicate the magnetic repulsive forces F_m^r, fluidic drag F_d, and frictions F_{fr}, respectively. (c) Schematics of the behaviors of ring region. The grey particles are in the oscillating region, while the red ones are in the ring regions. Dipole-dipole magnetic interactions F_m^a are shown by the red arrows.

because long chains are formed; while along the long axis of the swarm, the flow speed is relatively lower. For a clear expression, the velocity distribution surrounding the swarm is obtained from Eq. (3.16) and is then demonstrated in Figure 3.3d. The size of the arrows represents the magnitude of the flow velocity. The blue and red arrows indicate the velocity distribution inside and outside the swarm core, respectively.

3.2.3 Reconfiguration Stage II: Magnetic Field-Induced

With the decrease of the applied field ratio γ, the strength along the short-axial direction of the elliptic field will further reduce. Therefore, in the process of chain disassembly (Figure 3.4a, Part 2), shorter chains will be formed. The fluidic interaction becomes weaker and the magnetic factor gradually becomes dominating in the swarm pattern elongation. Finally, if the small short-axial field strength is not capable of providing sufficient magnetic torque to disassemble the long chain due to the attractive particle–particle surface bonding forces, the long chains are stepped out, the reconfiguration process of the swarm enters stage II.

(1) Mechanisms of Reconfiguration: The mechanisms of this stage that dominates the swarm pattern reconfiguration are schematically shown in Figure 3.4a. Initially, an EPNS is formed with a relatively lower aspect ratio (Figure 3.4a, Part 3). When the magnetic field vector points along the long-axial direction of the elliptic field, long particle chains will be assembled. Then, with the rotation of the field, the field strength decreases significantly due to the small γ, which can hardly provide sufficient magnetic torques. Because surface forces exist to bond particles with each other, instead of the disassembly behavior, the long chains are stepped out with small magnetic torques, and they tend to oscillate with a small amplitude about the long axis of the elliptical field. It is noted that, the core part of the swarm is relatively compact compared with the region near its contour, and the particles are distributed with a high concentration. This enlarges the contact surface among the nanoparticles, making the particle clusters bulkier, which is also an important reason for the phenomenon that the step-out behavior happens. When the field strength increases again, magnetic repulsive forces among parallel nanoparticle chains will be induced, which is the critical reason for the swarm elongation behavior. As a result, after more cycles of the elliptical field, the EPNS with a significantly higher aspect ratio will be formed, as shown in Figure 3.4a, Part 4.

In Stage II, a stable EPNS can be divided into three regions.

(1) Oscillating region $r < (R_I)$: The nanoparticle chains keep oscillating in a small range about the short-axial direction of the swarm, as shown by the blue region in Figure 3.4a, Part 4. In this region, the particle chains are repelled from each other due to the repulsive magnetic interaction, and meanwhile, fluidic drag F_d, the friction F_{fr} between the particle chains and the substrate, and the fluidic vortex constraints provide the opposite inward forces to maintain the stability of the swarm. The schematics is shown in Figure 3.4b.

(2) Ring region $(R_I < r < R_{II})$: Smaller pieces of nanoparticle chains keeps orbiting the swarm center due to magnetic dipole–dipole interactions, as demonstrated in the red region in Figure 3.4a, Part 4. In the contour region of the swarm, the particles are distributed relative loosely compared with that in the core part, and free particle chains that can follow the applied field. Without losing generality, herein, we investigate the motion of two free short particle chains, as schematically shown in Figure 3.4c. The grey circles indicate the particles in the oscillating region, while the red circles represent the particles in Ring region. When the field points Y' -axis with high strength, the red chains are assembled with the grey ones due to the magnetic attractions. During the process that the field points from Y' -axis to X' -axis, the red chains first oscillate with the grey ones, and when the field strength further decreases, disassembly occurs, which is the major reason that leads the red chains to orbit the swarm core (oscillating region). Another reason could be that, reconfiguration stage II is induced subsequently from reconfiguration stage I, and a part of the fluidic vorticity can still exist, which provide fluidic forces (the blue arrow in Figure 3.4c) to actuate the red chains. After the field vector points along Y' -axis again, the red chains will be attracted by the neighboring grey chains to form a new assembly. As a result, the entire ring region will also rotate about the oscillating region withoutpattern deformation.

(3) Ambient region $(r > R_{II})$: The region of the surrounding fluid. In the following section, we will characterize the fluidic field induced in these three regions.

(2) Flow Field Induced by the EPNS: In the oscillating region, the chains keep performing step-out oscillation, and no stable flow can be formed. Meanwhile, in ring region, the flow is mainly induced by the rotation of the free chains, and thus the flow velocity is simplified to be proportional to the chain lengths. The induced flow field in

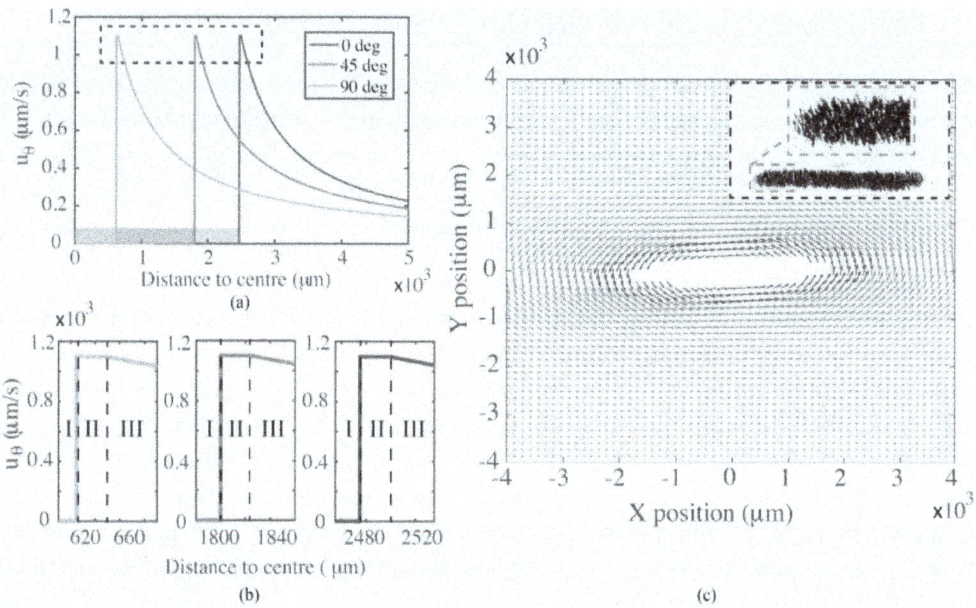

Figure 3.5 (a) Distribution of the tangential flow velocity u_θ with respect to the distance to the swarm center. (b) Details in the black dashed rectangle. (c) Clear expression of u_θ in 2D space. The blue and red arrows indicate the flow velocity inside and outside the vortex core, respectively. The size of the arrows represents the magnitude of the flow velocity. K_c is set as 1 in this case. The inset shows the chain-like structures inside the swarm region.

ambient region follows the domination of Eq. (3.14). Therefore, the flow distribution in the entire range can be expressed as

$$No\ stable\ flow \quad (r(\theta) < R_I(\theta)) \tag{3.17}$$

$$u_\theta = u_{II} = \pi K_c f L(\theta) \, (R_I(\theta) < r(\theta) < R_{II}(\theta)) \tag{3.18}$$

$$u_\theta = u_{II} \left[1 - \exp\left(-\frac{r(\theta)^2}{4vt}\right)\right] (r(\theta) > R_{II}(\theta)). \tag{3.19}$$

The flow distribution u_θ has been plotted in Figure 3.5a. The yellow, red, and blue regions indicate the oscillating regions corresponding to $\theta = 90°, \theta = 45°$, and $\theta = 0°$, respectively. In fact, due to the step-out oscillation of the chains, there is still flow induced. These colored regions only indicate that no calculable flow is generated. The details of the region highlighted by the black dashed rectangle are shown in Figure 3.5b, and the flow in different regions of the swarm is labeled. Moreover, for a clear express, the overall flow field has been demonstrated in Figure 3.5c. By applying a low field ratio (*e.g.*, 0.3), the chain-like structures can be observed, as shown in the inset in Figure 3.5c, which supports the mechanism proposed in Section 3.2.3. The analysis of the fundamental mechanism of swarm generation and induced flow field enhances the understanding of the elliptical swarms, and thus, helps construct an effective controller in the following sections.

3.3 EXPERIMENTAL SETUP AND MAGNETIC NANOPARTICLES

A three-axial Helmholtz electromagnetic coil setup is designed for generating dynamic magnetic fields. The magnetic field is determined by the superposition of each coil's contribution, which is linearly proportional to the current I_i applied

$$\mathbf{B}(\mathbf{P}) = \sum_{i=1}^{n} \mathbf{B}_i(\mathbf{P}) I_i \tag{3.20}$$

where n is the number of the electromagnetic coils, $\mathbf{B}_i(\mathbf{P}) \in \mathbb{R}^{3\times1}$ is a matrix depending on the measuring position in the workspace of the magnetic system, and $\boldsymbol{I}_i$ is a vector of the applied current in the ith coil. The control signals are generated by a PC, and then the current is amplified into the coils to generate magnetic fields in the workspace. We are able to use the numerically controlled setup to generate different magnetic fields with specific outputs. The magnetic actuation experiments are conducted in 1 wt.% Polyvinylpyrrolidone (PVP) solution, which has a viscosity of 1.3 cp. In the experiments, a piece of silicon wafer is used as the substrate, and with its polished surface upward, the imaging contrast for observation can be enhanced.

The synthesis of magnetite nanoparticles was previously reported in [38]. In our experiments, the diameter of the particles is approximately 100 nm. One drop of nanoparticle solution (4 μL, 3 mg/mL) is added into the tank filled with the PVP solution, and then the dispersed particles are first gathered using a magnetic field gradient. Then the nanoparticle clusters are transferred into the workspace of the electromagnetic setup. In order to create a uniform distribution of the nanoparticle chains, a 20 Hz-frequency dynamic magnetic field is applied to disassemble the particle clusters while spreading them [35], and after that, the nanoparticles are ready for further magnetic actuation process.

3.4 EXPERIMENTAL RESULTS

3.4.1 Reconfiguration of an EPNS

The generation of a circular vortex-like swarm is shown in Figure 3.6, and the elongation process of the EPNS is shown in Figures 3.7a–c. A circular VPNS is initially

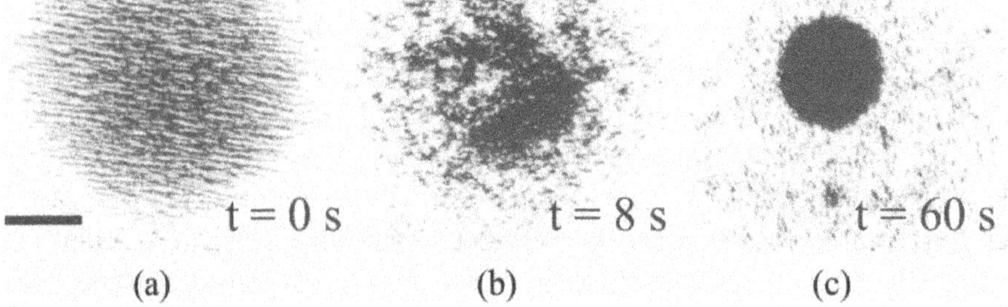

Figure 3.6 Experimental results of the generation of a vortex-like paramagnetic nanoparticle swarm (VPNS). The scale bar indicates 500 μm.

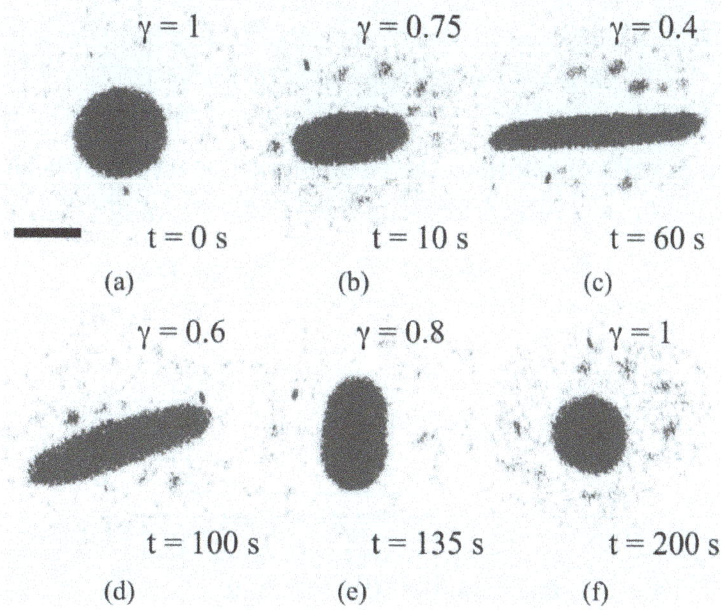

Figure 3.7 Reversible elongation process of an EPNS. The scale bar indicates 500 μm. The field strength applied is 8 mT, and the rotating frequency is 7 Hz.

formed at t = 0 s, and after the applied field ratio is decreased to 0.75, the swarm begin to elongate into an elliptical pattern. In this range, the fluidic factor dominates the reconfiguration process, and the swarm aspect ratio α is approximately 3. With the further decrease of the field ratio to 0.4, significant elongation of the swarm pattern can be observed ($\alpha \sim 7$). The reversible contraction of the swarm is demonstrated in Figures 3.7d–f. Fluidic inward interaction provided by induced vortices is the main factor for the contraction behavior. The contraction process needs more time to perform, *i.e.*, more than 100 s. Meanwhile, during the contraction, the long-axial direction of the swarm will change significantly, due to the increasing fluidic vortex and the reorganization of the particle chains. Finally, the swarm is capable to recover to the original circular pattern.

3.4.2 Omnidirectional Locomotion of an EPNS

Because the drag coefficient near a solid substrate is larger than that far from the substrate. By adding a small pitch angle (1°–6°), different parts of the swarm encounter drag inequality, and thus the swarm can be actuated to make locomotion. In this work, we propose an actuation algorithm to decouple the direction of locomotion and the long-axis direction of the swarm, and the swarm can perform omnidirectional locomotion with any specific long-axial directions. It is noted that this strategy is compatible with all kinds of mobile microrobotic swarms, as long as their triggering fields are known. The actuation elliptical field for generating an EPNS is expressed as

$$\boldsymbol{B_E} = [a\cos(2\pi ft) b\sin(2\pi ft) 0] \begin{bmatrix} x \\ y \\ 0 \end{bmatrix}. \tag{3.21}$$

By performing a series of rotation, the equation of the actuation field that enables the swarm with the capability of making omnidirectional locomotion can be given

$$\boldsymbol{B}_{\text{Omni}} = \boldsymbol{R_z}(\kappa) \cdot \boldsymbol{R_y}(\varphi) \cdot \boldsymbol{R_z}(\tau) \cdot \boldsymbol{B_E} \tag{3.22}$$

where

$$\boldsymbol{R_z}(\tau) = \underbrace{\begin{bmatrix} \cos\tau & -\sin\tau & 0 \\ \sin\tau & \cos\tau & 0 \\ 0 & 0 & 1 \end{bmatrix}}_{\text{Direction of swarm motion}} \tag{3.23}$$

$$\boldsymbol{R_y}(\varphi) = \underbrace{\begin{bmatrix} \cos\varphi & 0 & \sin\varphi \\ 0 & 1 & 0 \\ -\sin\varphi & 0 & \cos\varphi \end{bmatrix}}_{\text{Pitch angle}} \tag{3.24}$$

$$\boldsymbol{R_z}(\kappa) = \underbrace{\begin{bmatrix} \cos\kappa & -\sin\kappa & 0 \\ \sin\kappa & \cos\kappa & 0 \\ 0 & 0 & 1 \end{bmatrix}}_{\text{Long-axis direction}}. \tag{3.25}$$

In Eq. (3.22), $\boldsymbol{R_z}(\tau)$ decides the direction of motion of the swarm α, $\boldsymbol{R_y}(\varphi)$ adds a pitch angle φ to the rotating plane of the elliptical field, and $\boldsymbol{R_z}(\kappa)$ is for determining the long-axial direction of the swarm β, where $\beta = \tau + \kappa$.

The velocity profile of an EPNS actuated by $\boldsymbol{B}_{\text{Omni}}$ is presented in Figure 3.8. The blue and red curves indicate the cases that the actuation fields have a field ratio $\gamma = 0.7$ and $\gamma = 0.45$, respectively. The EPNS has a larger translational velocity when $|\beta - \tau|$, *i.e.*, the angle between the long-axis direction of the swarm and the moving direction, is smaller. When $|\beta - \tau| = 0°$ and $|\beta - \tau| = 50°$, the experimental results are shown in Figures 3.8a and 3.8b, respectively. When the applied field ratio γ is smaller, the velocities that the swarm can reach will be lower. A possible reason is that, the particle chains inside the swarm tends to step out when they are actuated by the fields with a smaller γ, and moreover, the fluidic interaction induced to coordinate the motion of the particle chains is weaker.

3.4.3 Adaptive Locomotion for Constrained Environments

The properties and advantages of a vortex-like paramagnetic nanoparticle swarm (VPNS) and an elliptical paramagnetic nanoparticle swarm (EPNS) differ in terms of locomotion capabilities. A VPNS, due to its circular shape, exhibits swift changes in moving direction with high locomotion dexterity. On the other hand, an EPNS, with its elliptical shape, is better suited for navigating highly constrained environments

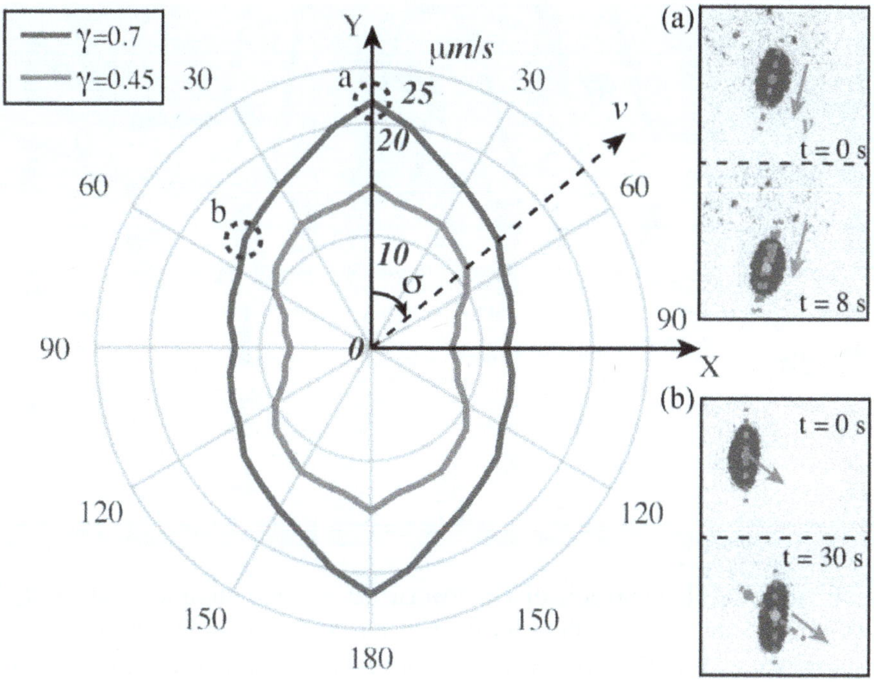

Figure 3.8 Omnidirectional velocity of a VPNS. The blue and red curved indicate the cases when the applied field ratio is 0.7 and 0.45, respectively. Herein, the short-axis and long-axis directions of the swarm are indicated using X- and Y-axis, respectively. The direction of swarm locomotion is indicated by σ. (a) and (b) show the experimental results when the angle between the locomotion direction and the swarm long-axial direction is 0° and 50°, respectively

such as narrow channels. By utilizing the swarm actuation strategy proposed in the article, efficient reversible elongation and contraction between a VPNS and an EPNS can be achieved. The article demonstrates the capability of the swarm to pass through a channel with a sharp turn and a narrowed space. The experiments detailing the process are shown in Figure 3.9, where a1–a4 and c1–c4 illustrate the experimental setup and b1–b4 and d1–d4 depict the real-time locomotion of the swarm inside the channel, indicated by the red spots.

In the presented scenario, the swarm is initially generated in the left reservoir and enters the entrance of the channel. As it navigates inside the channel, it encounters a sharp channel that poses a challenge for navigation. An EPNS, due to the restricting channel walls, is unable to perform a U-turn to pass through this narrow section, as shown in Figure 3.9a5. However, the VPNS, with its circular shape and high locomotion dexterity, can efficiently change its direction on-demand. When the VPNS approaches the narrowed space on the right half of the channel, it undergoes pattern reconfiguration and transforms into an EPNS, allowing it to pass through the constrained area. Once the swarm exits the channel, it can revert back to a VPNS configuration. It is important to note that if a VPNS were to attempt passing through the narrowed channel without undergoing pattern reconfiguration, it may collide with

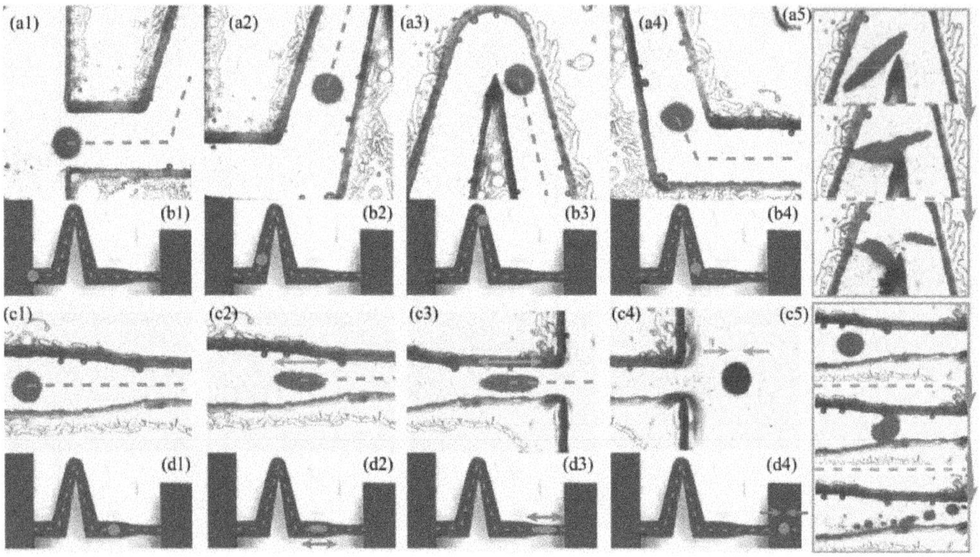

Figure 3.9 Adaptive locomotion of the swarm in a microchannel. (a1)–(a4) VPNS passes through a sharp turn. The red dashed curves indicate the desired trajectory. (a5) Failure case if an EPNS with a high aspect ratio is applied to pass the same turn. (b1)–(b4) Overall view of the channel. The red spots shows the realtime location of the swarm. (c1)–(c4) EPNS is formed to pass through the narrowed channel. The green arrows indicate the swarm pattern changing. (c5) Failure case when a VPNS is used for the narrowed environment. (d1)–(d4) Realtime location of the swarm. The pattern reconfiguration of the swarm is schematically shown by the red spots and ellipses.

the channel wall, as shown in Figure 3.9c5. Therefore, by combining the capabilities of VPNS and EPNS, the swarm exhibits enhanced motion dexterity, particularly in complex environments where precise navigation is required.

3.5 CHARACTERIZATIONS OF SWARM FEATURES

In this section, we examine and consolidate various crucial characteristics of an EPNS (elliptical paramagnetic nanoparticle swarm) that could pose challenges for achieving effective control using conventional algorithms. Additionally, we propose that these identified features might also be applicable to other microrobotic swarms generated through fluidic interactions. The outcomes presented in this section aim to enhance our comprehension of reconfigurable swarms, laying the groundwork for the development of advanced control strategies and algorithms that can effectively address the distinct behaviors and limitations exhibited by such swarms.

3.5.1 Feature I: Time Delay

Due to the nature of fluidic-induced interactions in an EPNS, the modulation of the entire swarm, including orientation change and reconfiguration, is not immediately

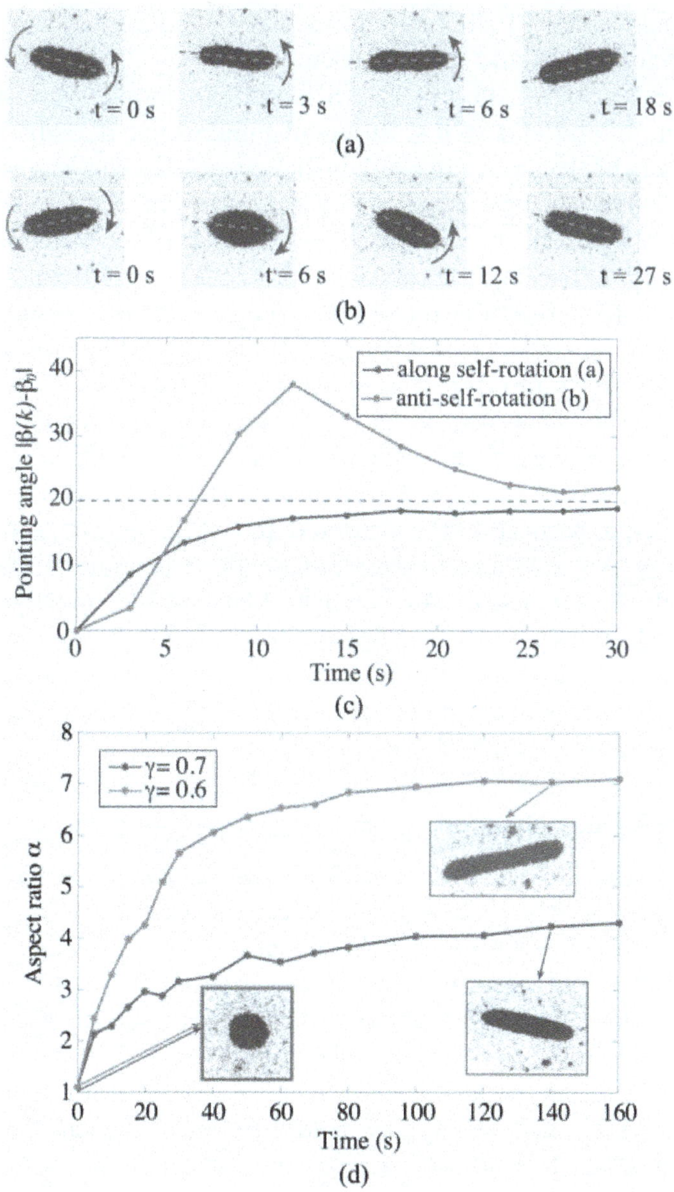

Figure 3.10 Time-delay property of an EPNS. (a) EPNS's long-axial direction tuned 20° anticlockwise, aligned with chain rotation (red arrows) and swarm rotation (blue arrows). (b) EPNS is tuned 20° clockwise against the rotation direction of the particle chains. (c) Relationship between the turning angle $|\beta(k) - \beta_0|$ and time. (d) Time delay in tuning the aspect ratio of the swarm.

effective. The response of the nanoparticle chains within the swarm needs time to propagate and synchronize, resulting in a time delay in the overall behavior of the EPNS. The characterization of this time delay in an EPNS is presented in Figure 3.10, focusing on two aspects: the delay in orientation change (Figures 3.10a-c) and the delay in ratio change (Figure 3.10d). These investigations provide insights into the temporal dynamics of an EPNS and help us understand and address the challenges associated with its control and manipulation.

In Figures 3.10a and 3.10b, an EPNS is initially formed with a specific long-axis orientation β_0, and at t = 0 s, an angular increment of $\pm 20°$ is applied. The rotation behaviors of the swarm depend on the directions of swarm rotation and the self-rotation of particle chains. When the swarm rotates in the same direction as the particle chains, the swarm initially twists and then gradually recovers its elliptical shape (Figure 3.10a). The angle of rotation $\Delta\beta = |\beta(k) - \beta_0|$ increases rapidly within 5 seconds ($\Delta\beta \approx 12°$), then the rotational velocity decreases, resulting in a slower increase in $\Delta\beta$ from 6 s to 18 s ($\Delta\beta \approx 6°$). After t = 18 s, the orientation stabilizes, but there is a steady-state error of approximately 2° (Figure 3.10c). On the other hand, in Figure 3.10b, when the swarm rotates against the direction of the chains, a reorganization process occurs, and the pattern shifts into an ellipse with a significant change in aspect ratio at t = 6 s. Subsequently, the swarm gradually recovers its initial circular shape. Analysis of the measured data (Figure 3.10c) shows that $Delta\beta$ initially increases ($\Delta\beta \approx 38°$) and then gradually decreases until a steady-state error of approximately 3° is reached. Furthermore, Figure 3.10d investigates two EPNS with different field ratios, $\gamma = 0.7$ and $\gamma = 0.6$, respectively, starting from circular patterns. Without a control algorithm, it takes a long time (over 100 s) for the aspect ratio to reach a steady state. Therefore, there is a need to significantly reduce the convergence time for stabilizing the swarm.

3.5.2 Property II: Reorganization

When the input field undergoes rapid and significant changes, the EPNS may exhibit reorganization and splitting behaviors, as illustrated in Figures 3.11a and 3.11b. In Figure 3.11a, when the orientation of the actuation elliptical field shifts by 90°, the EPNS loses stability and splits into several subswarms. The sudden change in agent-agent magnetic interactions disrupts the dynamic equilibrium that was gradually established through fluidic interactions. The overall fluidic field is unable to maintain the integrity of the entire swarm pattern, resulting in pattern reorganization. Similarly, in Figure 3.11b, when the applied field ratio is significantly reduced, splitting also occurs. Increasing the field ratio strengthens and regularizes the vortices induced by the rotating particle chains, leading to localized particle gathering. Consequently, the originally elongated pattern loses its cohesion as a single dynamic entity, and the strong fluidic interactions divide the swarm into multiple parts.

3.5.3 Property III: Translational Drifting

In experiments, the substrate we used has been set with a tilted angle of 3°, which will lead to translational drifting of the entire swarm. An EPNS is first generated and maintained using inplane elliptical magnetic field. Its drifting distance is presented in Figure 3.12. The drifting velocity is approximately 5 μm/s in this case.

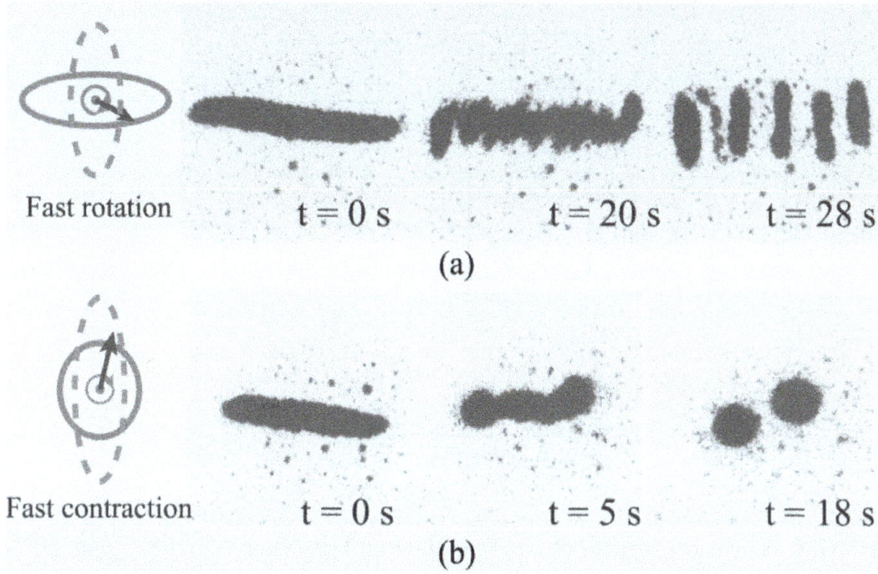

Figure 3.11 Swarm tends to reorganize when the parameters of the external magnetic field changes significantly. (a) When the orientation of the input elliptical field changes fast, the EPNS will be twisted and split into several small subswarms due to the fluidic drag. (b) When the applied field ratio decreases significantly, split also occurs.

3.6 CONTROL STRATEGIES

3.6.1 Fuzzy Logic-Based Control Scheme

To address the challenges and exploit the advantages of human operators' experience, we have developed a fuzzy logic-based control architecture, as depicted in Figure 3.13. The control system focuses on regulating the swarm's aspect ratio and involves several components. Firstly, the desired aspect ratio $\gamma_d(k)$ is input into a model-based feedforward controller. This controller generates appropriate electromagnetic coil configurations for swarm generation, taking into account the desired aspect ratio. Next, the swarm is tracked using statistics-based imaging techniques to obtain important parameters related to aspect ratio control, such as sensitivity $s(\alpha(k))$, changing speed $v(\alpha(k))$, and tracking accuracy $C(\alpha(k))$. These parameters are fed into a fuzzy logic controller for further processing. The fuzzy logic controller utilizes the collected data to make intelligent decisions and provide control signals for the aspect ratio regulation loop. It takes into account the sensitivity, changing speed, and tracking accuracy to determine the optimal control strategy. In addition to aspect ratio control, the control architecture also incorporates feedback control for the long-axis orientation $\beta(k)$ and the position of the swarm $P(x(k), y(k))$. These components ensure comprehensive control over the swarm's behavior. By combining model-based feedforward control, fuzzy logic-based decision-making, and feedback control, our proposed architecture aims to enhance the control performances of the swarm, leveraging the expertise and intuition of human operators. The blue region in Figure 3.13 represents the control strategy employed for the long-axis orientation and position control of the swarm.

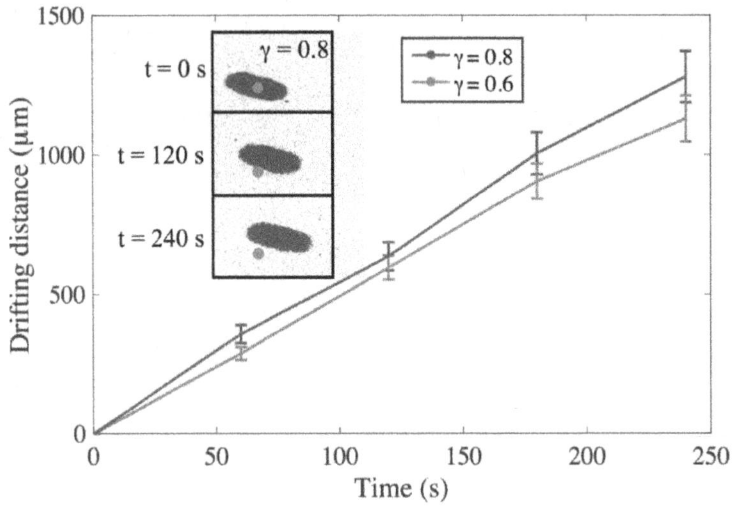

Figure 3.12 Calibration results of the translational drifting velocity of the EPNS. Two field ratios are applied, *i.e.*, 0.8 and 0.6. The red spots indicate the original location of the swarm center. The error bars indicate the standard deviation calculated from 3 times of measurements.

The feedforward controller generates a preset control input based on the $\gamma - \alpha$ model, which is fitted by the experimental characterization data in Figure 3.14.

$$\gamma = \begin{cases} (3.639\alpha_d^4 - 90.84\alpha_d^3 + 815.6\alpha_d^2 - 3498\alpha_d + 12830) \\ \times 10^{-4}, \alpha(k) \leq \alpha_d \\ (3.489\alpha_d^4 - 108\alpha_d^3 + 926.1\alpha_d^2 - 3378\alpha_d + 12730) \\ \times 10^{-4}, \alpha(k) > \alpha_d \end{cases} \tag{3.26}$$

where α_d and $\alpha(k)$ are the desired shape ratio and real shape ratio at the time instant k, respectively. Since the characterized model varies in a range with different particle doses and ambient fluids, a feedback controller is necessary to compensate for the model error and enhance the convergence speed. A PI controller with varying gains is adopted for the feedback controller, which has the following expression:

$$\alpha_{fb}(k) = -W_p \cdot K_p(k) \cdot e(k) - W_i \cdot \frac{T_s}{K_i(k)} \sum_{k=1}^{k} e(k) \tag{3.27}$$

where T_s, $K_p(k) \in [1, 10]$ and $K_i(k) \in [1, 10]$ are the sampling time, proportional gain, and integral gain determined by the fuzzy logic controller, respectively. $T_s = 0.2$ s in this work. W_p and W_i are the constant weights for the control gains set as 0.1 and 0.02, respectively. $e(k)$ stands for the tracking error, *i.e.*, $e(k) = \alpha_d - \alpha(k)$.

In order to design an effective and efficient fuzzy controller, three inputs should be considered to tune the control gains.

(1) $s(\alpha(k))$: The sensitivity of $\alpha(k)$, which increases with the aspect ratio of the swarm $\alpha(k)$. At large aspect ratios, $\alpha(k)$ is sensitive to the change of control input $\gamma(k)$, meaning that a small change in γ would cause a large change in α. Therefore,

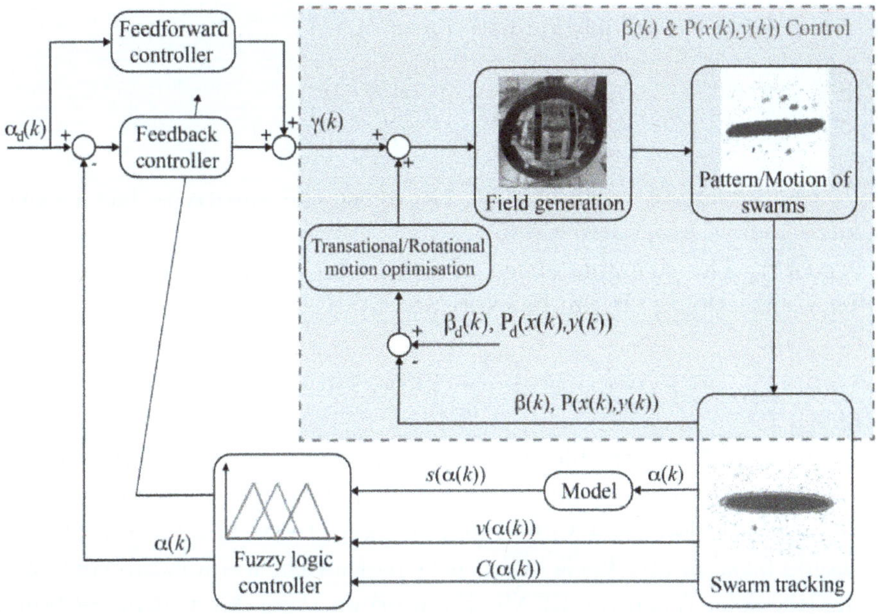

Figure 3.13 Control architecture for swarm pattern, orientation and position. The outer loop is for controlling the swarm pattern, while the inner loop (blue region) indicates the strategy to control the swarm long-axis orientation and position. The fuzzy logic controller is designed to dynamically tune the gains of the feedback controller. The model refers to the differentiation of the characterized $\gamma - \alpha$ relationship Eq. (3.26).

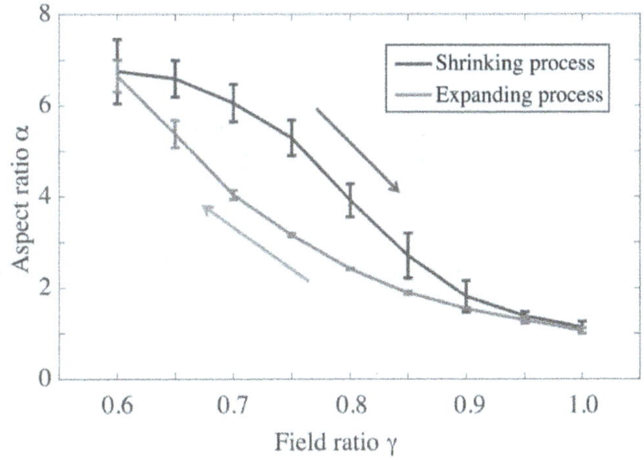

Figure 3.14 Fitted model describing the relationship between aspect ratio of the swarm α and input field ratio γ. The error bars indicate the standard deviation calculated from three times of measurements.

at this state, a small K_p should be set to prevent undesired elongation of the swarm. On the contrary, at small shape ratios, $s(\alpha(k))$ is low, and thus a large K_p is set to enhance the convergence speed. $s(\alpha(k))$ can be obtained by taking the derivative of the characterized $\gamma - \alpha$ model Eq. 3.26, *i.e.*,

$$s(\alpha(k)) = \frac{\gamma_f'(\alpha(k))}{\gamma_{f_{\max}}'} \tag{3.28}$$

where $\gamma_{f_{\max}}'$ is the largest norm of $\gamma_f'(\alpha(k))$, hence the sensitivity has a value range from 0 to 1.

(2) $v(\alpha(k))$: The changing speed of α(k), which reflects how fast the pattern elongation/contraction is. It can be expressed by

$$v(\alpha(k)) = \frac{1}{N \cdot v_{\max}} |\alpha(k) - \alpha(k - N)| \tag{3.29}$$

where the constant N is introduced considering that the shape deformation is a slow process, and $v_{\max}$ is the maximum speed of change that can also be obtained from Eq. (3.26). $v(\alpha(k))$ also has a value range of [0,1]. To set the fuzzy rules, small K_p and K_i should be set if $v(\alpha(k))$ is high, ensuring that the feedforward controller takes the dominating role. When the EPNS (Equilibrium Point Navigation System) comes to an equilibrium, large K_p and K_i take effect to regulate $\alpha(k)$ and eliminate the steady-state error.

(3) $C(\alpha(k))$: Tracked accuracy of $\alpha(k)$. During the pattern reconfiguration, the swarm cannot respond to the control input instantly due to its time-delay feature. With a high tracked accuracy, *i.e.*, $\alpha(k)$ is close to its targeted value, small K_p and K_i should be set to avoid inducing significant oscillations, and vice versa. $C(\alpha(k))$ is defined by

$$C(\alpha(k)) = \begin{cases} 1 - \frac{|\alpha(k)-\alpha_d(k)|}{\alpha_d(k)} & , \frac{|\alpha(k)-\alpha_d(k)|}{\alpha_d(k)} \leq 1 \\ 0 & , \frac{|\alpha(k)-\alpha_d(k)|}{\alpha_d(k)} > 1 \end{cases} \tag{3.30}$$

where $C(\alpha(k)) \in [0, 1]$. In order to avoid the improper error integration during the long-time convergence period, which can also cause the tracking oscillations, K_i is activated only when $C(\alpha(k)) \in [0.8, 1]$.

Two fuzzy logic controllers with multiple inputs and a single output are designed for K_p and K_i, respectively. Inputs of the fuzzy controller for K_p are $s(\alpha(k))$, $v(\alpha(k))$, and $C(\alpha(k))$, and those for the K_i controller are $v(\alpha(k))$ and $C(\alpha(k))$. Considering the strategy of tuning K_i, the membership function in the controller for tuning K_i is designed as shown in Figure 3.15a. Fuzzy sets and membership functions for all the remaining inputs and outputs are shown in Figures 3.15b and 3.15c, respectively. Then, fuzzy control rules are designed [39], and by adopting the centroid defuzzification method, nonlinear relationships between the outputs and inputs of the two fuzzy logic controllers are obtained (Figure 3.15e). From the designed fuzzy rules, it can be observed that K_p has large values for low tracked accuracy, while when the tracked accuracy is high, K_p will decrease. This improves the convergence speed and avoids large overshoot (or instability of the swarm). Meanwhile, when the sensitivity or changing speed is high, K_p is assigned a small value to avoid unnecessary elongation, and K_p is large when the sensitivity/changing speed is low to accelerate the convergence process. For K_i, the integration procedure only takes effect when the

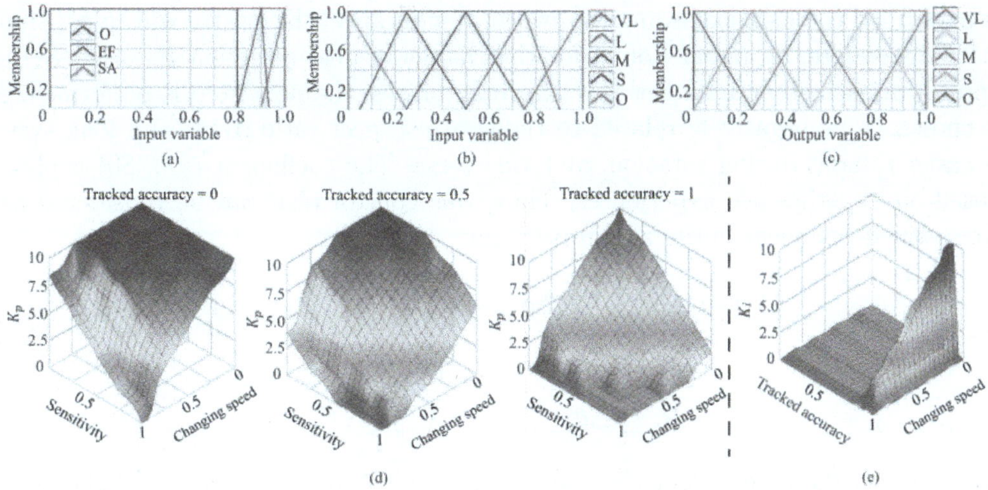

Figure 3.15 (a) Membership function in the controller for tuning K_i. (b) and (c) Fuzzy sets and membership functions for all the remaining inputs and all the outputs. (d) and (e) Nonlinear relationships between the outputs and inputs of the two fuzzy logic controllers for tuning K_p and K_i after adopting centroid defuzzification, respectively.

tracked accuracy is higher than 0.8, in which stage the steady-state error exists, and the value of K_i is negatively related to the changing speed. Therefore, the results validate that the designed fuzzy logic controllers have the same rule as human operation experiences.

3.6.2 Long-Axis Orientation and Motion Optimization

Besides the fuzzy logic-based ratio control, we have proposed optimization methods to control the long-axis orientation and position of the swarm (blue region, Figure 3.13). Three schemes are defined based on the positions and poses of the desired and current swarm patterns. Scheme I takes effect when $D_r > a$, where a is the half length of the short axis of the desired elliptical pattern, and

$$D_r = \sqrt{P_d^2(x_d, y_d) - P^2(x(k), y(k))} \tag{3.31}$$

where $P_d(x_d, y_d)$ and $P(x(k), y(k))$ are the desired and current swarm centers, respectively. In this case, the goal is to actuate the swarm to make its center coincide with that of the desired pattern (within 10 pixels). The moving direction of the swarm is defined to coincide with its long axis, which maximizes the translational velocity (Figure 3.8). The azimuth angle of the desired location with respect to the current location of the swarm is calculated by

$$\sigma_r = \arctan\left(\frac{y_d - y}{x_d - x}\right). \tag{3.32}$$

The current long-axis orientation of the swarm is defined as $\beta(k)$, and as a result, the angle that the swarm needs to rotate is $\Delta\sigma = \beta(k) - \sigma_r$. However, if the rotation is performed too fast, exceeding the swarm's endurance, the swarm will split (Figure 3.11). Therefore, an upper bound for the change of field direction $B_u = 80/\alpha(k)$ is applied in each step, and after the swarm stabilizes, the next step is performed. B_u is chosen to be negatively related to the swarm aspect ratio $\alpha(k)$, as a long swarm is easier to split during rotation, and vice versa. The coefficient (*i.e.*, 80) is chosen based on experimental experiences. Thus, this control task can be considered as a constrained nonlinear optimization problem

$$D_r = \min_{\Delta\theta} \Big[(x + T(\Delta\sigma)v \cdot \cos(\beta(k) + \Delta\theta) - x_d)^2 + (y + T(\Delta\sigma)v \cdot \sin(\beta(k) + \Delta\theta) - y_d)^2 \Big] \tag{3.33}$$

$$-B_u \le \Delta\theta \le B_u \tag{3.34}$$

where $\Delta\theta$ is the turning angle in each step, v is the moving velocity of the swarm with a specific pitch angle, and $T(\Delta\sigma)$ is a function deciding the moving direction.

$$\begin{cases} T = 1 & (\Delta\sigma \le 90^\circ \text{ or } \Delta\sigma \ge 270^\circ) \\ T = -1 & (90^\circ < \Delta\sigma < 270^\circ) \end{cases}. \tag{3.35}$$

Finally, the control input is decided as

$$u = u^- + \Delta\theta \tag{3.36}$$

where u^- is the control input at the former time step.

After the position of the swarm center coincides with the desired one, Scheme II is activated, which is for controlling the long-axis orientation and aspect ratio. When the error of long-axis orientation $e_\beta = \beta_d - \beta(k)$ (β_d is the desired orientation) is larger than (or equal to) B_u, the input order is to rotate the swarm with a step of B_u; while when $e_\beta < B_u$, an integral term is applied to eliminate the steady-state error. The strategy can be expressed as:

$$\beta(k) = \begin{cases} \beta(k-1) + B_u & (e_\beta > 15^\circ) \\ \beta(k-1) + K_{i\beta} \cdot e_\beta & (e_\beta < 15^\circ) \end{cases} \tag{3.37}$$

where $\beta(k-1)$ is the long-axis orientation at the previous time step $k-1$, $K_{i\beta}$ is set to be 0.1. Finally, Scheme III is designed for counterbalancing the influence of drifting. When the entire swarm drifts from the desired location, the omnidirectional locomotion of the swarm is activated (Figure 3.12). In this case, the moving direction σ_r is still fully defined by Eq. (3.32), while the long-axis orientation keeps being controlled as desired by the fuzzy controller.

3.6.3 Control Results

To verify the efficacy of our proposed control strategies, we systematically carried out three types of sequential experiments: (1) Pattern control, where the goal was to regulate the aspect ratio ($\alpha(k) \to \alpha_d(k)$). (2) Pattern-angle control, involving the regulation of both the aspect ratio ($\alpha(k) \to \alpha_d(k)$) and the long-axis orientation

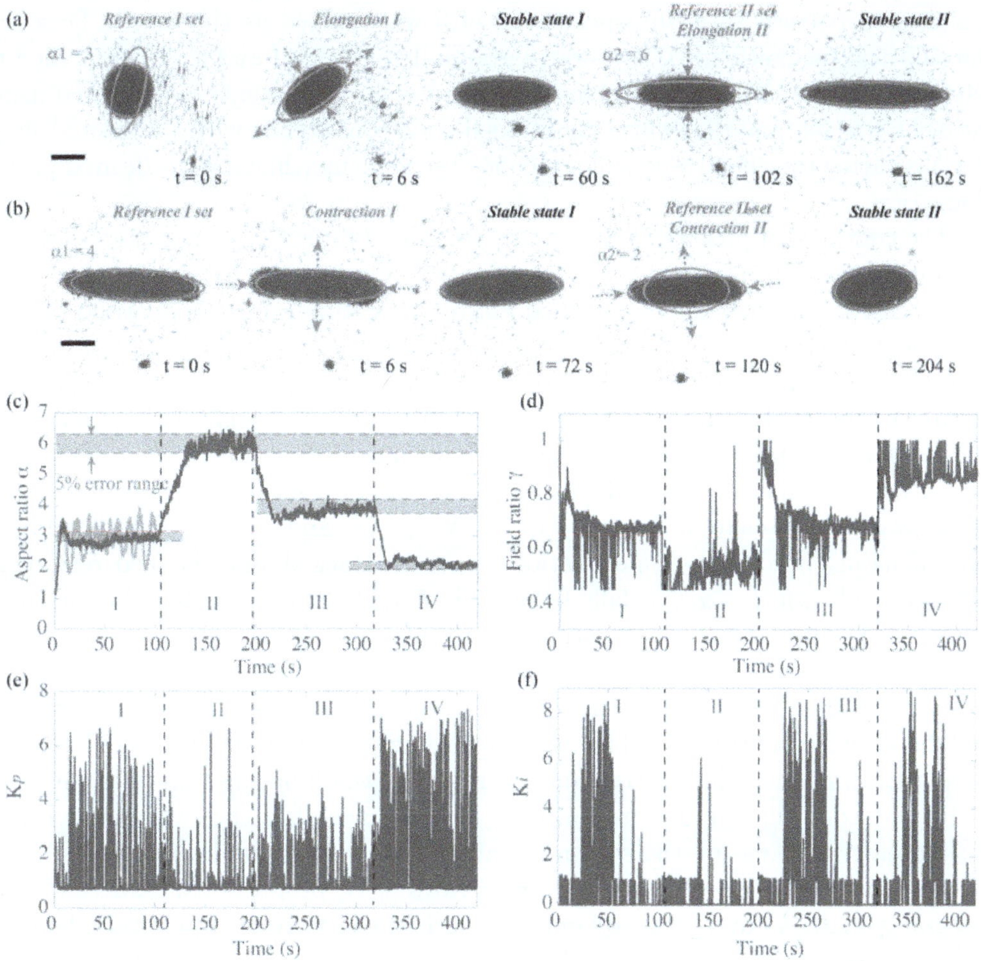

Figure 3.16 Control results of the aspect ratio $\alpha(k)$ of an EPNS. (a) and (b) Experimental results of the swarm elongation and contraction control, respectively. The green and red ellipses indicate the desired and current swarm pattern, respectively. The red dotted arrows represent the deformation directions of the swarm at specific locations. The scale bar indicates 500 µm. (c) Change in swarm aspect ratio $\alpha(k)$ with time. The red regions indicate the error range with 5% of the referenced aspect ratios. (d) Change in applied field ratio $\gamma(k)$ with time. (e) and (f) indicate the relationships between K_P , K_i and time, respectively. In (c)–(f), region I–IV are labeled corresponding with each other.

$(\beta(k) \rightarrow \beta_d(k))$. (3) Pattern-angle-position control, aiming to regulate the aspect ratio $(\alpha(k) \rightarrow \alpha_d(k))$, long-axis orientation $(\beta(k) \rightarrow \beta_d(k))$, and position coordinates $(P(x(k), y(k)) \rightarrow P_d(x(k), y(k)))$.

(1) Morphology Control for EPNS: The control scheme was initially implemented to regulate the aspect ratio of an EPNS. In this scenario, the long-axis orientation of the elliptical magnetic field remained fixed, and no feedback control was employed to adjust the orientation. The experimental results showcasing pattern elongation are presented in Figure 3.16a. At the beginning, a VPNS was generated, and at t = 0 s, a desired pattern with an aspect ratio of 3 was defined as the target. Driven by the elliptical magnetic field, the swarm gradually elongated and closely matched the reference contour. Subsequently, in the second stage of elongation, a desired aspect ratio of 6 was set, and the swarm maintained good consistency with the desired shape, demonstrating the effectiveness of the control scheme in achieving the desired pattern elongation.

The contraction process of the swarm presents different characteristics compared to the elongation process. During contraction, significant reorganization of nanoparticles occurs, resulting in a prolonged convergence time and a high time delay in response to field input. Moreover, if the input order ($\gamma(k)$) undergoes a sudden and large change during contraction control, the swarm may split into multiple parts. To ensure swarm stability throughout the contraction process, small intermediate steps ($\Delta\alpha = 0.5$) are employed. For instance, when transitioning from an aspect ratio of 6 to a desired aspect ratio of 4, instead of directly targeting an aspect ratio of 4, progressive intermediate references ($\alpha_r = 5.5$, $\alpha_r = 5$, and $\alpha_r = 4.5$) are introduced. The changing speed of the aspect ratio, $v(\alpha(k))$, is tracked, and the next reference is activated only when $v(\alpha(k))$, falls below 5% of $\alpha(k)$, indicating that the intermediate target has been reached. Experimental results showcasing swarm contraction are depicted in Figure 3.16b. Following the last state of the elongation process (Figure 3.16a, t = 162 s), where the swarm has an aspect ratio of 6, desired aspect ratios of 4 and 2 are set for contraction. The final pattern aligns well with the desired patterns, demonstrating successful contraction control. It is worth noting that in Figure 3.16a and b, the controlled actuation continues for over 50 s after the swarm matches the desired pattern to ensure the swarm remains in a dynamic equilibrium state.

The changes in aspect ratio $\alpha(k)$, field ratio $\gamma(k)$, proportional gain $K_p(k)$, and integral gain $K_i(k)$ over time are depicted in Figures 3.16c-f, respectively. Four distinct regions, I-IV, represent steady states at $\alpha = 3$, $\alpha = 6$, $\alpha = 4$, and $\alpha = 2$, respectively. In all regions, the steady-state errors are maintained within 5% of α(k), confirming the effectiveness of the pattern control scheme for an EPNS. When the aspect ratio is 3 (region I), the change in swarm ratio resulting from field input tuning is relatively small, leading to low sensitivity $s(\alpha(\text{k}))$. Conversely, in region II where the swarm pattern has an aspect ratio of 6, it is more sensitive to field inputs and disturbances. Consequently, the input signal γ exhibits significant oscillations in region I, whereas in region II, it needs to be constrained within a small range (Figure 3.16d). The same reasoning applies to the pattern of proportional gain K_p in regions I and II (Figure 3.16e). In region I, where $s(\alpha(\text{k}))$ is low, a sufficiently large K_p is required to achieve the desired pattern deformation. Conversely, in region II, where $s(\alpha(\text{k}))$ is high, a smaller K_p is employed to prevent significant overshooting and instability. In region I of Figure 3.16c, a steady-state error of approximately 0.4 persists for more than 35 s. During this period, the error and the low changing speed of α(k) activate the integration term in the control scheme, resulting in large values of K_i (Figure 3.16f), which brings α within the 5% error range. It is important to note that a lower limit of γ(k) is set to 0.45 to ensure the effectiveness of reversible elongation and contraction of the EPNS. With a γ(k) lower than 0.45, the swarm may elongate with an aspect ratio higher than 7, hindering effective contraction. In

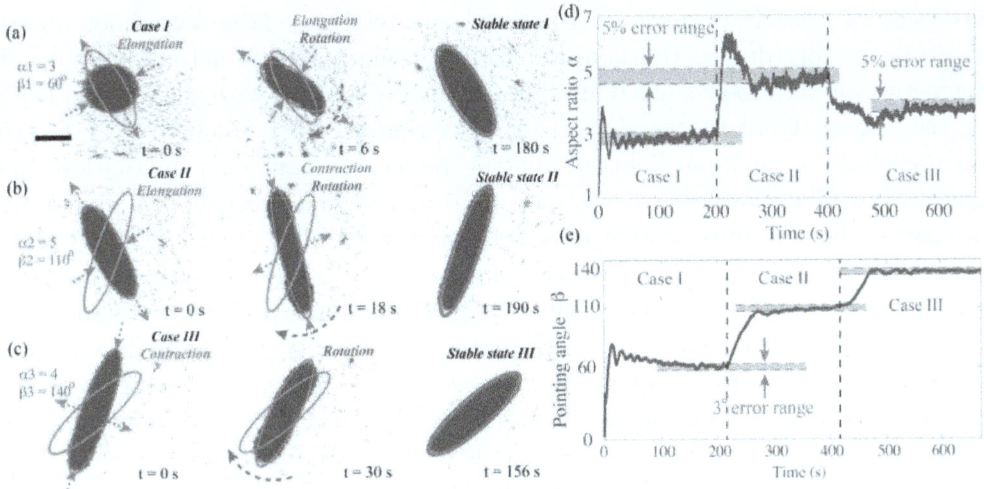

Figure 3.17 Experimental results of simultaneously control the aspect ratio $\alpha(k)$ and the long-axis orientation $\beta(k)$ of an EPNS. (a)–(c) Control process of the EPNS with three different pairs of desired aspect ratio and long-axis orientation. The green and red ellipses indicate the desired and current swarm pattern, respectively. The red dotted arrows represent the deformation directions of the swarm at specific locations. The scale bar indicates 500 μm. (d) Change in swarm aspect ratio $\alpha(k)$ with time. The red regions indicate the error ranges with 5% of the desired aspect ratios. (e) Relationship between the pointing angle of the EPNS $\beta(k)$ and time. The red regions represent the ±3° error ranges. The sections for each cases have been labeled accordingly.

comparison, a PID controller with fixed parameters is unable to successfully control the swarm. The control performance is represented by the green curve in Figure 3.16c, exhibiting significant oscillations with a large amplitude. Additionally, when a new order ($\alpha_d = 6$) is set, the controller fails to guarantee swarm stability, resulting in the swarm splitting into multiple parts.

(2) Pattern-Angle ($\alpha - \beta$) Control for EPNS: To simultaneously control the aspect ratio α(k) and long-axis orientation γ(k) of the EPNS, the strategy described in Section 3.6.2, Scheme II is employed. Three control targets are defined: (1) $\alpha 1 = 3$, $\beta 1 = 60°$; (2) $\alpha 2 = 5$, $\beta 2 = 110°$; (3) $\alpha 3 = 4$, $\beta 3 = 140°$. The experimental results are depicted in Figures 3.17a–c accordingly. Initially, a circular VPNS is used as the starting state. After setting the first target, the aspect ratio and orientation of the swarm are simultaneously controlled. If the current pattern's aspect ratio is smaller than the target, the swarm will elongate and rotate (t = 6 s, Figure 3.17a). Conversely, if the current aspect ratio is larger than the target, the swarm will contract and rotate (t = 18 s, Figure 3.17b). When α(k) matches α_d, only the direction tuning is effective (t = 30 s, Figure 3.17c). Eventually, the EPNS successfully aligns with the desired patterns in all three cases. Each equilibrium state is maintained for over 100 s to ensure the swarm is fully under control.

The change in aspect ratio over time is depicted in Figure 3.17d. In all three cases, the steady-state errors of the aspect ratio remain below 5% of $\alpha(k)$. Additionally, the control of the pointing angle is effective, with a steady-state error within 3°.

However, in Case II (Figure 3.17b), there is a relatively large overshoot observed in $\alpha(k)$, possibly due to the non-uniformity of the magnetic actuation setup. The magnetic field may vary slightly in different directions, and with the high α_d in Case II, the sensitivity of the swarm $s(\alpha(\mathrm{k}))$ is elevated. As a result, during rotation, slight changes in the input field parameters can lead to significant fluctuations in the aspect ratio. The change in orientation ($\beta(\mathrm{k})$) with time is illustrated in Figure 3.17e. In Case I, there is an overshoot of approximately 20° at t = 14 s, which might be influenced by the self-rotation behavior of the swarm. In this scenario, the integration term plays a crucial role in correcting the pointing angle back to the desired range of 3°. In both Case II and Case III, the rotational velocity of the EPNS is within an appropriate range, such as approximately 50° in 55 s (Case II), which helps prevent swarm splitting and confirms the effectiveness of the proposed optimized algorithm. In the steady states of these two cases, the overshooting and steady-state error are negligible, and combining with the results in Figure 3.17d, it can be concluded that the α - β control scheme is capable of well controlling the EPNS.

(3) $\alpha(k)-\beta(k)-P(x(k),y(k))$ Control for EPNS: To address the challenges of controlling an EPNS, including its aspect ratio $\alpha(\mathrm{k})$, long-axis orientation $\beta(\mathrm{k})$, and position in 2D space $P(x(k),y(k))$, we extend our control scheme. In addition to the inherent features of the swarm discussed earlier, such as time delay, reorganization behaviors, and drifting, we must also consider another critical challenge. Ensuring the cohesive movement of the swarm, without significant particle loss or splitting, from its initial location $P(x(k_0),y(k_0))$ to the desired location $P(x_d,y_d)$, requires an optimized actuation strategy. Furthermore, the substrate on which the swarm operates is tilted at an angle of 3°, leading to the drifting effect. Therefore, we employ the three previously discussed schemes (outlined in subsection 3.6.2) to address these challenges.

To validate the proposed schemes for the $\alpha(k)-\beta(k)-P(x(k),y(k))$ control of the EPNS, we perform three cases, as shown in Figures 3.18a–c, respectively. In the first case, a circular VPNS is initially actuated toward the desired location using Scheme I. When the distance between the swarm center and the center of the desired pattern is less than 10 pixels, Scheme II is triggered to control the aspect ratio and pointing angle of the swarm. At 114 s and 138 s, the swarm undergoes simultaneous elongation and rotation. Once the aspect ratio falls within the acceptable error range, pure rotation takes place. However, due to the drifting effect caused by the tilted substrate, a deviation between the EPNS and the desired pattern occurs. To correct this position error, Scheme III is activated, leveraging the omnidirectional locomotion of the swarm. The final result is achieved at t = 228 s, demonstrating a successful match between the EPNS and the desired pattern. Similar good matches are achieved in the second and third cases, indicating the effectiveness of the proposed strategy for the $\alpha(k)-\beta(k)-P(x(k),y(k))$ control of the EPNS. Each equilibrium state is maintained for over 100 s to ensure full control over the swarm.

The change of $\alpha(k)$ is shown in Figure 3.19a. In all three cases, the steady-state error of $\alpha(k)$ remains within the 5% α_d range. However, Case III exhibits larger oscillation amplitude and steady-state errors compared to the other two cases. This can be attributed to the experimental plane not being perfectly horizontal, combined

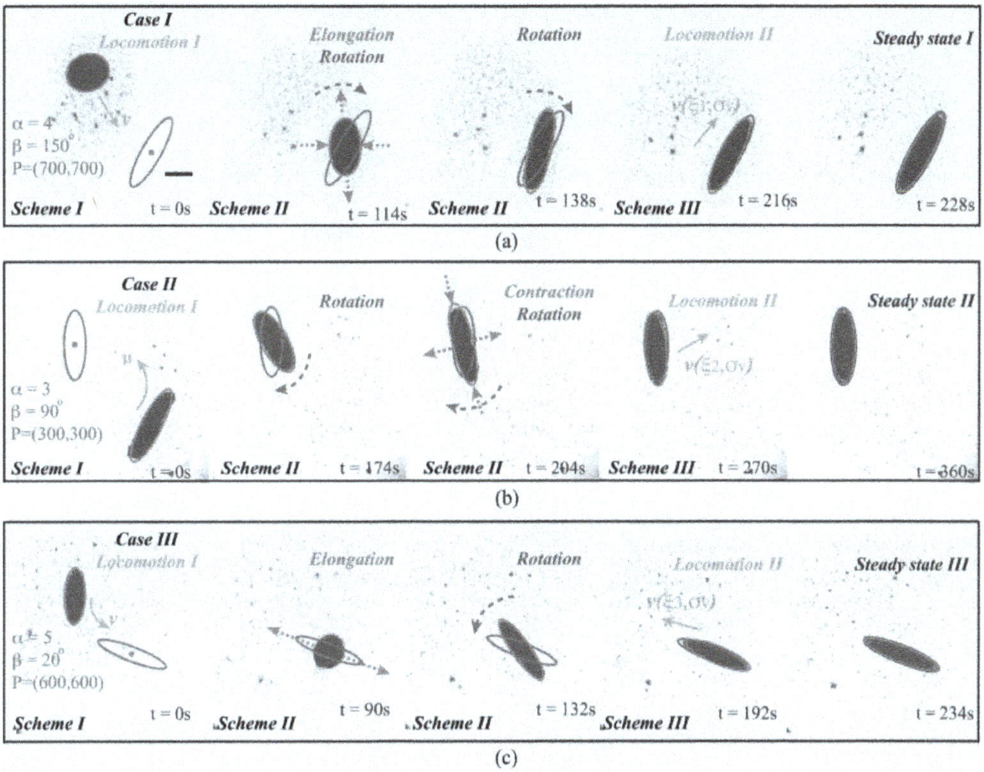

Figure 3.18 Experimental results of simultaneously control the aspect ratio $\alpha(k)$, the long-axis orientation $\beta(k)$ and the position $P(x(k), y(k))$ of an EPNS. (a) Control process when $\alpha_1 = 4$, $\beta_1 = 150°$ and $P(x_1, y_1) = (700, 700)$. (b) Control process when $\alpha_2 = 3$, $\beta_2 = 90°$ and $P(x_2, y_2) = (300, 300)$. (c) Control process when $\alpha_3 = 5$, $\beta_3 = 20°$ and $P(x_3, y_3) = (600, 600)$. The green and red ellipses indicate the desired and current swarm pattern, respectively. The red dotted arrows represent the deformation directions of the swarm at specific locations, the yellow arrows indicate the moving direction, and the blue dashed arrows show the rotating direction of the swarm. The scale bar indicates 500 μm.

with the fact that the aspect ratio of the swarm is set to 5, which has the highest sensitivity among the three cases. It is worth noting that in our control strategy, Scheme II (for $\alpha(k)$ and $\beta(k)$ control) and Scheme III (for $P(x(k), y(k))$ control) are independent and executed in series. This configuration represents the optimized strategy for the challenges discussed in this section. During the omnidirectional locomotion, the swarm may undergo slight pattern reconfiguration, resulting in the oscillation of $\alpha(k)$. In Figure 3.19a, the significant drop observed at the beginning of Cases II and III is due to the pattern reconfiguration induced by the locomotion during Scheme I. Once the EPNS approaches the target region, the aspect ratio is rapidly adjusted to the desired value.

The pointing angle of the EPNS is presented in Figure 3.19b. In all three cases, the pointing angle remains within the $\pm 3°$ range of β_d in the steady states. However,

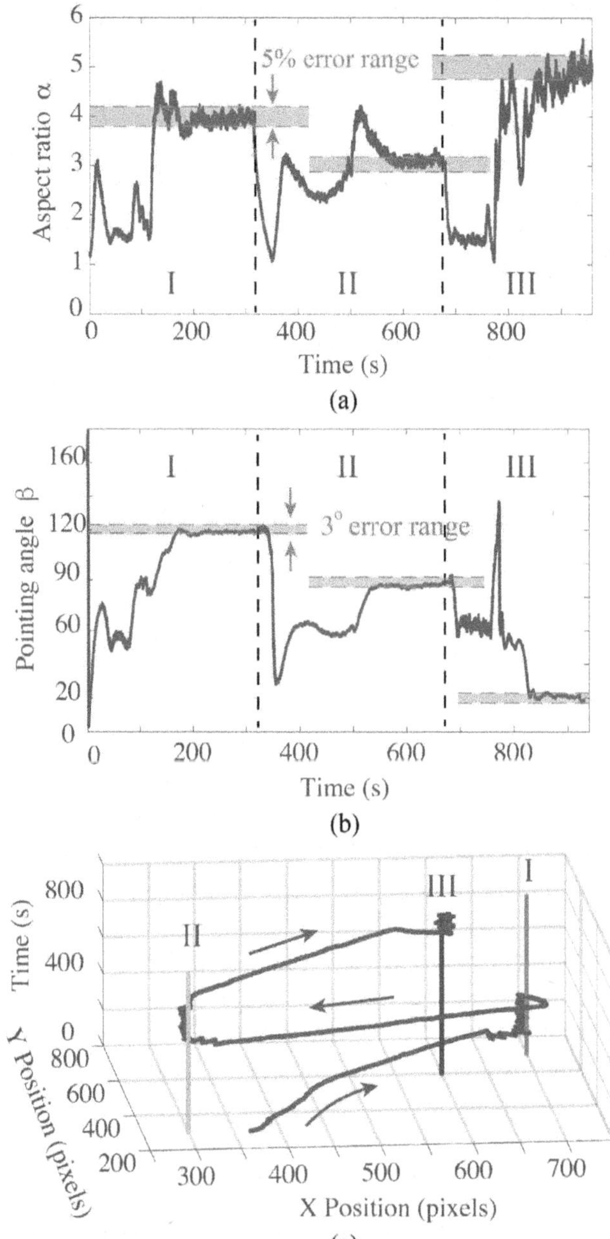

Figure 3.19 (a) EPNS aspect ratio change ($\alpha(k)$) during control. Red regions: 5% error range. (b) Long-axis orientation change $\beta(k)$ over time. Red regions: $\pm 3°$ error ranges. Labeled as regions I, II, and III for respective cases. (c) EPNS point-to-point position control results. Blue curve: swarm trajectory. Blue arrows: motion direction. Colored pillars: desired locations.

during the locomotion phase (Scheme I), the fast moving velocity applied to the swarm tends to compress it along its long axis, leading to a decrease in the aspect ratio and a change in the long axis of the patterns. This explains the significant drop in

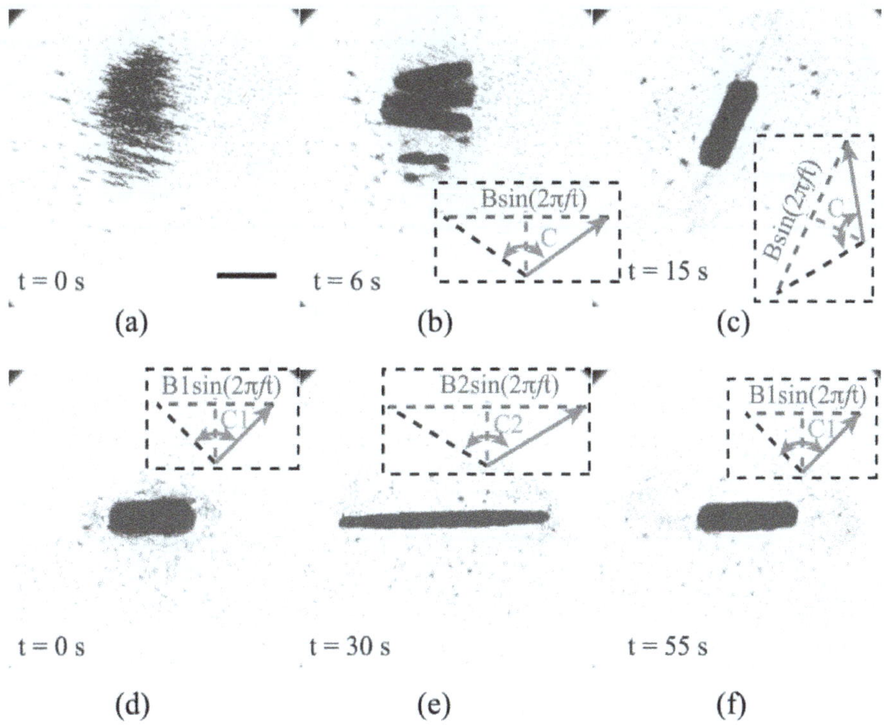

Figure 3.20 (a)–(c) Generation of a ribbon-like paramagnetic nanoparticle swarm (RPNS). (d)–(f) Reversible elongation process of the RPNS. The applied oscillating magnetic fields are schematically demonstrated. In order to realize the swarm elongation, a larger amplitude ratio needs to be applied, *i.e.*, $C_2 > C_1$. The scale bar indicates 500 μm.

$\beta(k)$ observed in Case II. The locomotion trajectory of the EPNS is depicted in Figure 3.19c. It can be observed that the position of the EPNS is well controlled during the point-to-point navigation. The positioning accuracy achieved is generally within 10 pixels, indicating the effectiveness of the control strategy in achieving accurate positioning of the EPNS.

(4) Control for Ribbon-Like Paramagnetic Nanoparticle Swarm (RPNS): The proposed control strategy is further validated using a different type of microrobotic swarm known as ribbon-like paramagnetic nanoparticle swarms (RPNS) [27]. The generation process of RPNS is demonstrated in Figures 3.20a-c. Initially, nanoparticle clusters are spread irregularly, and when a magnetic field is applied, ribbon-like swarming patterns are formed instantaneously. To induce swarm behavior, oscillating magnetic fields are utilized, as shown in the insets of Figures 3.20b and 3.20c. In one direction, a sinusoidal field $B_s = Bsin(2\pi ft)$ is applied (represented by the blue dashed line), while in the perpendicular direction, the field remains constant at C (represented by the green dashed line). Consequently, the resulting field is an oscillating field. Unlike EPNS, where the interaction between magnetic particles is primarily responsible for swarm generation, the magnetic agent-agent interactions

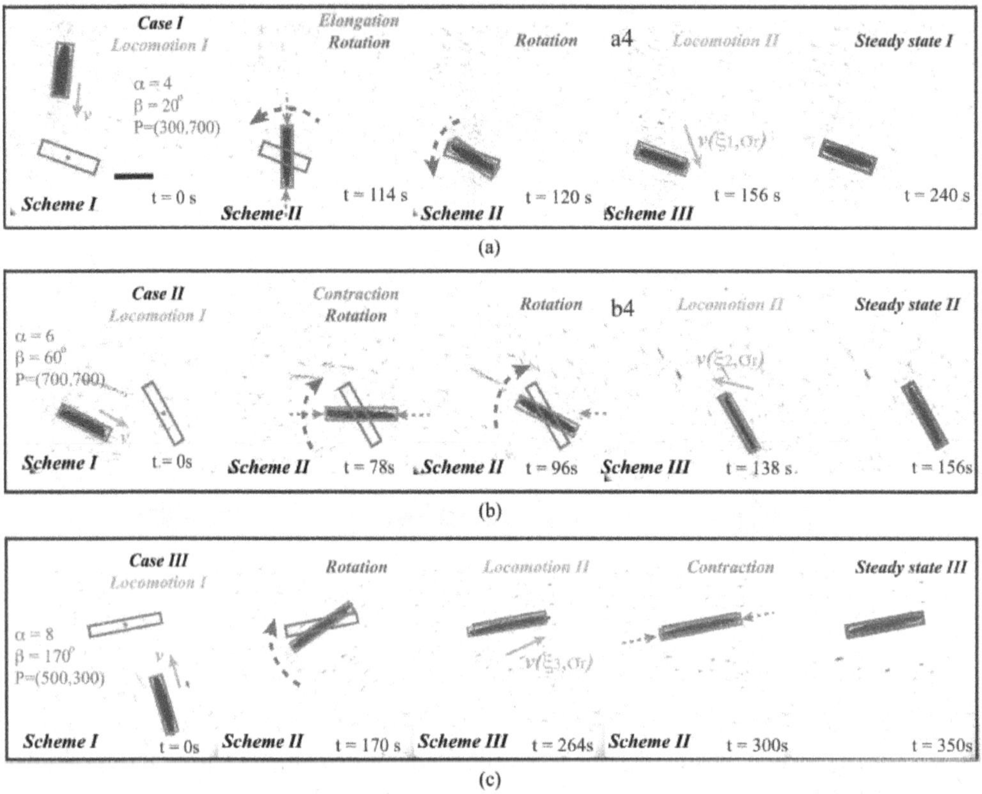

Figure 3.21 Experimental results of simultaneously control the aspect ratio α(k), the long-axis orientation β(k) and the position $P(x(k), y(k))$ of a RPNS. (a) $\alpha_1 = 4$, $\beta_1 = 20°$ and $P(x_1, y_1) = (300, 700)$. (b) $\alpha_2 = 6$, $\beta_2 = 60°$ and $P(x_2, y_2) = (700, 700)$. (c) $\alpha_3 = 8$, $\beta_3 = 170°$ and $P(x_3, y_3) = (500, 300)$. The green and red rectangles indicate the desired and current swarm patterns, respectively. The red dotted arrows represent the deformation directions of the swarms, the yellow arrows indicate the moving direction, and the blue dashed arrows show the rotational direction of the swarm. The scale bar indicates 1000 μm.

play a significant role in the formation of RPNS. As a result, the magnetic response of RPNS is faster. Additionally, RPNS can undergo reversible elongation and contraction by adjusting the amplitude ratio $\psi = B/C$, as depicted in Figures 3.20d-f.

To validate the effectiveness of the proposed control scheme, we apply RPNS actuated by oscillating magnetic fields. The actuation method is changed while keeping the control architecture, controllers, and experimental conditions unchanged. The experimental results are shown in Figure 3.21, where three representative cases are presented along with information about the targeted patterns. In Case I (Figure 3.21a), the control process is depicted. Initially, Scheme I is applied when the swarm is far from the desired pattern to maximize locomotion efficiency. As the swarm approaches the central region of the target pattern, Scheme II is activated to adjust the swarm's aspect ratio and long-axis direction. Due to the non-horizontal experimental substrate, drifting effect occurs, leading to positioning deviations. To ensure accuracy and keep the RPNS within the targeted region, Scheme III is triggered. The processes in Cases II and III are demonstrated in Figures 3.21b and 3.21c, respectively. In all three trials, the aspect ratios of the swarms have a maximum error of 10% of α_d, and the pointing angles exhibit steady-state errors within $\pm 3°$. Furthermore, the RPNS can be effectively maintained at the desired position with a deviation of approximately 10 pixels. These results demonstrate the capability of the proposed control scheme to successfully control the RPNS in terms of aspect ratio, pointing angle, and position accuracy.

3.7 CONCLUSION

Microrobotic swarms have the potential to revolutionize targeted drug delivery missions by offering advantages such as enhanced drug loading, high targeting resolution, and the ability to perform pattern reconfiguration. In this study, we presented an actuation method to induce the formation of elliptical and ribbon-like swarms, which exhibit adaptive behavior in confined and complex environments, enabling them to access hard-to-reach regions. However, swarms exhibit distinct characteristics compared to monolithic microrobots, and operating swarms consisting of millions of nanoparticles requires trained human operators with sufficient experience. To address this, we proposed a strategy for automatic control of the aspect ratio, long-axis orientation, and position of elliptical and ribbon-like swarms. The control errors were effectively minimized in all cases, demonstrating the efficiency and effectiveness of our strategy for controlling microscopic colloidal swarms. In addition to magnetic swarms, other types of micromotors, such as catalytic and light-propelled micromotors, can form functional and therapeutic microrobotic swarms. These micromotors have recently found success in environmental and biomedical applications. By integrating magnetic shells, they can also be utilized in conjunction with our proposed programmable control strategy. Our control strategy serves as a prototypical paradigm for effectively controlling various swarm behaviors and opens up possibilities for adaptive path planning and pattern formation of active matter in complex environments in a fully autonomous manner. Looking ahead, artificial intelligence (AI) holds promise in assisting the control of challenging-to-model microrobotic swarms, enabling adaptive pattern and motion control based on the swarms' interactions with their ambient environments. Additionally, incorporating 3D visual information analysis can provide further insights into swarm behavior and contribute to a better understanding of this field.

Bibliography

[1] Bradley J Nelson, Ioannis K Kaliakatsos, and Jake J Abbott. Microrobots for minimally invasive medicine. *Annual Review of Biomedical Engineering*, 12:55–85, 2010.

[2] Qianqian Wang, Kai Fung Chan, Kathrin Schweizer, Xingzhou Du, Dongdong Jin, Simon Chun Ho Yu, Bradley J Nelson, and Li Zhang. Ultrasound doppler-guided real-time navigation of a magnetic microswarm for active endovascular delivery. *Science Advances*, 7(9):eabe5914, 2021.

[3] Metin Sitti, Hakan Ceylan, Wenqi Hu, Joshua Giltinan, Mehmet Turan, Sehyuk Yim, and Eric Diller. Biomedical applications of untethered mobile milli/microrobots. *Proceedings of the IEEE*, 103(2):205–224, 2015.

[4] Yue Dong, Lu Wang, Ke Yuan, Fengtong Ji, Jinhong Gao, Zifeng Zhang, Xingzhou Du, Yuan Tian, Qianqian Wang, and Li Zhang. Magnetic microswarm composed of porous nanocatalysts for targeted elimination of biofilm occlusion. *ACS Nano*, 15(3):5056–5067, 2021.

[5] Li Zhang, Jake J Abbott, Lixin Dong, Kathrin E Peyer, Bradley E Kratochvil, Haixin Zhang, Christos Bergeles, and Bradley J Nelson. Characterizing the swimming properties of artificial bacterial flagella. *Nano Letters*, 9(10):3663–3667, 2009.

[6] Bumjin Jang, Emiliya Gutman, Nicolai Stucki, Benedikt F Seitz, Pedro D Wendel-García, Taylor Newton, Juho Pokki, Olgaç Ergeneman, Salvador Pané, Yizhar Or, et al. Undulatory locomotion of magnetic multilink nanoswimmers. *Nano Letters*, 15(7):4829–4833, 2015.

[7] Yabin Zhang, Lin Zhang, Lidong Yang, Chi Ian Vong, Kai Fung Chan, William KK Wu, Thomas NY Kwong, Norman WS Lo, Margaret Ip, Sunny H Wong, et al. Real-time tracking of fluorescent magnetic spore–based microrobots for remote detection of c. diff toxins. *Science Advances*, 5(1):eaau9650, 2019.

[8] Sylvain Martel and Mahmood Mohammadi. Using a swarm of self-propelled natural microrobots in the form of flagellated bacteria to perform complex microassembly tasks. In *2010 IEEE International Conference on Robotics and Automation*, pages 500–505. IEEE, 2010.

[9] Ouajdi Felfoul, Mahmood Mohammadi, Samira Taherkhani, Dominic De Lanauze, Yong Zhong Xu, Dumitru Loghin, Sherief Essa, Sylwia Jancik, Daniel Houle, Michel Lafleur, et al. Magneto-aerotactic bacteria deliver drug-containing nanoliposomes to tumour hypoxic regions. *Nature Nanotechnology*, 11(11):941–947, 2016.

[10] Sylvain Martel, Mahmood Mohammadi, Ouajdi Felfoul, Zhao Lu, and Pierre Pouponneau. Flagellated magnetotactic bacteria as controlled mri-trackable propulsion and steering systems for medical nanorobots operating in the human microvasculature. *The International Journal of Robotics Research*, 28(4):571–582, 2009.

[11] Mariana Medina-Sánchez and Oliver G Schmidt. Medical microbots need better imaging and control. *Nature*, 545(7655):406–408, 2017.

[12] Jinxing Li, Berta Esteban-Fernández de Ávila, Wei Gao, Liangfang Zhang, and Joseph Wang. Micro/nanorobots for biomedicine: Delivery, surgery, sensing, and detoxification. *Science Robotics*, 2(4):eaam6431, 2017.

[13] Ania Servant, Famin Qiu, Mariarosa Mazza, Kostas Kostarelos, and Bradley J Nelson. Controlled in vivo swimming of a swarm of bacteria-like microrobotic flagella. *Advanced Materials*, 27(19):2981–2988, 2015.

[14] Jiangfan Yu, Qianqian Wang, Mengzhi Li, Chao Liu, Lidai Wang, Tiantian Xu, and Li Zhang. Characterizing nanoparticle swarms with tuneable concentrations for enhanced imaging contrast. *IEEE Robotics and Automation Letters*, 4(3):2942–2949, 2019.

[15] Lidong Yang, Jiangfan Yu, and Li Zhang. Statistics-based automated control for a swarm of paramagnetic nanoparticles in 2-d space. *IEEE Transactions on Robotics*, 36(1):254–270, 2019.

[16] Xiaoguang Dong and Metin Sitti. Controlling two-dimensional collective formation and cooperative behavior of magnetic microrobot swarms. *The International Journal of Robotics Research*, 39(5):617–638, 2020.

[17] Hui Xie, Mengmeng Sun, Xinjian Fan, Zhihua Lin, Weinan Chen, Lei Wang, Lixin Dong, and Qiang He. Reconfigurable magnetic microrobot swarm: Multimode transformation, locomotion, and manipulation. *Science Robotics*, 4(28):eaav8006, 2019.

[18] Igor S Aranson. Collective behavior in out-of-equilibrium colloidal suspensions. *Comptes Rendus Physique*, 14(6):518–527, 2013.

[19] Qian Chen, Sung Chul Bae, and Steve Granick. Directed self-assembly of a colloidal kagome lattice. *Nature*, 469(7330):381–384, 2011.

[20] Xiaoming Mao, Qian Chen, and Steve Granick. Entropy favours open colloidal lattices. *Nature Materials*, 12(3):217–222, 2013.

[21] Jérôme J Crassous, Adriana M Mihut, Erik Wernersson, Patrick Pfleiderer, Jan Vermant, Per Linse, and Peter Schurtenberger. Field-induced assembly of colloidal ellipsoids into well-defined microtubules. *Nature Communications*, 5(1):5516, 2014.

[22] Fuduo Ma, Sijia Wang, David T Wu, and Ning Wu. Electric-field–induced assembly and propulsion of chiral colloidal clusters. *Proceedings of the National Academy of Sciences*, 112(20):6307–6312, 2015.

[23] Jeremie Palacci, Stefano Sacanna, Asher Preska Steinberg, David J Pine, and Paul M Chaikin. Living crystals of light-activated colloidal surfers. *Science*, 339(6122):936–940, 2013.

[24] Jing Yan, Moses Bloom, Sung Chul Bae, Erik Luijten, and Steve Granick. Linking synchronization to self-assembly using magnetic janus colloids. *Nature*, 491(7425):578–581, 2012.

[25] M Belkin, A Snezhko, IS Aranson, and W-K Kwok. Driven magnetic particles on a fluid surface: Pattern assisted surface flows. *Physical Review Letters*, 99(15):158301, 2007.

[26] Alexey Snezhko and Igor S Aranson. Magnetic manipulation of self-assembled colloidal asters. *Nature Materials*, 10(9):698–703, 2011.

[27] Jiangfan Yu, Ben Wang, Xingzhou Du, Qianqian Wang, and Li Zhang. Ultra-extensible ribbon-like magnetic microswarm. *Nature Communications*, 9(1):3260, 2018.

[28] Xingzhou Du, Jiangfan Yu, Dongdong Jin, Philip Wai Yan Chiu, and Li Zhang. Independent pattern formation of nanorod and nanoparticle swarms under an oscillating field. *ACS Nano*, 15(3):4429–4439, 2021.

[29] Jiangfan Yu, Lidong Yang, and Li Zhang. Pattern generation and motion control of a vortex-like paramagnetic nanoparticle swarm. *The International Journal of Robotics Research*, 37(8):912–930, 2018.

[30] Daniel Ahmed, Thierry Baasch, Nicolas Blondel, Nino Läubli, Jürg Dual, and Bradley J Nelson. Neutrophil-inspired propulsion in a combined acoustic and magnetic field. *Nature Communications*, 8(1):770, 2017.

[31] Frank Cichos, Kristian Gustavsson, Bernhard Mehlig, and Giovanni Volpe. Machine learning for active matter. *Nature Machine Intelligence*, 2(2):94–103, 2020.

[32] Edward B Steager, Mahmut Selman Sakar, Ceridwen Magee, Monroe Kennedy, Anthony Cowley, and Vijay Kumar. Automated biomanipulation of single cells using magnetic microrobots. *The International Journal of Robotics Research*, 32(3):346–359, 2013.

[33] Antoine Barbot, Dominique Decanini, and Gilgueng Hwang. Local flow sensing on helical microrobots for semi-automatic motion adaptation. *The International Journal of Robotics Research*, 39(4):476–489, 2020.

[34] Xinyu Wu, Jia Liu, Chenyang Huang, Meng Su, and Tiantian Xu. 3-d path following of helical microswimmers with an adaptive orientation compensation model. *IEEE Transactions on Automation Science and Engineering*, 17(2):823–832, 2019.

[35] Jiangfan Yu, Tiantian Xu, Zheyu Lu, Chi Ian Vong, and Li Zhang. On-demand disassembly of paramagnetic nanoparticle chains for microrobotic cargo delivery. *IEEE Transactions on Robotics*, 33(5):1213–1225, 2017.

[36] A Lecuona, U Ruiz-Rivas, and J Nogueira. Simulation of particle trajectories in a vortex-induced flow: application to seed-dependent flow measurement techniques. *Measurement Science and Technology*, 13(7):1020, 2002.

[37] Sheldon Green. *Fluid Vortices*, volume 30. Springer Science & Business Media, 2012.

[38] Hong Deng, Xiaolin Li, Qing Peng, Xun Wang, Jinping Chen, and Yadong Li. Monodisperse magnetic single-crystal ferrite microspheres. *Angewandte Chemie International Edition*, 44(18):2782–2785, 2005.

[39] Ebrahim H Mamdani and Sedrak Assilian. An experiment in linguistic synthesis with a fuzzy logic controller. *International Journal of Man-Machine Studies*, 7(1):1–13, 1975.

CHAPTER 4

Dynamic Path Planning and Motion Control of Collective Nanorobots for Mobile Target Tracking

4.1 INTRODUCTION

The use of milli/microrobots, controlled remotely by magnetic fields, has generated considerable interest due to their potential biomedical applications [1, 2, 3, 4, 5, 6, 7, 8, 9]. Various types of milli/microrobots have been explored, including spherical [10, 11, 12], helical [13, 14, 15], and bio-hybrid milli/microrobots [16, 17, 18]. These robots exhibit different modes of locomotion, such as crawling, walking, rolling, translation, rotation, and chiral rotating [19, 20, 21]. While a range of milli/microrobots have been developed, microrobotic swarms are particularly promising for addressing challenges in minimally invasive therapies like targeted drug delivery and in-situ sensing [22, 23]. Drawing inspiration from collective behaviors observed in nature, various types of mirorobotic swarms have been investigated, including vortex-like, ribbon-like, elliptical, and tornado-like swarms [24, 25, 26, 27]. Since microrobotic swarms are typically not equipped with onboard sensors and circuits, closed-loop control is crucial for achieving controlled locomotion and pattern adaptive reconfiguration, particularly in confined environments [26]. Additionally, tracking mobile targets using microrobotic swarms holds further significance. In this chapter, dynamic path planning and motion control are critical steps for achieving the intended objectives.

Path planning serves as the initial stage in mobile target tracking. Previous studies have explored various path planning methods for microrobots to track stationary targets. Examples include a gradient-based path planner designed for cluttered environments with triangular obstacles [28], an informed rapidly-exploring random tree star (Informed RRT*) path generator applicable to environments featuring rectangular obstructions [29], and an obstacle-weighted rapidly exploring random tree (RRT)

 DOI: 10.1201/9781032665788-4

algorithm employed in simulated vascular networks [30]. These approaches share a common characteristic: once the trajectory is planned, it remains fixed as the target position is static. However, when tracking a mobile target, the position of the target constantly changes, posing a challenge for the path planner to adapt in real-time. Consequently, there is a need for dynamic path planning methods that can accommodate the tracking of mobile targets.

Another critical aspect is the motion control of swarms to precisely regulate their direction and velocity. Two main categories of control methods are model-based and model-free approaches. Model-based control techniques leverage mathematical models to navigate microrobots with enhanced accuracy. For example, a novel model predictive controller has been developed for targeted delivery using magnetic spore-based microrobots [31], and an MRI-based control method has been devised for endovascular navigation of magnetic microcapsules [32]. On the other hand, model-free control methods become crucial when obtaining accurate models of microrobots is challenging. A model-free trajectory tracking control approach, which does not rely on complex dynamics models, has been demonstrated to navigate a two-particle magnetic microrobot with high tracking accuracy [33]. However, there is still ongoing research required to develop effective and efficient control strategies specifically tailored for microrobotic swarms [34, 35].

The realization of mobile target tracking using microrobotic swarms poses challenges in both dynamic path planning and motion control. Further investigation is needed to develop effective dynamic path planning methods. The simultaneous movement of the microrobotic swarm and the target adds complexity to the path planning process, making it difficult to achieve a high updating frequency for adapting to rapid changes in the positions of the swarm and target. Additionally, efficient motion control of microrobotic swarms requires additional research. The changes in external physical inputs can significantly impact the interactions among swarm agents, affecting the stability of swarm patterns [26]. Furthermore, the interactions and motion of swarm agents are complex, and obtaining a precise mathematical model for swarms is challenging [36]. Therefore, there is a need to explore an effective and efficient strategy that considers dynamic path planning and motion control to track a mobile target using microrobotic swarms.

This study presents a novel control strategy for a group of small robotic units to track a mobile target. The proposed approach involves an advanced algorithm called Enhanced Bidirectional Rapidly-Exploring Random Tree Star (EB-RRT*) for generating optimal paths in real-time while avoiding collisions with obstacles. To achieve precise tracking, a combination of a direction controller and a Genetic Algorithm-based Linear Quadratic Regulator (GA-LQR) velocity controller is integrated into an image-guided motion controller. This controller effectively manages both the swarm's movement direction and velocity. Additionally, a Targeted Bursting Algorithm is introduced to cater to the tracking of high-speed mobile targets. The performance and reliability of the control scheme are evaluated through simulations and experiments conducted in various environments, including ones with virtual obstacles and micromazes with virtual walls. These tests confirm the efficacy and robustness of the proposed control scheme.

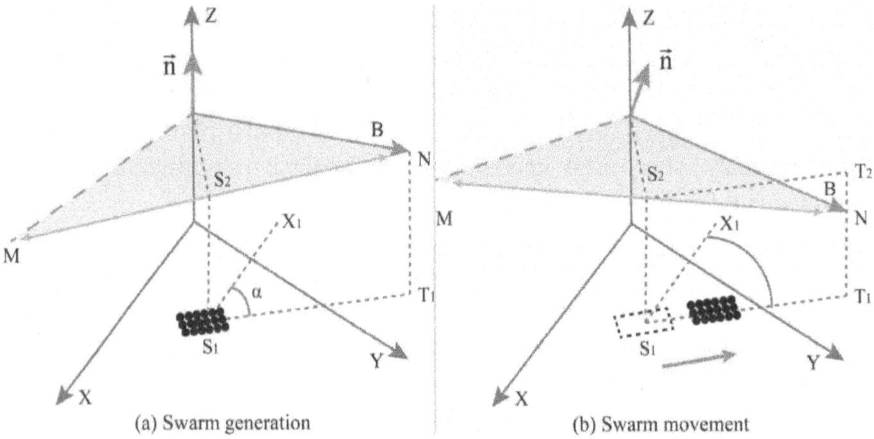

Figure 4.1 The schematics of the swarm generation and movement actuated by oscillating magnetic fields. (a) Swarm generation. (b) Swarm movement actuated by an oscillating field with a pitch angle. The green, red and orange arrows denote the movement direction of the swarm, the magnetic field vector and the oscillation of the field, respectively. The normal vector of the magnetic field is indicated by $\vec{n}$, while the green triangle with the blue dotted boundary represents the magnetic field plane. The direction angle and pitch angle of the magnetic field are indicated by α, γ.

4.2 MODELING

4.2.1 Magnetic Actuation

Earlier studies have documented the existence of swarm formations characterized by ribbon-like structures [25]. Figure 4.1 presents a visual representation of the process involved in generating and guiding such swarms using an oscillating magnetic field. Specifically, the figure illustrates the mechanism of swarm generation induced by an oscillating magnetic field, as depicted in Figure 4.1a. By introducing a slight pitch angle, typically ranging from 2° to 6°, the swarm exhibits translational motion, as depicted in Figure 4.1b. The pitch angle, denoted by γ, represents the angle between the normal vector $\vec{n}$ of the magnetic field plane and the Z axis. In Figure 4.1b, the oscillation of the field is depicted by the line MN, and its projection in X-Y plane is represented by the line S_1T_1. The line S_1X_1 is parallel to the X-axis. By adjusting the direction angle α, which is the angle between the line S_1T_1 and the line S_1X_1, the moving direction of the swarm can be altered. The input actuation oscillating magnetic field can be expressed as

$$B = \begin{bmatrix} B_x \\ B_y \\ B_z \end{bmatrix} = \begin{bmatrix} A\cos(\alpha)\cos(\gamma)\sin(2\pi ft) - C\sin(\alpha) \\ A\sin(\alpha)\cos(\gamma)\sin(2\pi ft) + C\cos(\alpha) \\ -A\sin(\gamma)\sin(2\pi ft) \end{bmatrix} \tag{4.1}$$

where B_x, B_y, B_z denote the corresponding component of the magnetic field in X, Y, Z axis, respectively.

To achieve complete control over the motion of the swarm, it is necessary to accurately adjust three crucial parameters: the oscillating frequency $f(t)$, the direction angle $\alpha(t)$, and the pitch angle $\gamma(t)$. These parameters need to be precisely tuned in order to manipulate the movement of the swarm effectively.

4.2.2 Analytical Model

Establishing an accurate analytical model for the swarm presents a challenge due to the large number of swarm agents and the complex interactions among them, such as magnetic and hydrodynamic interactions. In this chapter, we employ the following model:

$$\begin{cases} \dot{C}_x(t) = c_i g[f(t), \gamma(t)] \cos(\alpha(t)) \\ \dot{C}_y(t) = c_i g[f(t), \gamma(t)] \sin(\alpha(t)) \end{cases} \tag{4.2}$$

where $C[C_x(t), C_y(t)]$ is the position of the swarm *i.e.*, the centroid of the swarm contour, $\dot{C}_x(t)$ and $\dot{C}_y(t)$ are the derivatives of $C_x(t)$ and $C_x(t)$, respectively. The resultant factor $g[f(t), \gamma(t)]$ considering magnetic field frequency $f(t)$ and pitch angle $\gamma(t)$ affects the swarm velocity. As previously reported [36], the swarm velocity is mainly determined by the pitch angle $\gamma(t)$, and has a minor correlation with the input frequency $f(t)$. The linear function considering the above factors can thus be expressed as:

$$\begin{cases} \dot{C}_x(t) = c_v \gamma(t) \cos(\alpha(t)) \\ \dot{C}_y(t) = c_v \gamma(t) \sin(\alpha(t)) \end{cases} \tag{4.3}$$

where c_v is a positive constant that can be calibrated by experiments.

4.3 PATH PLANNING AND MOTION CONTROL

4.3.1 Dynamic Path-Planning Algorithm

(1) EB-RRT* Path Planning Algorithm: Herein, we apply an enhanced bidirectional rapidly-exploring random tree star (EB-RRT*) algorithm as the path planner and its schematics is shown in Figure 4.2. Without losing any generality, tree T_a is taken as an example, and the dynamic path planning procedure is described as following steps.

As shown in Figure 4.2a, EB-RRT* starts from the initial node ξ_i and a random node ξ_{randi} is sampled from the free space χ_{free}. It is noted that, node ξ_{randi} will not be sampled from the region of obstacles. Based on ***Algorithm 1***, the nearest node ξ_{neari} of the random node ξ_{randi} with the shortest distance is selected by **NearestNode**, and meanwhile, a new node ξ_{newi} is chosen by the **Steer** function ***Algorithm 1***. In Figure 4.2b, because $|\xi_{neari}\vec{\xi}_{randi}|$, *i.e.*, the norm of vector $\xi_{neari}\vec{\xi}_{randi}$ (a vector connecting node ξ_{neari} and node ξ_{randi}), is larger than the predefined step length l_{step}, node ξ_{newi} is selected as the new node. However, if $|\xi_{neari}\vec{\xi}_{randi}|$ is smaller than the step length l_{step}, the new node will be node ξ_{randi}. The proposed algorithm then utilizes **CollisionCheck** in ***Algorithm 1*** to check whether there is any collision between the vector $\xi_{neari}\vec{\xi}_{newi}$, *i.e.*, the vector connecting node ξ_{neari} and node ξ_{newi}, and obstacles. If collision is detected, the node ξ_{newi} will be discarded. A successful extension of tree T_a is shown in Figure 4.2c. By using the **NearArea** function in ***Algorithm 1***, a circle is generated, with its center locating in node ξ_{new1} and its

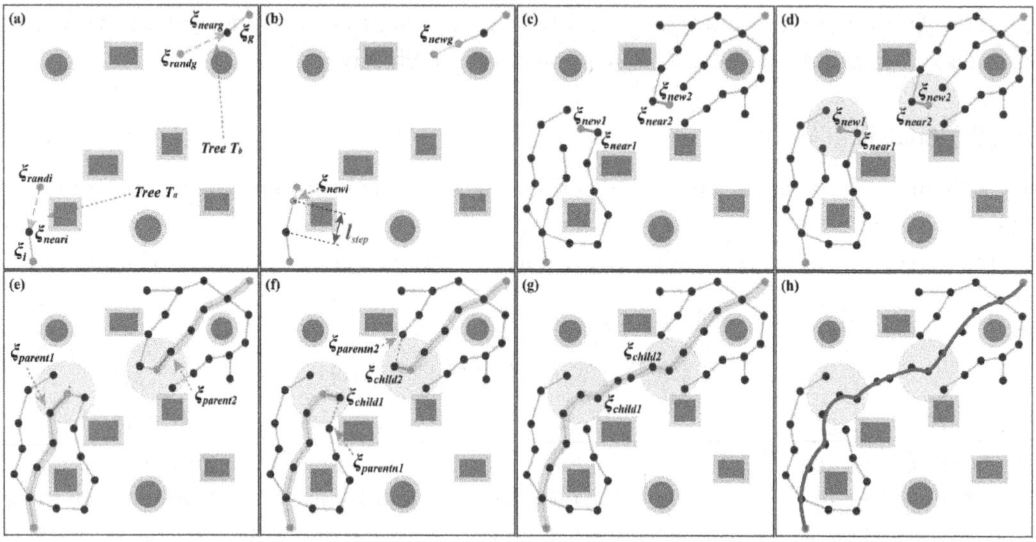

Figure 4.2 The schematic illustration of the EB-RRT* dynamic path planning algorithm. (a) Random nodes sampling. The node ξ_{randi} and node ξ_{randg} are randomly sampled from two separate trees T_a and T_b, respectively. The nearest nodes of ξ_{randi} and ξ_{randg} are marked by ξ_{neari} and ξ_{nearg}, respectively. (b) Steering procedure. New nodes ξ_{newi} and ξ_{newg} are sampled after the process of steering, while l_{step} is the predefined step length. (c) Node extension. The current nodes of the two trees are represented by ξ_{new1} and ξ_{new2}, while their nearest nodes are ξ_{near1} and ξ_{near2}. (d) Definition of neighboring regions. The neighboring areas are marked by the orange circles whose center are the new nodes, *e.g.*, ξ_{new1}. (e) New parent node creation. $\xi_{parent1}$ and $\xi_{parent2}$ are the new parent nodes. (f) Rewiring procedure. The new child nodes are denoted by ξ_{child1} and ξ_{child2}, while their previous parent nodes are denoted by $\xi_{parentn1}$ and $\xi_{parentn2}$. (g) The connection of the two trees. (h) Path smoothing. The pink dots denote the starting nodes ξ_i and ξ_g, and the current nodes are represented by the green dots. The dark blue dots are the general nodes. The grey regions are the obstacles, and the surrounding light-grey regions are the collision buffer layers.

radius of $r_{na} = \varepsilon \left(\frac{log_k}{k}\right)^{\frac{1}{d}}$ [37], where $\epsilon \in [50, 60]$ is an independent constant, κ is the number of nodes in tree T_a, and d is the dimension of the space, *i.e.*, $d = 2$. The circle is regarded as the neighboring region of node ξ_{new1}, which is shown by the orange circle in Figure 4.2d. Once the neighboring area is generated, the new parent node can be determined by **ChooseParent** function in ***Algorithm 1***, which is represented by:

$$\begin{gathered} Cost_p^i = \sum_{j=1}^{J_i-1} Dist(\xi_p^j, \xi_p^{j+1}) + Dist(\xi_p^{J_i}, \xi_{new1}) \\ \xi_{parent1} \leftarrow min\{Cost_p^1, ..., Cost_p^i, ..., Cost_p^I\} \end{gathered} \tag{4.4}$$

where $i \in [1, I], j \in [1, J_i], J_i \in [J_1, J_I]$, p denotes the factors relevant to the

Algorithm 1: EB-RRT* Algorithm

```
CollisionBufferLayer();
T_a ← InitTree();
T_b ← InitTree();
T_a ← InsertNode(ξ_init, T_a);
T_b ← InsertNode(ξ_goal, T_b);
for k = 1 to K do:
    ξ_rand ← Sample(k);
    ξ_near ← NearestNode(ξ_rand, T_a);
    ξ_new ← Steer(ξ_rand, ξ_near);
    if(CollisionCheck(ξ_near, ξ_new) then:
        ξ_na ← NearArea(ξ_new, T_a, r);
        ξ_parent ← ChooseParent(ξ_na, ξ_near, ξ_new);
        T_a ← InsertNode(ξ_parent, ξ_new, T_a);
        T_a ← Rewire(ξ_na, x_parent, ξ_new, T_a);
        ξ'_near ← NearestNode(ξ_new, T_b);
        ξ'_new ← Steer(ξ_new, ξ'_near);
        if(CollisionCheck(ξ'_near, ξ'_new) then:
            ξ'_na ← NearArea(ξ'_new, T_b, r);
            ξ'_parent ← ChooseParent(ξ'_na, ξ'_near, ξ'_new);
            T_b ← InsertNode(ξ'_parent, ξ'_new, T_b);
            T_b ← Rewire(ξ'_na, x'_parent, ξ'_new, T_b);
if |T_a| < |T_b| then:
    Swap(T_a, T_b)
    PathSmoothing(T_a, T_b)
return T_a, T_b
```

ChooseParent function, ξ_p^j is the j-th node, $Cost_p^i$ is the i-th distance cost function, $\xi_{parent1}$ is the new parent node, and particularly, $\xi_p^1 = \xi_i$. As shown in Figure 4.2e, the connection of node ξ_{new1} and node ξ_{near1} (red dotted line) will be discarded. Subsequently, node $\xi_{parent1}$ inside the circular boundary is chosen as the new parent node and the red line denotes the new connection. After the new parent node is selected, the rewiring process is performed based on **Rewire** function in ***Algorithm 1***, which is demonstrated in Figure 4.2f. The mathematical expression of **Rewire** is shown as:

$$\begin{aligned} Cost_r^e &= Cost_p^P + Dist(\xi_{new1}, \xi_p^e) \\ &= \sum_{j=1}^{J_P-1} Dist(\xi_p^j, \xi_p^{j+1}) + Dist(\xi_p^{J_P}, \xi_{new1}) \\ &\quad + Dist(\xi_{new1}, \xi_p^e) \\ \xi_{child1} &\leftarrow min\{Cost_r^1, ..., Cost_r^e, ..., Cost_r^{J_I}\} \end{aligned} \tag{4.5}$$

where $j \in [1, J_P], e \in [J_1, J_P) \cup (J_P, J_I]$, r denotes the factors relevant to **Rewire** function, ξ_p^e is e-th node of the remaining nodes in neighboring region, $Cost_p^e$ is the

e-th distance cost function, ξ_{child1} is the new child node, and particularly, $\xi_p^{J_P} = \xi_{parent1}$. In this process, the green node ξ_{new1} is regarded as the new parent node. The current node ξ_{new1} selects node ξ_{near1} as its new child node since the Euclidean distance between them is the shortest. This leads to the disconnection between ξ_{near1} and its previous parent node $\xi_{parentn1}$, which is represented by the red dotted line in Figure 4.2f. Therefore, node ξ_{near1} is replaced by node ξ_{child1}. The other tree T_b will be formed starting from the goal node ξ_g, with the same processes shown in Figures 4.2a - 4.2f. Finally, two trees are connected with each other and the whole path is marked by the blue region shown in Figure 4.2g. The static planned path σ_p consists p_N pairs of nodes, with their positions represented by:

$$\begin{aligned}\sigma_p =&\{(x_c, y_c), (x_{p_1}, y_{p_1}), ..., (x_{p_n}, y_{p_n}), ...,\\&(x_{p_N}, y_{p_N}), (x_r, y_r)\}\end{aligned} \tag{4.6}$$

where $p_n \in [p_1, p_N], (x_{p_n}, y_{p_n})$ is the n-th point of the static planned path, $C(x_c, y_c)$ and $R(x_r, y_r)$ represent the positions of the swarm and the mobile target, respectively. However, since the swarm and the target are moving during the target tracking process, the dynamic updating of the planned path σ_p^t is demanded, and it is defined as:

$$\begin{aligned}\sigma_p^t =&\{(x_c^t, y_c^t)|t, (x_{p_1}^t, y_{p_1}^t)|t, ..., (x_{p_n}^t, y_{p_n}^t)|t, ...,\\&(x_{p_N}^t, y_{p_N}^t)|t, (x_r^t, y_r^t)|t\}\end{aligned} \tag{4.7}$$

where $t \in [t_1, t_T], p_n \in [p_1, p_N], (x_{p_n}^t, y_{p_n}^t)$ is the n-th point of the dynamic planned path at moment t, $C^t(c_x^t, c_y^t)$ and $R^t(r_x^t, r_y^t)$ are the swarm and target position at moment t, respectively. Because swarms may lose dynamic stability upon sudden shift of moving direction, the generated path shall be smoothened. The smoothed static path σ_s is shown in Figure 4.2h.

(2) Collision Buffer Layers: Using the aforementioned method, even though the generated path avoids all obstacles, a swarm may still collide with the obstacles if their physical sizes are ignored. Therefore, the factor is taken into account by adding collision buffer layers surrounding the obstacles accordingly. By detecting the real-time shape and dimension of the swarm, the thickness of the collision buffer can be correspondingly tuned. For different shapes of obstacles, the collision buffer layer can be determined by:

$$\delta_k = c_k \frac{l_s^t}{2} \tag{4.8}$$

where l_s^t represents the length of the detected swarm at moment t, δ_k denotes the thickness of the collision buffer layer surrounding the k-th obstacle, and c_k is the secure constant to compensate the experimental error, including detection error. The range of the secure constants calibrated by preliminary experiments are [1.5, 2].

The comparison between the cases without and with collision buffer layers is shown in Figure 4.3. If no buffer layers are created, as shown in Figure 4.3a, collision between the swarm and obstacles will occur since the swarm has a physical size. By adding collision buffer layers, the updated planned path can guarantee that the swarm will not collide with the obstacles, as shown in Figure 4.3b.

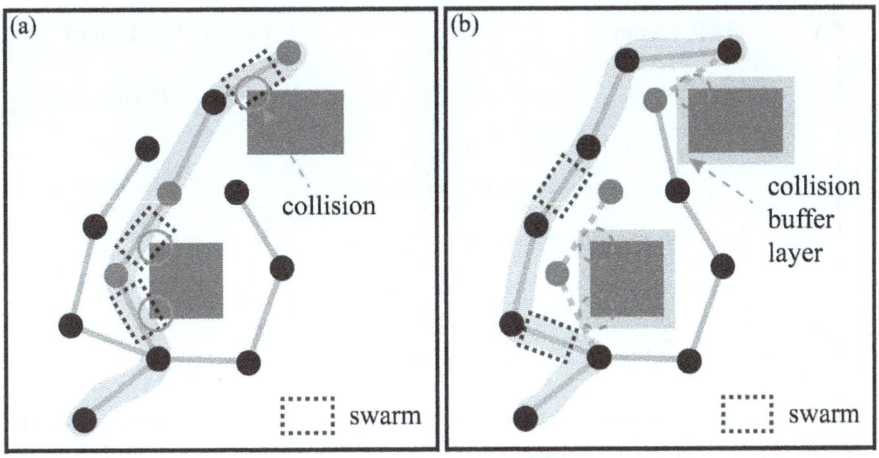

Figure 4.3 The design of collision buffer layers. (a) The planned path without considering the collision buffer layers. The grey square and rectangle represent the obstacles. (b) The planned path considering the collision buffer layer. The light grey areas surrounding the grey obstacles are the collision buffer layers. The red circles indicate the regions of the collision between the swarm and obstacles, while the red dotted circles show that there is no collision by considering the collision buffer layers. The dotted orange lines denote the disconnection between nodes, whereas the orange lines are the connections between nodes. The dark blue dots are the general nodes belonging to the tree. The green dots are effective in (a) but invalid in (b). The final planned path is covered by the blue area. The dotted rectangles represent the swarms.

(3) Path Smoothing: In order to improve the smoothness of the planned path, B-spline is applied and the smoothed static path σ_s represented by the blue curve in Figure 4.2h is expressed as [38]:

$$\sigma_s = \sum_{n=1}^{N} \Phi_{n,m}(u)\sigma_{p_n} \tag{4.9}$$

where σ_{p_n} denotes n-th point of the planned path σ_p, $\Phi_{n,p}(u)$ represents the n-th B-spline basis function of degree m and u is a normalized curve knot. The first order and higher orders basis functions can be defined by these two equations, respectively [39]:

$$\Phi_{n,0} = \begin{cases} 1, & u \in [\hat{u}_n, \hat{u}_{n+1}) \\ 0, & else \end{cases} \tag{4.10}$$

$$\begin{aligned} \Phi_{n,m}(u) = & \frac{u - \hat{u}_n}{\hat{u}_{n+m} - \hat{u}_n} \Phi_{n,m-1}(u) \\ & + \frac{\hat{u}_{n+m+1} - u}{\hat{u}_{n+m+1} - \hat{u}_{n+1}} \Phi_{n+1,m-1}(u) \end{aligned} \tag{4.11}$$

where $\hat{u}_i$ is the knot vector of i-th knot u_i. Subsequently, the smoothed dynamic path

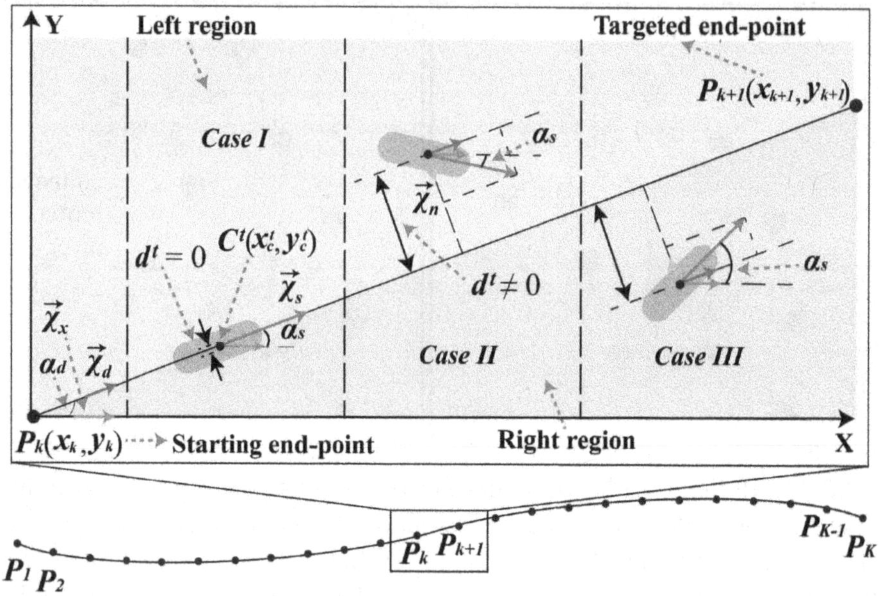

Figure 4.4 The schematic diagram of swarm direction control. Three cases are presented, *i.e.*, the swarm locates on the line, in the left and right regions of the line. The rounded rectangles denote the swarm. The starting end-point and targeted end-point of the line segment P_kP_{k+1} are represented by P_k and P_{k+1}, respectively. The blue arrow $\vec{\chi}_x$ is a unit vector parallel to the X axis, while the green arrow $\vec{\chi}_d$ is a unit vector parallel to line segment P_kP_{k+1}. The angle between line segment P_kP_{k+1} and X axis is denoted by α_d. The red arrow $\vec{\chi}_s$ denotes the unit vector of the swarm moving direction. The direction angle between $\vec{\chi}_s$ and $\vec{\chi}_x$ is denoted by α_s. The orange arrow $\vec{\chi}_n$ denotes the unit vector that is perpendicular to $\vec{\chi}_d$. The distance between the swarm center and the current path segment P_kP_{k+1} at the moment t is denoted by d^t.

σ_s^t at moment t is then represented by:

$$\sigma_s^t = \sum_{n=1}^{N} \Phi_{n,m}(u)\sigma_{p_n}^t \tag{4.12}$$

where $\sigma_{p_n}^t$ denotes n-th point of the dynamic planned path σ_p^t at moment t. The smoothed dynamic path guarantees the stability of the swarm during the target tracking process.

4.3.2 Image-Guided Motion Control

In order to precisely control the motion of the swarm, an image-guided motion controller is proposed, which controls the moving direction and velocity of a swarm.

(1) Direction Control: The method to determine the moving direction of a swarm is shown in Figure 4.4. The planned path generated by EB-RRT* is a sequence of key points, and each two adjacent points form a path segment. The procedure of target tracking is an iterative process. Each iteration ends if the distance $d^t_{C,P_{k+1}}$ between the swarm center C^t and the targeted end-point, *e.g.*, P_{k+1} in Figure 4.4, of the current path segment is smaller than a predefined threshold ϵ, where ϵ is a real constant close to zero, *e.g.*, 5% body length of the swarm. When the swarm lies on the desired path segment, as shown in **Case I** of Figure 4.4, the unit vector of swarm velocity $\vec{\chi}_s$ is equal to the unit vector of path segment $\vec{\chi}_d$, which ensures the low distance error during the target tracking process. In contrast, in **Case II** and **Case III**, the swarm is deviated from the desired path segment, and therefore, the unit vector of swarm velocity $\vec{\chi}_s$ is required to be modified to minimize the distance error d^t ($d^t \to 0$).

Given three points $P_k(x_k, y_k)$, $P_{k+1}(x_{k+1}, y_{k+1})$, and $C_t(x^t_c, y^t_c)$, the dynamic orientation coefficient c_{ori} can be obtained:

$$c_{ori} = det\begin{bmatrix} x^t_c - x_k & x^t_c - x_{k+1} \\ y^t_c - y_k & y^t_c - y_{k+1} \end{bmatrix}. \tag{4.13}$$

Therefore, the relative position of the swarm center C_t and the desired path segment P_kP_{k+1} can be determined: (1) If $c_{ori} < 0$, the swarm locates in the left region. (2) If $c_{ori} = 0$, the swarm lies on the line segment P_kP_{k+1}. (3) If $c_{ori} > 0$, the swarm locates in the right region.

Accordingly, the angle α_o between vector $\vec{\chi}_s$ and vector $\vec{\chi}_d$ can be determined, which is expressed as:

$$\alpha_o = \arccos\left(\frac{h\vec{\chi}_d \cdot ld^t\vec{\chi}_n}{|h\vec{\chi}_d||ld^t\vec{\chi}_n|}\right) \tag{4.14}$$

where h is a stable constant to maintain the low distance error when the swarm is close to the path segment, ld^t is a dynamic coefficient to guarantee a quick converge of distance error, l is the scale factor to ensure that vector $\vec{\chi}_d$ and vector $\vec{\chi}_n$ have the same order of magnitude. If $h/ld^t > 1$, the distance error tends to converge slowly but the swarm moves smoothly. On the contrary, a quicker convergence of distance error can be achieved if $h/ld^t < 1$. In this case, the moving direction of the swarm will be suddenly changed, which weakens the stability of the swarm. A suitable h can maintain the balance between the convergence speed and the tracking accuracy. Finally, the direction vector $\vec{\chi}_s$ is modified using the following formula:

$$\vec{\chi}_s = \begin{cases} Rot(Z, \alpha_d - \alpha_o)\vec{\chi}_d, & c_{ori} < 0 \\ \vec{\chi}_d, & c_{ori} = 0 \\ Rot(Z, \alpha_o - \alpha_d)\vec{\chi}_d, & c_{ori} > 0 \end{cases} \tag{4.15}$$

where $\alpha_d = \arccos(\frac{\vec{\chi}_d \cdot \vec{\chi}_x}{|\vec{\chi}_d| \cdot |\vec{\chi}_x|})$ is the angle between vector $\vec{\chi}_d$ and vector $\vec{\chi}_x$, and $Rot(\bullet)$ represents the rotation matrix of vector $\vec{\chi}_d$ around the Z axis.

Instead of the unit direction vector $\vec{\chi}_s$, the angle α_s between vector $\vec{\chi}_s$ and vector $\vec{\chi}_x$ will be used in experiments to tune the moving direction of the swarm, which is

Algorithm 2: Genetic Algorithm Based Linear-Quadratic Regulator (GA-LQR) Velocity Control

input : *a LQR specification* (A, B, Q, R);
output : *an optimal feedback* $U^*(k)$;
backward pass:
  for $k = 1$ **to** K **do:**
    $min\ J \leftarrow \sum_{k=o}^{\infty}[X^T(k)QX(k) + U^T(k)RU(k)]$;
    $Q_g, R_g \leftarrow GA\ optimization$;
    $H_k \leftarrow Q_g + A^T H_{k+1} A - [A^T H_{k+1} B] \cdot [R_g + B^T H_{k+1} B]^{-1} [B^T H_{k+1} A]$;
    $L_k \leftarrow [R_g + B^T H_{k+1} B]^{-1} B^T H_{k+1} A$;
forward pass:
  for $k = 1$ **to** K **do:**
    $U_k^* \leftarrow - L_k X_k$
    $X_{k+1} \leftarrow AX_k + BU_k$
return U_k^*

described as:

$$\alpha_s = \begin{cases} \arccos(\frac{\vec{X}_x \cdot Rot(Z, \alpha_d - \alpha_o)\vec{X}_d}{|\vec{X}_x||Rot(Z, \alpha_d - \alpha_o)\vec{X}_d|}), & c_{ori} < 0 \\ \arccos(\frac{\vec{X}_x \cdot \vec{X}_d}{|\vec{X}_x||\vec{X}_d|}), & c_{ori} = 0 \\ \arccos(\frac{\vec{X}_x \cdot Rot(Z, \alpha_o - \alpha_d)\vec{X}_d}{|\vec{X}_x||Rot(Z, \alpha_o - \alpha_d)\vec{X}_d|}), & c_{ori} > 0 \end{cases}. \tag{4.16}$$

Therefore, the moving direction of the swarm can be determined by Eq. (4.16).

(2) GA-LQR Velocity Control: In order to reduce the distance error during the locomotion of the swarm, a Linear Quadratic Regulator velocity controller with Genetic Algorithm (GA-LQR) is developed. The discrete-time state space equation of the system can be represented by:

$$\begin{cases} X_{k+1} & = AX_k + BU_k \\ Y_k & = CX_k \end{cases} \tag{4.17}$$

where X is the system state, U is the control feedback, Y is the system output,

$$A = \begin{bmatrix} 0 & 0 \\ 0 & 0 \end{bmatrix}, B = \begin{bmatrix} c_v & 0 \\ 0 & c_v \end{bmatrix}, C = \begin{bmatrix} 1 & 0 \\ 0 & 1 \end{bmatrix}, \tag{4.18}$$

and c_v is a positive constant that can be calibrated by experiments. As shown in ***Algorithm 2***, the GA-LQR velocity control is applied for generating the optimal linear feedback $U_k = -L_k X_k + X_d$ (*i.e.*, the control input of the magnetic system), where X_d is the desired state. The optimal feedback U_k is further used to minimize the quadratic cost function, which is expressed as:

$$J = \sum_{k=0}^{K}(X_k^T Q X_k + U_k^T R U_k) \tag{4.19}$$

Algorithm 3: Genetic Algorithm

```
input : population I_k; size K; initialize, k = 0;
output : best population I_b;
while k ≤ k_desire do:
    Use p_s(I_k) to select parents I_1, I_2;
    Inject crossover sites with probability p_c(I_k);
    Perform mutation under probability p_m(I_k);
    Evaluate individuals with F(I_k);
    Generate offspring;
    if any doubles or misses then:
        Eliminate doubles;
        Eliminate misses;
    end
    k = k + 1;
end
return best population I_b
```

where K is the time horizon, $Q > 0$ and $R > 0$ are weighting matrices. Because X_d serves as the external input of the GA-LQR control system, and it has negligible effect on the system stability [40], the simplified feedback $U_k = -L_k X_k$ is used in our experiments. The input U_k of the GA-LQR control loop is relevant to the feedback gain L_k, as shown in ***Algorithm 2***, and U_k will be further affected by the weighting matrices Q and R. The system with a large value of Q, *e.g.*, $Q \in [1000, 5000]$, can ensure a smaller distance error, but the swarm could be unstable during locomotion. On the contrary, the system with $R \in [1000, 2000]$ may reduce the sudden change of the swarm velocity, which ensures the stability of a swarm. However, the higher value of R may cause low tracking accuracy. Therefore, in order to find the optimal values of Q and R, the Genetic Algorithm in ***Algorithm 3*** is introduced to tackle the optimization problem. The specific ranges are defined: $Q \in (0, Q_l]$, $R \in [R_s, R_l]$. With K numbers, an initial population of chromosomes which contains k gene bit is randomly chosen from the set $\Omega = \omega_1, \omega_2, \ldots, \omega_x$. The fitness function is described as follows:

$$F(I_k) = X_k^T Q X_k + U_k^T R U_k \tag{4.20}$$

where $k \in [1, K]$ and K is the maximum number of iterations. The function $F(I_k)$ is used to evaluate the fitness of each individual in the population. The individuals with suitable fitness values are stochastically selected from the current population to form a new generation, whereas the other individuals will be discarded. In this case, the selection probability of each chromosome I_k is inversely proportional to their fitness, which is defined as [41]:

$$p_s(I_k) = \frac{F(I_k)}{\sum\limits_{k=1}^{K} F(I_k)} \tag{4.21}$$

where $k \in [1, K]$ and K is the maximum number of iterations. Therefore, the chromosomes with a low fitness value are more likely to be selected for the offspring. The crossover sites of genes are chosen and exchanged among the independent gens. The adaptive process promises a higher crossover probability in the parent generation, which can be expressed as [34]:

$$p_c(I_k) = \begin{cases} p_c(I_1),\ if\ k = 1 \\ \dfrac{k}{K}[p_c(I_1) - \dfrac{\sum_{u=1}^{k} p_c(I_u)}{k}],\ if\ k > 1 \end{cases} \tag{4.22}$$

where $k \in [1, K]$ and $p_c(I_1)$ is a constant, *e.g.*, 0.01. After crossover between individual samples, the mutation process occurs. Replacing individuals of population on random gene segments with certain mutation probability is the key operation of mutation. The procedure can be analytically expressed as [35]:

$$p_m(I_k) = \begin{cases} p_m(I_1),\ if\ k = 1 \\ \dfrac{F(I_k) - F_{mean}(I_k)}{F_{max}(I_k) - F_{mean}(I_k)},\ if\ k > 1 \end{cases} \tag{4.23}$$

where $k \in [1, K]$ and $p_m(I_1)$ is a constant, *e.g.*, 0.01, $F_{mean}(I_k)$ and $F_{min}(I_k)$ are the mean and minimum fitness value, respectively. The process of selection, crossover and mutation is repeated until the maximum number of iterations is reached. After the optimization process using the Genetic Algorithm, the optimal Q_g and R_g are selected. By substituting Q_g and R_g into the previous equations, *i.e.*, Eq. (4.17) and Eq. (4.19), the solution of the discrete-time algebraic Riccati equation of GA-LQR is defined as:

$$\begin{aligned} H_k = Q_g + A^T H_{k+1} A - [A^T H_{k+1} B]\cdot \\ [R_g + B^T H_{k+1} B]^{-1} [B^T H_{k+1} A] \end{aligned} \tag{4.24}$$

where the transient matrix is H. Therefore, the feedback gain L_k and optimal control input U_k^* in ***Algorithm 2*** are represented by:

$$\begin{cases} L_k = [R_g + B^T H_{k+1} B]^{-1} [B^T H_{k+1} A] \\ U_k^* = -L_k X_k \end{cases}. \tag{4.25}$$

Subsequently, the discrete-time input parameters of the magnetic field are described as:

$$\begin{cases} \gamma_k = sel(\sqrt{(U_{k_x}^*)^2 + (U_{k_y}^*)^2},\ \gamma_{max}) \\ \alpha_k = \alpha_s \end{cases} \tag{4.26}$$

where $sel(a, b)$ is a selection function [33], which returns the smaller value between a and b:

$$sel(a, b) = \begin{cases} a, & a \leq b \\ b, & a > b \end{cases} \tag{4.27}$$

4.3.3 Targeted Bursting Algorithm

In order to improve the tracking accuracy, the GA-LQR velocity control method will cause the decrease of velocity when the swarm is close to the targeted endpoint of each path segment, which may cause the failure of tracking a high-speed

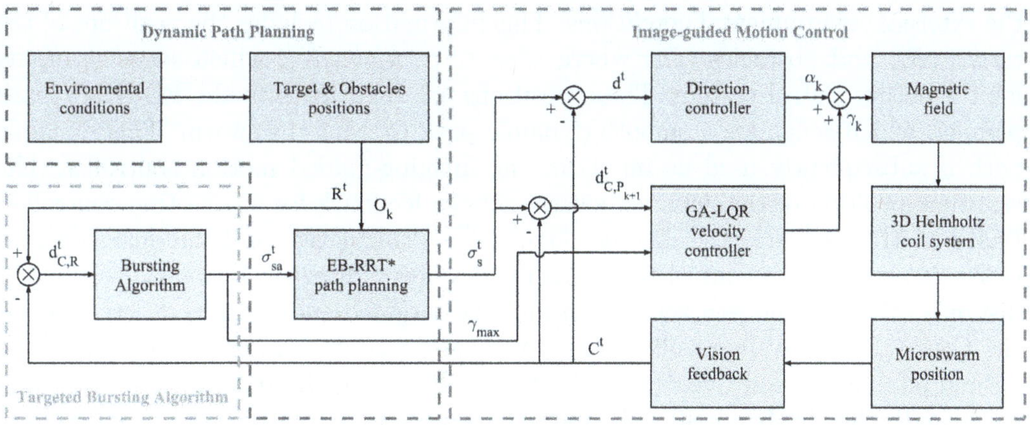

Figure 4.5 The system diagram consisting of the dynamic path planning unit, the image-guided motion control unit and the targeted bursting unit. The positions of the swarm and the target are represented by C^t and R^t, respectively. The position of k-th obstacle is denoted by O_k. The distance between the swarm and the line segment P_kP_{k+1}, *i.e.*, the distance error, at moment t is d^t. The distance between the swarm and the target at moment t is $d^t_{C,R}$. The distance between the swarm and the targeted end-point at moment t is $d_{C,P^t_{k+1}}$. The paths generated by the EB-RRT* path planning algorithm and the bursting algorithm are represented by σ^t_s and $\sigma_s a^t$, respectively. The desire direction angle generated by the direction controller is indicated by α_k, while the desire pitch angle generated by the GA-LQR velocity controller is denoted by γ_k. The largest pitch angle that the swarm can still maintain its stability is labeled by γ_{max}.

mobile target. Herein, we further modify the control scheme by tailoring the targeted bursting algorithm. Considering the morphology of the target, we define a circular region surrounding it, *i.e.*, the bursting region, with its radius of $r_{ba} = c_{bu}r_T$, where r_T is the radius of the circular target, and $c_{bu} \in [1.2, 1.5]$ is a constant to enlarge the circular region of the mobile target. The bursting region and the circular target share the same center. When the swarm reaches the bursting region, the path σ^t_s is replaced by a new one σ^t_{sa}, which is expressed as:

$$\sigma^t_{sa} = \begin{cases} \{(x^t_c, y^t_c)\,|\,t), (x^t_r, y^t_r)\,|\,t)\}, & 0 < d^t_{C,R} \leq \dfrac{r_{ba}}{2} \\ \{(x^t_c, y^t_c)\,|\,t, (x^t_m, y^t_m)\,|\,t, (x^t_r, y^t_r)\,|\,t\}, & \dfrac{r_{ba}}{2} < d^t_{C,R} \leq r_{ba} \end{cases} \tag{4.28}$$

where $t \in [t_1, t_G]$, $d^t_{C,R}$ is the distance between the swarm $C^t(x^t_c, y^t_c)$ and the mobile target $R^t(x^t_r, y^t_r)$ at the moment t, $x^t_m = (x^t_c + x^t_r)/2$ and $y^t_m = (y^t_c + y^t_r)/2$. Morever, during the bursting process, the pitch angle γ_k generated by the image-guided motion controller is replaced by the largest pitch angle γ_{max} that the swarm can still maintain its stability.

Figure 4.5 illustrates the comprehensive control diagram, which comprises three main units: the dynamic path planning unit, the imaging-guided motion control unit, and the targeted bursting unit. Initially, the dynamic path planning unit identifies the external environmental conditions. This information includes the positions of the target (R_t) and obstacles (O_k, where $k = 1, \ldots, n, \ldots, N$), which serve as inputs for the entire control system. These positions are then fed into the EB-RRT* path planner, which generates a smooth dynamic path (σ_s^t) for the swarm. This dynamic path is subsequently used as input for the imaging-guided motion controller. The real-time position of the detected swarm acts as feedback for the motion controller. Based on the feedback, the distance error (d^t) is calculated, and the direction controller is activated to control the swarm's movement direction. Simultaneously, the distance ($d^t_{C,P_{k+1}}$) between the swarm and the targeted end-point is determined for the GA-LQR velocity controller. This information guides the determination of the desired pitch angle and velocity for the swarm. Using the desired direction angle and pitch angle, the 3D Helmholtz coil system generates an oscillating field to actuate the swarm. This field facilitates the swarm's movement according to the desired parameters. To meet the tracking requirements of a high-speed mobile target, a targeted bursting algorithm is designed. The position of the detected swarm again serves as feedback for the bursting process, enabling efficient coordination and adaptation of the swarm's behavior.

4.4 SIMULATION

Simulations are conducted to validate the effectiveness of the EB-RRT* path planning, motion control, and targeted bursting algorithm by tracking mobile targets that exhibit bouncing behavior upon contact with obstacles and walls.

4.4.1 Formation of Trees

The simulation results depicted in Figure 4.6 showcase the planned paths and branch configurations. Figures 4.6a and 4.6b display the results when the swarm and target are in close proximity in environments with obstacles and a micromaze. These simulations demonstrate that the path planner generates paths with minimal branching and explores only a small region, highlighting the high efficiency of the path planner in complex environments. Conversely, when the starting position is far from the target position in an environment with obstacles and a micromaze, the path planner still generates well-planned paths that avoid collisions by extending the branches, as depicted in Figures 4.6c and 4.6d. These simulation results underscore the robustness of the EB-RRT* path planner.

4.4.2 Dynamic Path Planning and Mobile Target Tracking

We initially conducted simulations of the EB-RRT* dynamic path planning in an environment with virtual circular, square, and rectangular obstacles. The results are depicted in Figure 4.7. In Figure 4.7a, a low-speed mobile target (12 μm/s) is utilized. The swarm, with a translational velocity of 16 μm/s, is actuated to approach and track the target at $t = 6$ s and $t = 18$ s, respectively. Notably, in this scenario, the swarm successfully tracks the bouncing target before it makes contact with the boundaries or obstacles, thereby avoiding sudden shifts in the target's motion direction. To further evaluate the effectiveness of the dynamic path planning algorithm

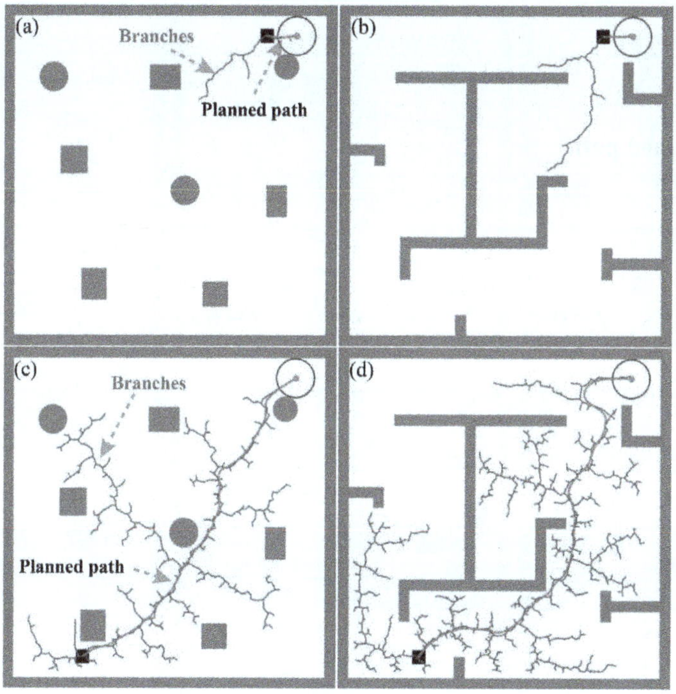

Figure 4.6 The formation of trees with different external conditions. (a) The tree configuration when the simulated swarm is close to the target in an environment with obstacles. (b) The tree configuration when the simulated swarm is close to the target in a micromaze. (c) The tree configuration when the simulated swarm has a large distance to the target in an environment with obstacles. (d) The tree configuration when the simulated swarm has a large distance to the target in a micromaze. The black squares denote the simulated swarms while the dark blue circles represent the targets. The tree branches are marked by green curves, and the final paths are outlined with a red curve.

when the target encounters multiple bounces with obstacles or boundaries, we introduced a high-speed mobile target (20 μm/s). In this case, the target's moving direction changes frequently, resulting in a complex target trajectory. However, as demonstrated in Figure 4.7b, the EB-RRT* algorithm generates dynamic paths without any collision with obstacles. Moreover, the motion control and bursting algorithm are also validated in this scenario. When the simulated swarm reaches the predefined bursting region, the targeted bursting process is triggered. During this process, the swarm is accelerated to track the mobile target with a re-planned path, utilizing the maximum velocity that allows the swarm to maintain stability. Consequently, the simulated swarm successfully tracks the high-speed mobile target.

The simulation results comparing the tracking of 541 and 542 high-speed mobile targets using three different path planning algorithms, namely Enhanced Bidirectional Rapidly-Exploring Random Tree (EB-RRT), Bidirectional Rapidly-Exploring Random Tree Star (B-RRT*), and Enhanced Rapidly-Exploring Random Tree Star (E-RRT*), are presented in Figure 8. Despite generating non-optimal paths, the

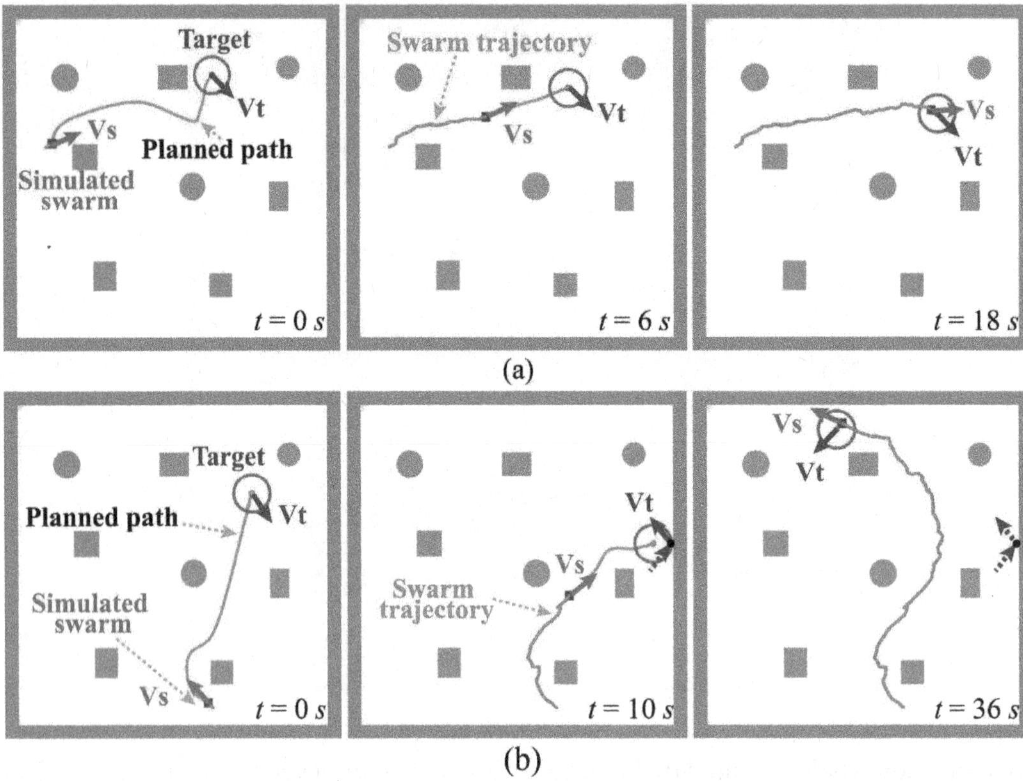

Figure 4.7 The simulation results of mobile target tracking. (a) The tracking of a low-speed target with EB-RRT* path planning algorithm in an environment with obstacles. (b) The tracking of a high-speed target with EB-RRT* path planning algorithm in an environment with obstacles. The velocities of the swarm and the target are represented by V_s and V_t, respectively. The blue curve is the dynamic planned path and the red curve shows the trajectory of the swarm. The dotted blue arrows show the previous bounces, and the black dots are the bouncing points.

EB-RRT algorithm successfully tracks the mobile target. However, the swarm requires a longer distance to reach the target, resulting in a longer completion time of 68 seconds, compared to the EB-RRT* algorithm which takes only 36 seconds. Applying the B-RRT* algorithm neglects the physical size of the swarm and lacks collision buffer layers around obstacles, leading to collisions between the simulated swarm and obstacles. On the other hand, when the E-RRT* algorithm is employed, the swarm fails to reach the current position of the mobile target. The E-RRT* algorithm takes more time to generate a planned path as it only deploys a single tree. Consequently, the planned path only connects the swarm to the previous position of the mobile target, rendering the algorithm unable to adapt to rapid changes in the swarm and target position. These results demonstrate that the EB-RRT* algorithm is effective and efficient in generating desired collision-free paths during mobile target tracking.

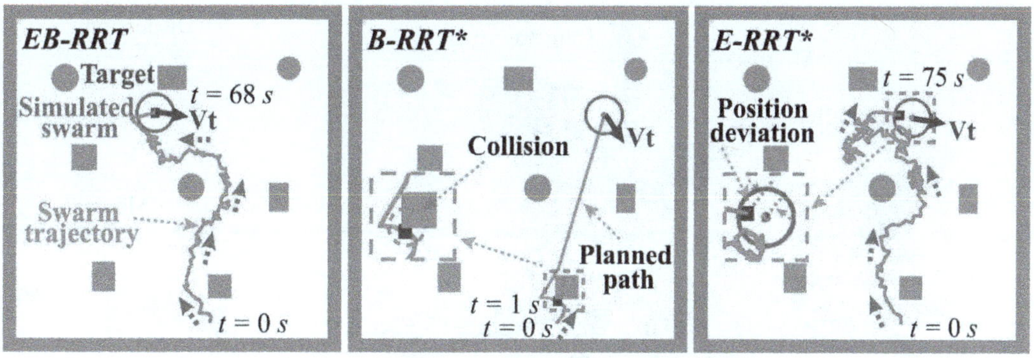

Figure 4.8 The simulated results of tracking high-speed targets with EB-RRT, B-RRT* and E-RRT* path planning algorithms in an environment with obstacles. The velocity of the target is represented by V_t. The blue curve is the dynamic planned path and the red curve shows the trajectory of the swarm. The dotted green arrows show the moving direction of the simulated swarm. The enlarged insets provide clear observations of collision and position deviation in experiments.

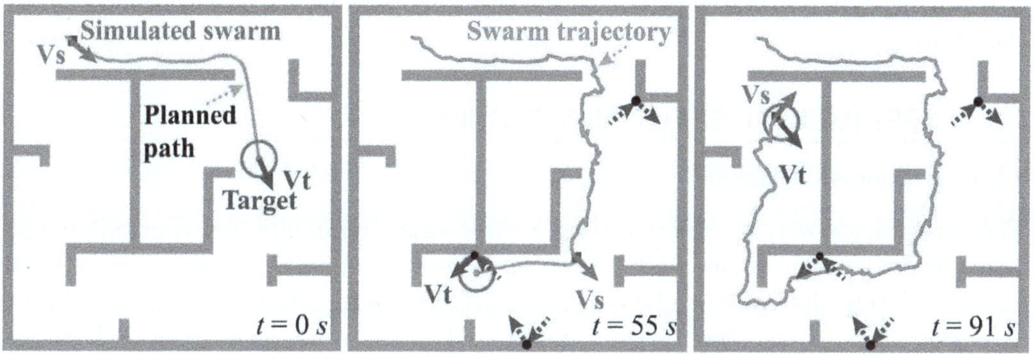

Figure 4.9 The simulation results of tracking a high-speed target with EB-RRT* path planning algorithm in a micromaze. The velocities of the swarm and the target are represented by V_s and V_t, respectively. The blue curve is the dynamic planned path and the red curve shows the trajectory of the swarm. The dotted blue arrow pairs show the previous bounces and the black dots are the bouncing points.

4.4.3 Mobile Target Tracking in a Micromaze

To further validate the proposed control scheme, we deployed a micromaze as a highly constrained environment. As shown in Figure 4.9, the mobile target's moving trajectory becomes irregular due to bouncing off the walls of the micromaze. However, even in this challenging scenario, the simulated swarm successfully tracks the high-speed mobile target, demonstrating the effectiveness of the proposed method in constrained environments. These simulations provide evidence that the proposed control scheme is effective in tracking both low-speed and high-speed targets using the swarm in various environments, including those with obstacles and micromazes.

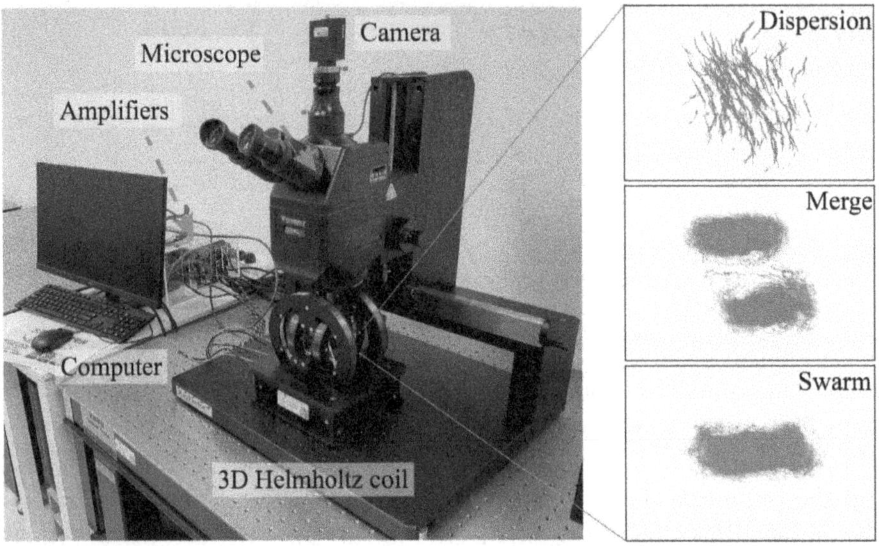

Figure 4.10 The three-axial Helmholtz electromagnetic coil setup. The zoomed-in insets show different states of the magnetite nanoparticles, *i.e.*, dispersion, merge and swarm.

4.5 EXPERIMENTAL SETUP AND RESULTS

4.5.1 Experimental Setup

The experiments were conducted using a three-axial Helmholtz electromagnetic coil setup, as depicted in Figure 4.10. The setup consists of an optical microscope (Model PS888, SEIWA Optical CO., LTD.), an sCMOS camera (Model GS3-U3-41C6C-C, Teledyne FLIR LLC.), and a host computer. The control signals generated by the host computer are amplified by servo amplifiers (Model JSP-180-10, Analogic Corporation). The amplified signals are then fed into the coils, generating the desired magnetic fields. In the experiments, the magnetic field strength and frequency were maintained at 10 mT and 10 Hz, respectively. The camera operated at a frame rate of 10 frames per second (fps). A silicon wafer was used as the substrate during the experiments. The polished surface of the silicon wafer facing upwards enhanced the imaging contrast, providing clear visual feedback for the closed-loop control system.

Magnetite nanoparticles with an average diameter of 50 nm are dispersed in deionized (DI) water. One drop of nanoparticle suspension (2 μL, 1 mg/ml) is added into a tank. The tank is filled with DI water with the addition of 20 μL Tween 20 solution. The particles are gathered into clusters by applying a magnetic field gradient, and then, the particle clusters are put into the workspace of the magnetic coils for further actuation and control.

4.5.2 Experimental Results

(1) Mobile Target Tracking With Obstacle Avoidance: The proposed control scheme was also applied to track mobile targets in an environment with virtual obstacles. The mobile targets in this case were circular objects that exhibited bouncing behavior

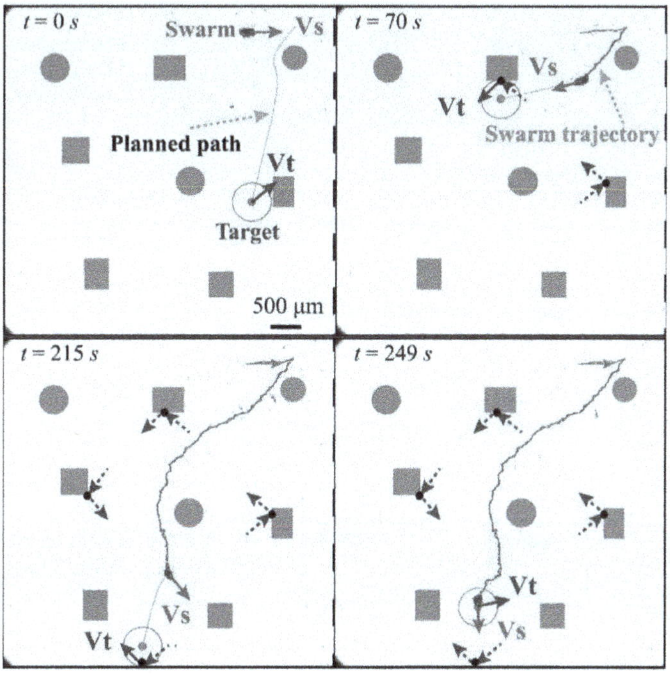

Figure 4.11 Tracking slow mobile target amidst obstacles: Experimental results. Swarm tracking results. Swarm velocity: V_s, target velocity: V_t. Dotted blue arrow pairs indicate previous bounces, black dots represent bouncing points. Scale bar: 500 μm.

when they came into contact with obstacles or walls. The control scheme was designed to effectively track and navigate these targets while avoiding collisions with the virtual obstacles.

1) Low-Speed Mobile Target Tracking: The results of tracking a low-speed (12 μm/s) mobile target are depicted in Figure 4.11. Despite the sudden changes in the target's moving direction caused by bouncing, the EB-RRT* dynamic path planning algorithm, with a sufficiently high updating frequency of 1.7-2.4 Hz, successfully generates a desired path that avoids collisions with the virtual obstacles. The path is represented by the blue curves, and the points where bouncing occurs are marked by black dots.

Following the successful validation of dynamic path planning, the effectiveness of the proposed image-guided motion control method is further tested. This method combines the dynamic path planning unit, the direction controller, and the GA-LQR velocity controller to control both the velocity and direction of the swarm. The results, as shown in Figure 4.11, illustrate the tracking process of a mobile target with initial positions of the swarm and target at $t = 0$ s. Due to the presence of obstacles and the bouncing boundary condition, the target's trajectory is complex and unpredictable, posing a challenge for the controller. At certain instances, such as $t = 70$ s and $t = 117$ s, the target makes contact with rectangular obstacles, resulting in sudden changes in its direction. However, through multiple bouncing processes, the target eventually approaches the bottom boundary at $t = 215$ s. The swarm

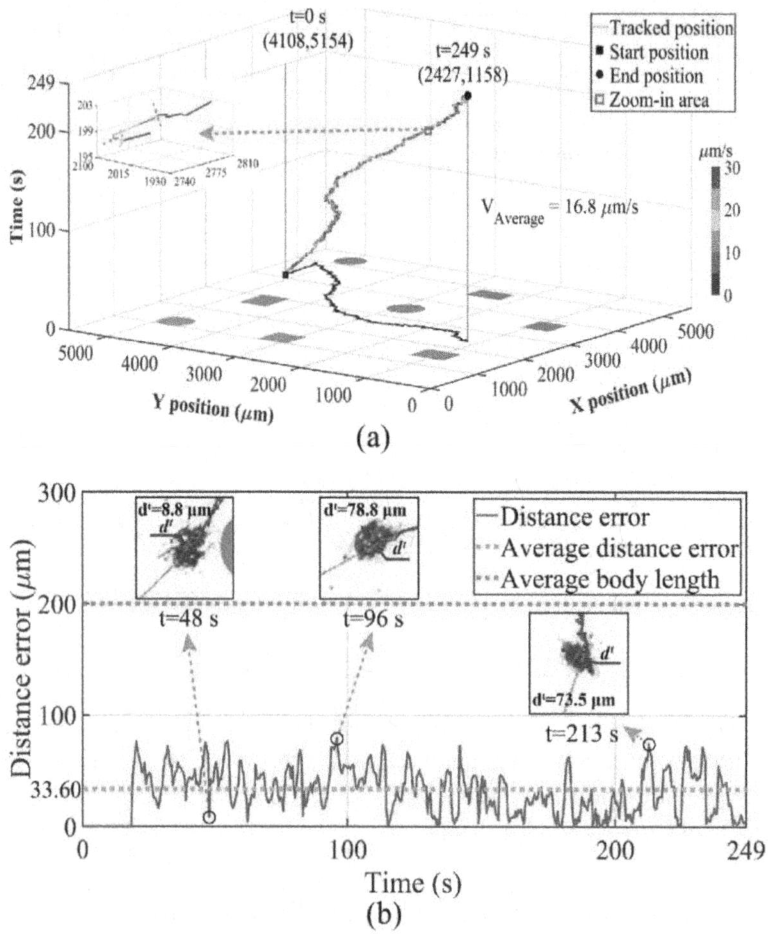

Figure 4.12 Tracking slow mobile target amidst obstacles: Experimental results. (a) Trajectory plot over time. Colors represent swarm speed distribution. Grey areas: obstacles. Black path: 2D swarm trajectory. Starting position marked by black square, terminal position by circle. Red dotted lines separate iterations. (b) Target tracking distance error. Enlarged insets provide clear observations of distance error in experiments. Average swarm body length: 200 µm. Scale bar: 500 µm.

continuously adjusts its motion to track the target, following dynamically planned trajectories that avoid collisions with obstacles. Finally, at t = 249 s, the mobile target is successfully tracked by the swarm. Notably, the trajectory of the swarm (represented by the red curve) closely aligns with the planned path toward the mobile target (represented by the green curve) in Figure 4.11, indicating a small distance error. The locomotion trajectory over time is depicted in Figure 4.12a. The swarm's initial position is (4108, 5154) µm, and it has an average velocity of 16.8 µm/s. In the inset, the color transitions from yellow to blue within one iteration, and this color change repeats periodically throughout the tracking process. This color variation indicates that the swarm's velocity decreases as it approaches the targeted end-point in each iteration. This demonstrates the successful control of swarm velocity by the

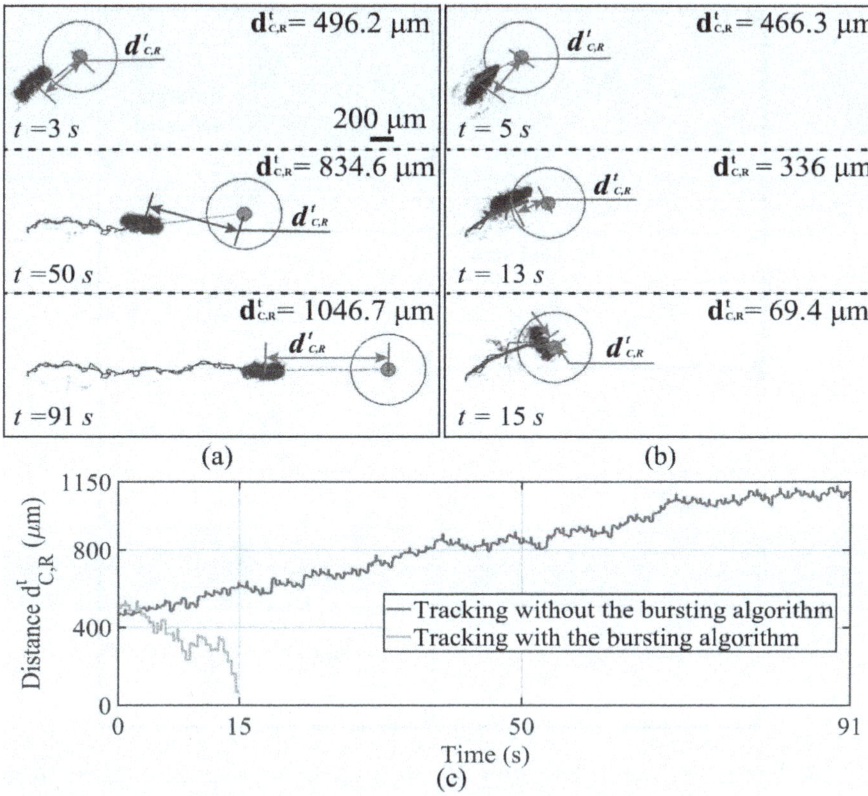

Figure 4.13 The validation of the targeted bursting algorithm. (a) The results of tracking a high-speed mobile target without applying the bursting algorithm. (b) The results of tracking a high-speed mobile target with applying the bursting algorithm. (c) The results of distance $d^t_{C,R}$ between the swarm center and the target. The scale bar is 200 μm.

GA-LQR velocity controller. The distance error between the swarm and the target is displayed in Figure 4.12b. The highest distance error is 78.8 μm, which accounts for 39% of the average body length of the swarm (200 μm). The average distance error is 33.6 μm, representing 17% of the swarm's body length. The amplitude oscillation of the distance error remains within a reasonable range. These results highlight that the proposed image-guided motion control method, with the GA-LQR velocity controller, ensures high accuracy in tracking the mobile target.

2) High-Speed Mobile Target Tracking: As discussed in 4.3.3, the swarm's velocity decreases as it approaches the targeted end-point in each iteration. To overcome this drawback and meet the requirements of tracking a high-speed mobile target, the use of the targeted bursting algorithm in the tracking control scheme is necessary. For comparisons, the control scheme without the bursting algorithm is also applied, keeping the other units of the control scheme (*i.e.*, the EB-RRT* path planner, the direction controller, and the GA-LQR velocity controller) the same. The effectiveness of the bursting algorithm is first validated by tracking a high-speed mobile target in a free space, as shown in Figure 4.13. Swarms controlled by the control scheme without

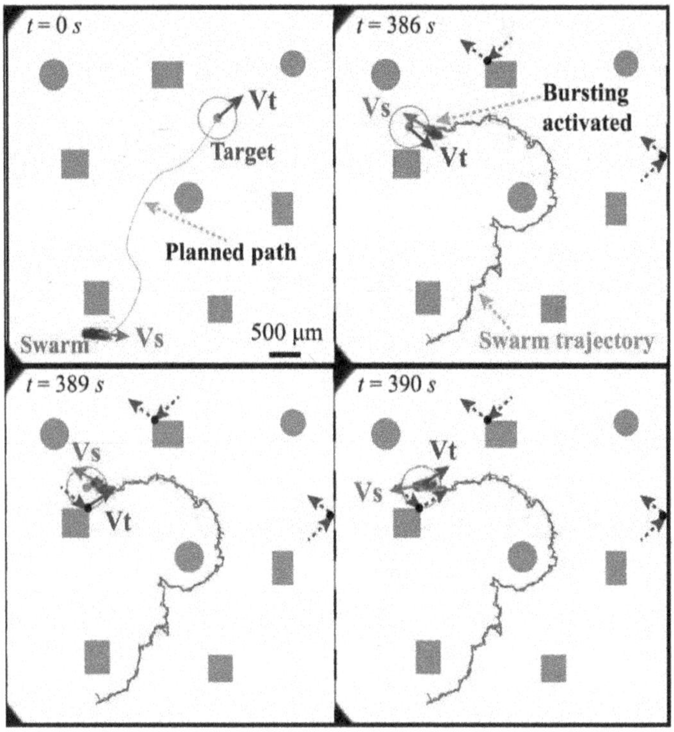

Figure 4.14 The experimental results of tracking a high-speed mobile target with applying the bursting algorithm using EB-RRT* path planning algorithm in an environment with obstacles. The velocities of the swarm and the target are represented by V_s and V_t, respectively. The dotted blue arrow pairs show the previous bounces and the black dots are the bouncing points. The scale bar is 500 μm.

and with the bursting algorithm are deployed to track high-speed mobile targets in a similar experimental setup. In Figure 4.13a, it can be observed that the distance ($d^t_{C,R}$) between the swarm and the target increases because the swarm's velocity decreases when it approaches the targeted end-point in each iteration. Consequently, the swarm fails to reach the target in this case. Conversely, by activating the bursting unit, the swarm successfully tracks the high-speed mobile target within a short time period, as shown in Figure 4.13b. The bursting process is triggered when the swarm reaches the bursting region of the mobile target. A comparison between these two cases is presented in Figure 4.13c, where the distance between the swarm and the target continuously increases over time when the bursting algorithm is not applied, whereas it rapidly decreases when the bursting algorithm is applied, indicating the effectiveness of the bursting algorithm in achieving successful tracking.

To further validate the effectiveness of the bursting algorithm, experiments are conducted to track a high-speed (20 μm/s) mobile target in an environment with obstacles. By utilizing the proposed bursting algorithm, the control results are shown in Figure 4.14. Initially, the swarm is guided to follow the planned path to track the mobile target. The bursting region surrounding the mobile target is activated, and when the swarm reaches the bursting region at t = 386 s, the bursting behavior is

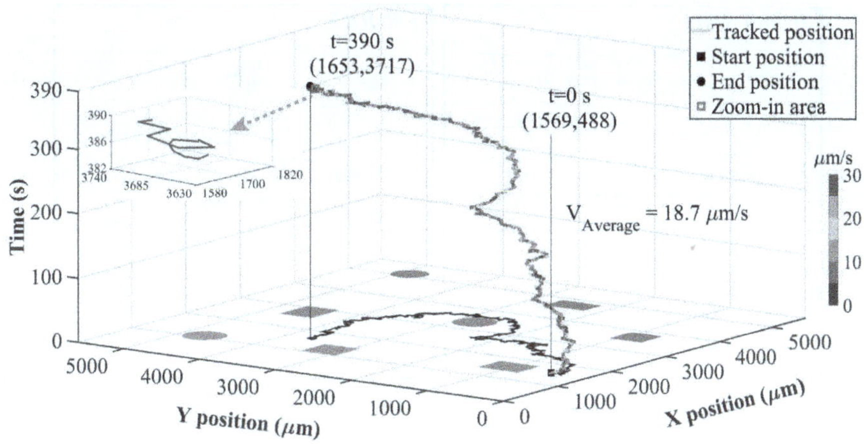

Figure 4.15 The plots of trajectory over time using GA-LQR velocity control algorithm. Different colors indicate the speed distribution of the swarm over time. The grey areas represent the obstacles and the black path denotes the 2D trajectory of the swarm. The starting position and terminal position are marked by red square and circle, respectively.

triggered. The path toward the target is re-planned, and the swarm is accelerated due to the increased input pitch angle of the magnetic field. As a result, the target is successfully tracked within a short time period of 390 s. The locomotion trajectory over time using the proposed control scheme is depicted in Figure 4.15. The initial position of the swarm is (1569, 488) μm, and the average velocity of the swarm is 18.7 μm/s. By observing the enlarged inset, it can be seen that the swarm exhibits a yellowish color during the bursting process, which corresponds to the latter part of the trajectory and indicates an increased velocity of the swarm. These results confirm the effectiveness and high tracking efficiency of the proposed tracking control scheme.

To evaluate the performance of the EB-RRT* algorithm, three other path planning algorithms, namely enhanced bidirectional rapidly-exploring random tree (EB-RRT), bidirectional rapidly-exploring random tree star (B-RRT*), and enhanced rapidly-exploring random tree star (E-RRT*), are employed for comparison. The remaining units of the control scheme, including the direction controller, GA-LQR velocity controller, and bursting algorithm, are kept consistent across the experiments. The control results are presented in Figure 4.16, where the initial positions of the swarm and the target, as well as the locations of the obstacles, are maintained the same (Figure 4.16a). Figure 4.16b shows the tracking result when using the EB-RRT algorithm. Although the mobile target is successfully tracked, it requires a longer time period (519 s) compared to the proposed EB-RRT* algorithm (390 s). In the case of the B-RRT* algorithm (Figure 4.16c), a collision occurs between the swarm and a rectangular obstacle. This is due to the fact that the physical size of the swarm is ignored, resulting in the absence of collision buffer layers around the obstacles. Figure 4.16d depicts the tracking result using the E-RRT* algorithm, where the swarm can only reach the previous positions of the mobile target. This indicates that the planned

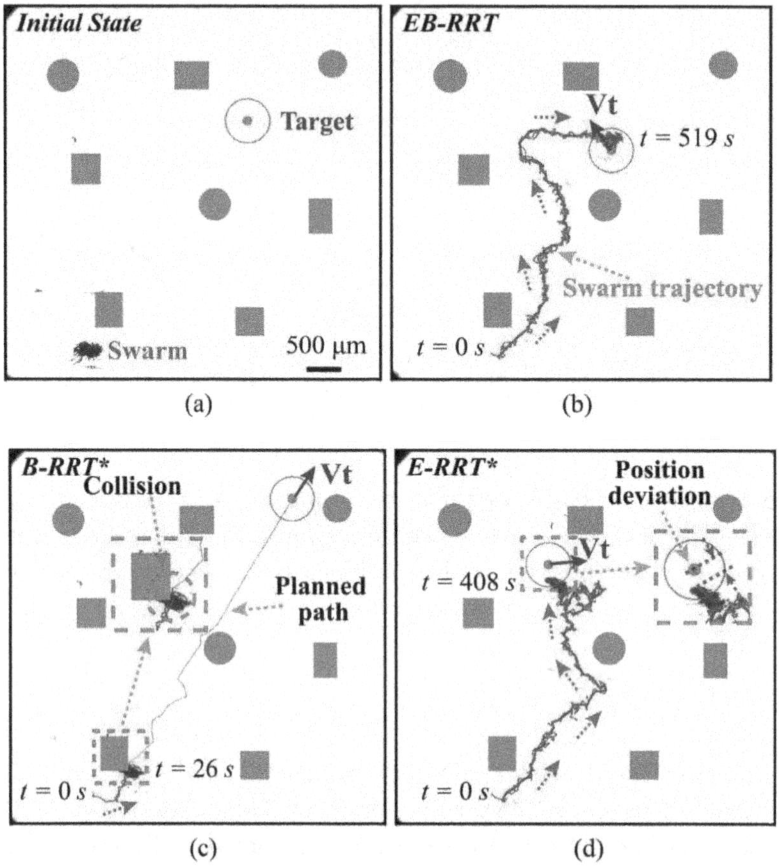

Figure 4.16 The experimental results of tracking a high-speed mobile target using different path planning algorithms in an environment with obstacles. (a) The initial positions of the swarm and the target. (b)–(d) The tracking results using EB-RRT, B-RRT* and E-RRT* algorithms, respectively. The velocity of the target is represented by V_t. The dotted green arrows show the moving direction of the simulated swarm. The enlarged insets provide clear observations of collision and position deviation in experiments. The scale bar is 500 μm.

path generated by the E-RRT* algorithm fails to adapt to the rapid changes of the swarm and target positions. The experimental results align well with the simulation results presented in Figure 4.8, affirming that the EB-RRT* algorithm ensures the shortest time cost during mobile target tracking.

To validate the performance of the Genetic Algorithm (GA) in the control scheme, the other units of the control scheme, including the EB-RRT* path planner, direction controller, and bursting algorithm, are applied equally. The experimental results are presented in Figures 4.17a and 4.17b. In Figure 4.17a, the proposed GA-LQR algorithm is utilized, and the Genetic Algorithm is employed to select optimal values for the weighting matrices (Q and R) to achieve the desired velocity. The average distance error is measured at 44.01 μm, which accounts for 22% of the swarm body length (200 μm). Furthermore, the oscillation amplitude of the distance error remains

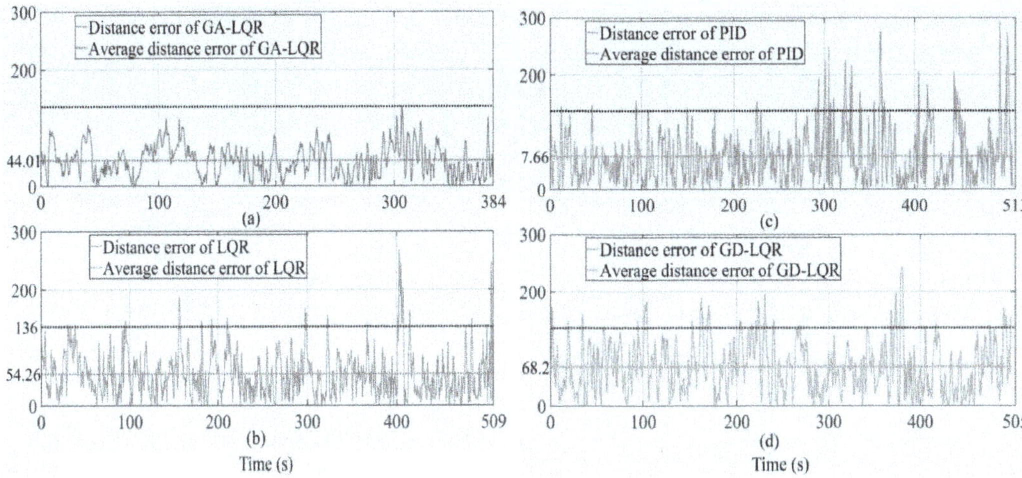

Figure 4.17 The distance error of the mobile target tracking using different velocity control algorithms. (a)-(d) Distance errors using GA-LQR, LQR, PID and GD-LQR velocity control algorithms, respectively. The average body length of the swarm is 200 μm.

within a relatively small range of 0–136 μm. On the other hand, Figure 4.17b demonstrates the experimental results using the LQR velocity controller, where the values of Q and R are determined through experiments. In this case, the highest distance error increases to 268 μm, and the average distance reaches 54.26 μm. These results indicate that the proposed Genetic Algorithm effectively ensures high tracking accuracy when compared to the LQR velocity controller, as the distance error is significantly reduced with the GA-LQR algorithm.

To compare the tracking performance with two other velocity control algorithms, namely PID and Gradient Descent-based Linear Quadratic Regulator (GD-LQR), the GA-LQR velocity control algorithm is evaluated. In this comparison, only the velocity control module differs, while the other parts of the control scheme, including the EB-RRT* path planner, direction controller, and bursting algorithm, remain the same. Figures 4.17c and 4.17d present the distance errors obtained using the two alternative velocity control algorithms. When using the PID velocity controller, the average distance error is measured at 57.66 μm, while the highest distance error significantly increases to 294 μm. This value is 2.16 times higher than the highest distance error achieved using the GA-LQR algorithm (136 μm), as shown in Figure 4.17c. In the case of the GD-LQR velocity controller, as demonstrated in Figure 4.17d, the highest distance error reaches 242 μm. The average distance error is 68.2 μm, which is the highest among the three trials. Furthermore, the oscillation amplitudes of the distance error in Figures 4.17c and 4.17d remain in an unsatisfactory range and may exceed the highest distance error obtained with the GA-LQR algorithm (136 μm) in Figure 4.17a. These results highlight that the GA-LQR velocity control algorithm ensures high tracking accuracy compared to the PID and GD-LQR velocity

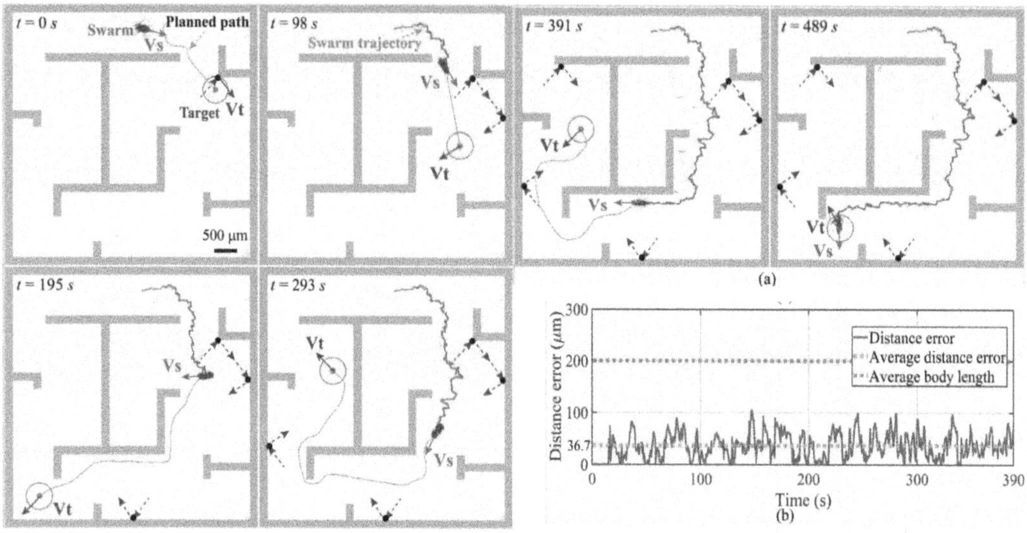

Figure 4.18 The experimental results of tracking a high-speed mobile target in a micromaze. (a) The trajectory tracking results of the swarm. The velocities of the swarm and the target are represented by V_s and V_t, respectively. The blue curve is the dynamic planned path and the red curve shows the trajectory of the swarm. The dotted blue arrow pairs show the previous bounces and the black dots are the bouncing points. (b) The distance error of the target tracking. The average body length of the swarm is 200 μm. The scale bar is 500 μm.

control algorithms. The GA-LQR algorithm yields lower average and highest distance errors, indicating superior tracking performance.

As a consequence, the EB-RRT* algorithm for path planning, along with the proposed motion control algorithm, encompassing the direction controller and the GA-LQR velocity controller, work in conjunction with the bursting algorithm to achieve both efficient path planning and precise tracking of mobile targets.

(2) Mobile Target Tracking in a Micromaze: When comparing environments with obstacles, it is observed that the presence of confined spaces, such as a micromaze with virtual walls, increases the likelihood of the target experiencing rebounds. Consequently, the trajectory of the target becomes more intricate. In this study, Figure 4.18a presents experimental outcomes of a swarm tracking a high-speed target within a micromaze. The swarm adeptly follows a path while avoiding collisions with the micromaze walls, ultimately succeeding in tracking the mobile target. Figure 4.18b illustrates the real-time and average distance errors. Remarkably, the average distance error measures 36.7 μm, which is significantly lower than the swarm's body length (approximately 200 μm). These results strongly suggest that the proposed tracking control scheme, incorporating the bursting algorithm, effectively tracks high-speed dynamic targets within a micromaze, achieving remarkable tracking accuracy.

4.6 CONCLUSION

This chapter presents a novel and efficient swarm control scheme for the purpose of tracking mobile targets. The proposed scheme combines three key components: an EB-RRT* path planning unit, an image-guided motion control unit, and a targeted bursting process. Initially, an EB-RRT*-based dynamic path planner is developed to iteratively plan real-time paths while avoiding obstacles in complex environments. Subsequently, an image-guided motion control algorithm, comprising a direction control algorithm and a GA-LQR-based velocity control algorithm, is introduced to regulate the swarm's moving direction and velocity. This control scheme ensures minimal distance errors throughout the tracking process. To cater to the tracking of high-speed mobile targets, a targeted bursting algorithm is implemented. Simulation and experimental results validate the efficacy of the proposed tracking control scheme, demonstrating successful tracking of both low-speed and high-speed mobile targets in environments with obstacles and micromazes, respectively. This research serves as a prototypical paradigm for other swarm types, enabling dynamic motion control tasks, while offering new opportunities for further insights in the field.

The proposed control scheme demonstrates high compatibility with additional modules to address complex conditions. For instance, when the swarm operates on a curved surface, the swarm's velocity may be affected. To mitigate this, adjustments can be made to the pitch angle or a velocity adjustment module can be incorporated to maintain the distance error within an acceptable range. External disturbances, such as adhesion, friction, and fluid flows in the environment, can also impact the swarm's moving direction and velocity. The proposed direction control algorithm effectively corrects the deviation angle, and a disturbance observer can be employed to compensate for velocity errors caused by disturbances. Furthermore, even when the swarm encounters physical obstacles, the stability and pattern can be maintained by guiding the swarm to approach the obstacles, as outlined in [25]. Thus, the proposed control scheme provides controllability over the swarm's moving direction and velocity. Moreover, various medical imaging techniques, including Ultrasound Doppler Imaging, Fluorescence Imaging, and Magnetic Resonance Imaging, hold potential for *in vivo* detection of the swarm and the mobile target.

Bibliography

[1] Qian Zou, Xingzhou Du, Yuezhen Liu, Hui Chen, Yibin Wang, and Jiangfan Yu. Dynamic path planning and motion control of microrobotic swarms for mobile target tracking. *IEEE Transactions on Automation Science and Engineering*, 2022.

[2] Bradley J Nelson, Ioannis K Kaliakatsos, and Jake J Abbott. Microrobots for minimally invasive medicine. *Annual Review of Biomedical Engineering*, 12:55–85, 2010.

[3] Metin Sitti, Hakan Ceylan, Wenqi Hu, Joshua Giltinan, Mehmet Turan, Sehyuk Yim, and Eric Diller. Biomedical applications of untethered mobile milli/microrobots. *Proceedings of the IEEE*, 103(2):205–224, 2015.

[4] Huaijuan Zhou, Carmen C Mayorga-Martinez, Salvador Pané, Li Zhang, and Martin Pumera. Magnetically driven micro and nanorobots. *Chemical Reviews*, 121(8):4999–5041, 2021.

[5] Zhiguang Wu, Ye Chen, Daniel Mukasa, On Shun Pak, and Wei Gao. Medical micro/nanorobots in complex media. *Chemical Society Reviews*, 49(22):8088–8112, 2020.

[6] Ben Wang, Kostas Kostarelos, Bradley J Nelson, and Li Zhang. Trends in micro-/nanorobotics: materials development, actuation, localization, and system integration for biomedical applications. *Advanced Materials*, 33(4):2002047, 2021.

[7] Chengzhi Hu, Salvador Pané, and Bradley J Nelson. Soft micro- and nanorobotics. *Annual Review of Control, Robotics, and Autonomous Systems*, 1:53–75, 2018.

[8] Yong Hu. Self-assembly of dna molecules: towards dna nanorobots for biomedical applications. *Cyborg and Bionic Systems*, 2021, 2021.

[9] Hao Wang, Jiacheng Kan, Xin Zhang, Chenyi Gu, and Zhan Yang. Pt/cnt micro-nanorobots driven by glucose catalytic decomposition. *Cyborg and Bionic Systems*, 2021, 2021.

[10] Dongdong Jin, Jiangfan Yu, Ke Yuan, and Li Zhang. Mimicking the structure and function of ant bridges in a reconfigurable microswarm for electronic applications. *ACS nano*, 13(5):5999–6007, 2019.

[11] Katherine Villa, Ludmila Krejčová, Filip Novotnỳ, Zbynek Heger, Zdeněk Sofer, and Martin Pumera. Cooperative multifunctional self-propelled paramagnetic microrobots with chemical handles for cell manipulation and drug delivery. *Advanced Functional Materials*, 28(43):1804343, 2018.

[12] TO Tasci, PS Herson, KB Neeves, and DWM Marr. Surface-enabled propulsion and control of colloidal microwheels. *Nature Communications*, 7(1):10225, 2016.

[13] Xiaopu Wang, Xiao-Hua Qin, Chengzhi Hu, Anastasia Terzopoulou, Xiang-Zhong Chen, Tian-Yun Huang, Katharina Maniura-Weber, Salvador Pané, and Bradley J Nelson. 3d printed enzymatically biodegradable soft helical microswimmers. *Advanced Functional Materials*, 28(45):1804107, 2018.

[14] Qian Zou, Xingzhou Du, Yuezhen Liu, Hui Chen, Yibin Wang, and Jiangfan Yu. Dynamic path planning and motion control of microrobotic swarms for mobile target tracking. *IEEE Transactions on Automation Science and Engineering*, 2022.

[15] Jinxing Li, Pavimol Angsantikul, Wenjuan Liu, Berta Esteban-Fernández de Ávila, Xiaocong Chang, Elodie Sandraz, Yuyan Liang, Siyu Zhu, Yue Zhang, Chuanrui Chen, et al. Biomimetic platelet-camouflaged nanorobots for binding and isolation of biological threats. *Advanced Materials*, 30(2):1704800, 2018.

[16] Haifeng Xu, Mariana Medina-Sánchez, Veronika Magdanz, Lukas Schwarz, Franziska Hebenstreit, and Oliver G Schmidt. Sperm-hybrid micromotor for targeted drug delivery. *ACS Nano*, 12(1):327–337, 2018.

[17] Veronika Magdanz, Islam SM Khalil, Juliane Simmchen, Guilherme P Furtado, Sumit Mohanty, Johannes Gebauer, Haifeng Xu, Anke Klingner, Azaam Aziz, Mariana Medina-Sánchez, et al. Ironsperm: Sperm-templated soft magnetic microrobots. *Science Advances*, 6(28):eaba5855, 2020.

[18] Yabin Zhang, Lin Zhang, Lidong Yang, Chi Ian Vong, Kai Fung Chan, William KK Wu, Thomas NY Kwong, Norman WS Lo, Margaret Ip, Sunny H Wong, et al. Real-time tracking of fluorescent magnetic spore–based microrobots for remote detection of c. diff toxins. *Science Advances*, 5(1):eaau9650, 2019.

[19] Xiong Yang, Wanfeng Shang, Haojian Lu, Yanting Liu, Liu Yang, Rong Tan, Xinyu Wu, and Yajing Shen. An agglutinate magnetic spray transforms inanimate objects into millirobots for biomedical applications. *Science Robotics*, 5(48):eabc8191, 2020.

[20] Stefano Palagi, Andrew G Mark, Shang Yik Reigh, Kai Melde, Tian Qiu, Hao Zeng, Camilla Parmeggiani, Daniele Martella, Alberto Sanchez-Castillo, Nadia Kapernaum, et al. Structured light enables biomimetic swimming and versatile locomotion of photoresponsive soft microrobots. *Nature Materials*, 15(6):647–653, 2016.

[21] S Yu, T Li, F Ji, S Zhao, K Liu, Z Zhang, W Zhang, and Y Mei. Trimer-like microrobots with multimodal locomotion and reconfigurable capabilities. *Materials Today Advances*, 14:100231, 2022.

[22] Zhiguang Wu, Jonas Troll, Hyeon-Ho Jeong, Qiang Wei, Marius Stang, Focke Ziemssen, Zegao Wang, Mingdong Dong, Sven Schnichels, Tian Qiu, et al. A swarm of slippery micropropellers penetrates the vitreous body of the eye. *Science Advances*, 4(11):eaat4388, 2018.

[23] Ania Servant, Famin Qiu, Mariarosa Mazza, Kostas Kostarelos, and Bradley J Nelson. Controlled in vivo swimming of a swarm of bacteria-like microrobotic flagella. *Advanced Materials*, 27(19):2981–2988, 2015.

[24] Jiangfan Yu, Lidong Yang, and Li Zhang. Pattern generation and motion control of a vortex-like paramagnetic nanoparticle swarm. *The International Journal of Robotics Research*, 37(8):912–930, 2018.

[25] Jiangfan Yu, Ben Wang, Xingzhou Du, Qianqian Wang, and Li Zhang. Ultra-extensible ribbon-like magnetic microswarm. *Nature Communications*, 9(1):3260, 2018.

[26] Qian Zou, Xingzhou Du, Yuezhen Liu, Hui Chen, Yibin Wang, and Jiangfan Yu. Dynamic path planning and motion control of microrobotic swarms for mobile target tracking. *IEEE Transactions on Automation Science and Engineering*, 2022.

[27] Fengtong Ji, Dongdong Jin, Ben Wang, and Li Zhang. Light-driven hovering of a magnetic microswarm in fluid. *ACS Nano*, 14(6):6990–6998, 2020.

[28] Hoyeon Kim, U Kei Cheang, Louis W Rogowski, and Min Jun Kim. Motion planning of particle based microrobots for static obstacle avoidance. *Journal of Micro-Bio Robotics*, 14:41–49, 2018.

[29] Jia Liu, Tiantian Xu, Simon X Yang, and Xinyu Wu. Navigation and visual feedback control for magnetically driven helical miniature swimmers. *IEEE Transactions on Industrial Informatics*, 16(1):477–487, 2019.

[30] Li Huang, Louis Rogowski, Min Jun Kim, and Aaron T Becker. Path planning and aggregation for a microrobot swarm in vascular networks using a global input. In *2017 IEEE/RSJ International Conference on Intelligent Robots and Systems (IROS)*, pages 414–420. IEEE, 2017.

[31] Lidong Yang, Yabin Zhang, Qianqian Wang, Kai-Fung Chan, and Li Zhang. Automated control of magnetic spore-based microrobot using fluorescence imaging for targeted delivery with cellular resolution. *IEEE Transactions on Automation Science and Engineering*, 17(1):490–501, 2019.

[32] Karim Belharet, David Folio, and Antoine Ferreira. Endovascular navigation of a ferromagnetic microrobot using mri-based predictive control. In *2010 IEEE/RSJ International Conference on Intelligent Robots and Systems*, pages 2804–2809. IEEE, 2010.

[33] Lidong Yang, Qianqian Wang, and Li Zhang. Model-free trajectory tracking control of two-particle magnetic microrobot. *IEEE Transactions on Nanotechnology*, 17(4):697–700, 2018.

[34] Xingzhou Du, Jiangfan Yu, Dongdong Jin, Philip Wai Yan Chiu, and Li Zhang. Independent pattern formation of nanorod and nanoparticle swarms under an oscillating field. *ACS Nano*, 15(3):4429–4439, 2021.

[35] Qian Zou, Yibin Wang, and Jiangfan Yu. Colloidal microrobotic swarms. *Field-Driven Micro and Nanorobots for Biology and Medicine*, pages 179–209, 2022.

[36] Lidong Yang, Jiangfan Yu, and Li Zhang. Statistics-based automated control for a swarm of paramagnetic nanoparticles in 2-d space. *IEEE Transactions on Robotics*, 36(1):254–270, 2019.

[37] Sertac Karaman and Emilio Frazzoli. Sampling-based algorithms for optimal motion planning. *The International Journal of Robotics Research*, 30(7):846–894, 2011.

[38] Mohamed Elbanhawi, Milan Simic, and Reza N Jazar. Continuous path smoothing for car-like robots using b-spline curves. *Journal of Intelligent & Robotic Systems*, 80:23–56, 2015.

[39] Iram Noreen. Collision free smooth path for mobile robots in cluttered environment using an economical clamped cubic b-spline. *Symmetry*, 12(9):1567, 2020.

[40] Richard M Murray et al. Optimization-based control. *California Institute of Technology, CA*, pages 111–128, 2009.

[41] SN Sivanandam, SN Deepa, SN Sivanandam, and SN Deepa. *Genetic Algorithms*. Springer, 2008.

CHAPTER 5

Collective Behavior of Reconfigurable Magnetic Droplets at Air-Liquid Interfaces

5.1 INTRODUCTION

Untethered small-scale robots powered by external sources have garnered attention due to their potential for biomedical applications and their ability to perform robotic manipulation tasks [1, 2, 3, 4, 5]. Several designs of small-scale robots actuated by magnetic fields have been presented, and various manipulation tasks have been reported. Through multiple actuation models, a soft millimeter-scale robot is capable of performing pick-and-place and cargo-release tasks [6]. A miniature magnetic robot can be actuated in two vibration modes, which have been effectively exploited for pushing and releasing millimeter-scale objects [7]. Recently, Jing *et al.* reported that a microrobot equipped with a sensing end-effector is capable of manipulating cells with force-sensing abilities [8]. Various manipulation strategies using small-scale robots have been reported, ranging from millimeter scale to micro/nanoscale [9, 10, 11]. However, as miniature robots are scaled down, their controllability and cargo delivery capability may become limited. To address these issues, it is worth investigating the introduction of collective behavior to robots, particularly at small scales. A group of agents can be assembled to work closely and enhance their capabilities, which can be difficult for individual agents to achieve [12, 13, 14]. Furthermore, the pattern of assembled agents can be adjusted by regulating the external energy input, which has been applied to perform cooperative tasks [15, 16, 17].

Interactions among building blocks are crucial for inducing collective behavior, and various energy sources, such as external fields, light, and chemical reactions, have been utilized to introduce complex interactions [18, 19, 20, 21, 22]. To achieve a stable assembled pattern within a practical timescale, self-assembly offers a range of options and results in two major systems: static and dynamic. In a static self-assembly

DOI: 10.1201/9781032665788-5

system, stability is achieved once it reaches global or local equilibrium, and it is usually difficult to adjust. In a dynamic self-assembly system, the assembled pattern dissipates energy, and the interactions among the building blocks dominate the pattern formation. The interactions can be adjusted by regulating the energy input, and the resulting structures are typically not achievable under equilibrium conditions [23, 24]. However, controlling the position of a dynamic pattern, particularly in a system energized by a global magnetic field, can be challenging. The time required for forming, positioning, and adjusting an assembled pattern is crucial for the time efficiency of manipulation tasks. Rapid formation and navigation of small-scale robotic patterns remain a challenge and require further investigation. In addition, controlling the locomotion of an assembled pattern is also an essential aspect. Simple locomotion control may not be sufficient to meet the demands of tasks in complex environments [25]. A strategy that combines effective locomotion control with pattern control is necessary.

In this chapter, a control strategy of forming and navigating collective patterns of magnetic droplets at air-liquid interfaces will be introduced. The microparticles inside our droplets differ from ferrofluid droplets that have homogeneous properties [23], and the microparticles are dynamically assembled into rotating particle chains under a precessing magnetic field, resulting in rotating droplets (Figure 5.1). By balancing the induced magnetic, hydrodynamic and capillary interactions among the droplets, a highly ordered pattern of droplets can be generated. The ordered pattern can be regarded as a dissipative structure and requires a continuous external energy supply to sustain. The structure of the pattern can be controlled by modulating the inner interactions between droplets, and the navigation and formation efficiency are increased by inducing field gradient near the pattern. Through simulations, we further investigate the hydrodynamic interactions and induced fluid flow by the ordered pattern, indicating that induced circular flows at the central and surrounding region of the pattern provide the trapping and caging of cargo with a mechanism. Moreover, we can use a magnetic field gradient to steer the assembled dynamic droplets as an entity in a controlled manner, and hence, achieve automated steering of the droplets. Herein, we will primarily introduce a micromanipulation strategy utilizing dynamically self-assembled magnetic droplets guided by an iron needle. The needle was magnetized by precessing magnetic fields generated from a three-axis Helmholtz coil system (Figure 5.2) mounted on a 3-DoF manipulator. By varying the number of magnetic droplets beneath the air-liquid interface, we formed various ordered dynamic patterns and modeled the interactions between the droplets and the induced field gradient around the needle. The induced field gradient significantly decreased the required time for forming an ordered pattern and enabled the determination of the center of the assembled pattern by the needle's position. We optimized the process of pattern formation based on real-time visual feedback and a Genetic algorithm. Additionally, we designed a PSO-based optimal path planner with obstacle-avoidance capability to guide the assembled pattern in multi-obstacle environments. The assembled droplets were able to be navigated along preplanned paths by following the magnetized needle, exhibiting reversible pattern expansion and shrinkage. Experimental

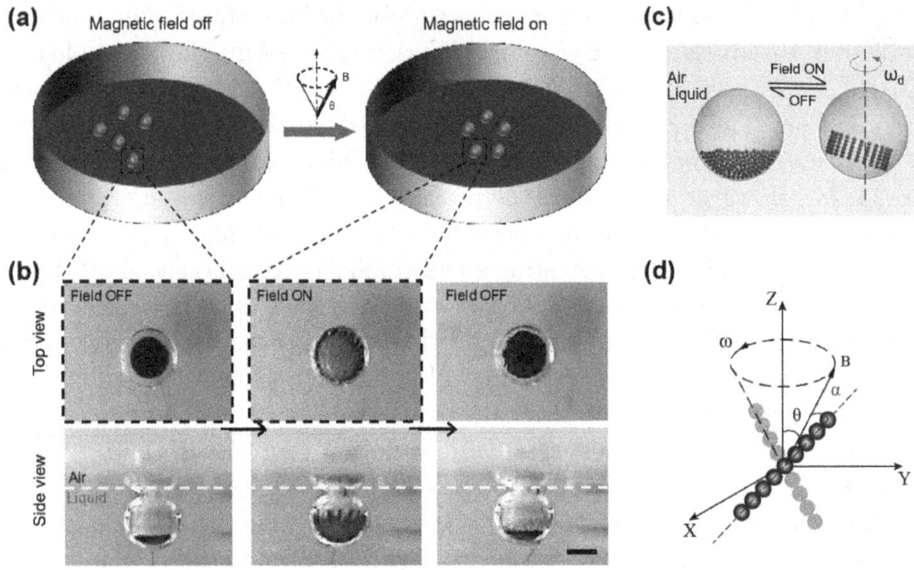

Figure 5.1 Magnetic droplets under a precessing magnetic field. (a) Schematic drawing of droplets in a Petri dish. They are gradually assembled into an ordered pattern under a precessing field. (b) Top view and corresponding side view of a droplet with or without a magnetic field. Under the magnetic field, these microparticles form chains and will sink to the bottom of the droplets with the field turned off. The scale bar is 1 mm. (c) A side view schematically shows the reversible assembly of separated rotating particle chains inside the droplet with a precessing magnetic field on or off. ω_d refers to the angular velocity of the rotating droplet. (d) Microparticle chains are formed under a precessing magnetic field with frequency ω, precession angle θ and field strength B. α refers to the phase lag and is defined as the angle between the external field and long axis of the chain.

results demonstrated the ability of the assembled pattern to trap and cage cargo, perform non-contact and contact transportation, and avoid obstacles.

5.2 EXPERIMENTAL SETUP AND METHODS

Magnetic actuation was achieved using a three-axis Helmholtz coil system (Figure 5.3a). The three pairs of coils were actuated by servo amplifiers (ADS 50/5 4-Q-DC, Maxon Inc.) and controlled by the control PC. The input field parameters were controlled by an I/O card (Model 826, Sensoray Inc.) through the controller box. The camera was used for video recording and real-time image acquisition, while the 3-DoF robotic manipulator was placed on the right side of the coils and was controlled by an Arduino Mega using a LabVIEW program. A gamepad was used to control the movement of the 3-DoF robotic manipulator in the X, Y, and Z directions via serial communication. The iron needle used in the experiment has a diameter of 0.6 mm and is gripped on the robotic manipulator. A glass Petri dish filled with dibenzyl

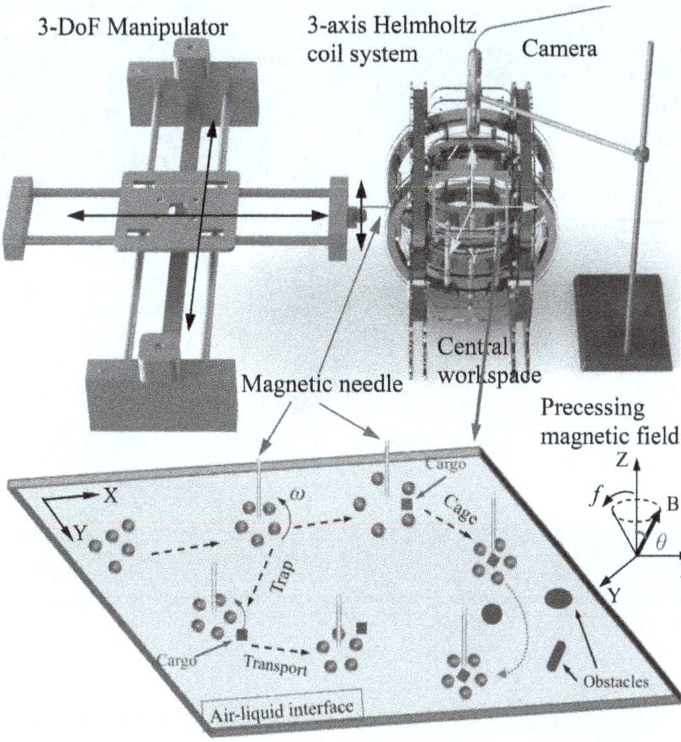

Figure 5.2 Schematic illustration of the experimental setup, the processes of pattern formation, cargo trapping, caging, and obstacle-avoidance transportation. The iron needle was controlled by a 3-DoF manipulator and magnetized by the Helmholtz coil. A precessing magnetic field was generated by the coil system, which had field parameters including strength (B), rotating frequency (f), and precession angle (θ). A camera was positioned on top to provide visual feedback. Self-assembled droplets were navigated by following the needle to perform micromanipulation tasks.

ether was put at the central workspace of the coil system. The needle was inserted into the central workspace of the Helmholtz coils through the middle space of the Z-pair coils. During the experiments, the needle tip was positioned perpendicular to the air-liquid interface, and the distance between the needle tip and the interface was adjusted as necessary. A droplet was obtained by pipetting one drop of carbonyl iron microparticles DI water suspension into the dibenzyl ether. Carbonyl iron microparticles (BASF, China) have an average diameter of 3 μm (Figure 5.3b), and they exhibit ferromagnetic properties based on their magnetic hysteresis loop. To ensure consistency in the magnetic properties of the droplets, the carbonyl iron microparticle suspension (with a concentration of 30 mg/mL) was stirred prior to being added into the Petri dish. Additionally, basic fuchsin dye (Aladdin, 2 mg/mL) was added to the suspension to facilitate better tracking of the droplets. After adding one drop (4 μL) of the suspension, a droplet with a radius of ~980 μm was formed beneath the air-liquid interface (Figure 5.3c).

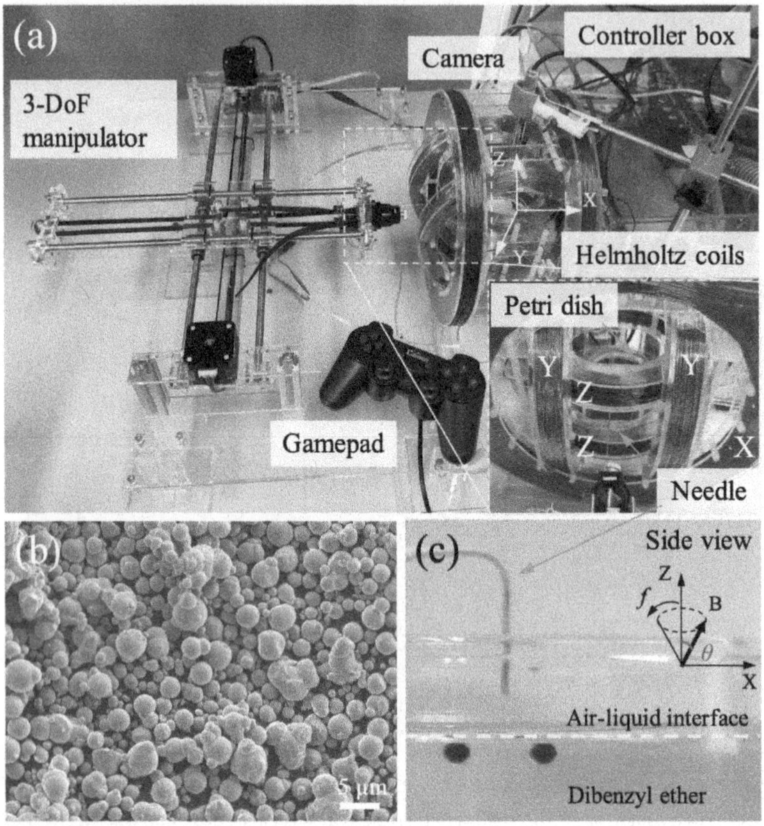

Figure 5.3 Experimental setup and materials. (a) The Helmholtz coil system was controlled by the controller box, and field parameters were adjusted via a control PC. The three coil pairs are labeled as X, Y, and Z. The iron needle was fixed on a copper holder, which was gripped by a robot arm positioned on the side. A camera was mounted on top for real-time image acquisition and video recording. (b) SEM image of the magnetic microparticles. (c) Magnetic droplets were located beneath the air-liquid interface and energized by a precessing magnetic field.

5.3 MATHEMATICAL MODELING AND SIMULATIONS

The self-assembled pattern was mainly influenced by the interplay of various factors such as magnetic, hydrodynamic, and capillary interactions among droplets. All droplets were attracted toward the magnetized needle due to the locally induced field gradient.

5.3.1 Induced Magnetic Field Gradient

The simulation of induced magnetic field distribution using COMSOL Multiphysics was performed to investigate the interactions between the magnetized needle and droplets. During experiments, a precessing magnetic field was generated to rotate droplets and magnetize the iron needle. After turning off the magnetic field, no

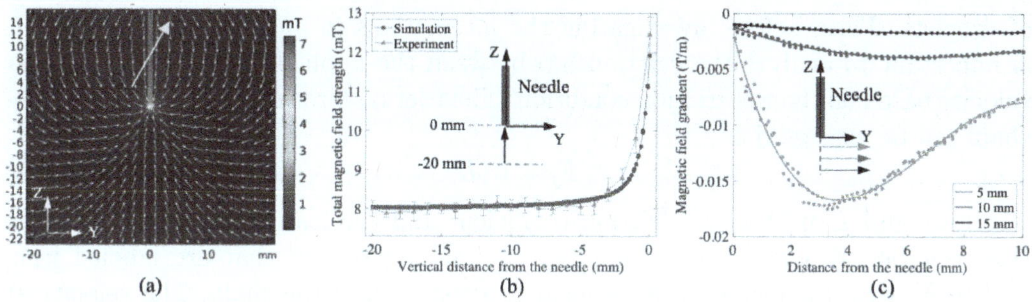

Figure 5.4 Simulation results of the induced magnetic field near the iron needle. (a) The yellow arrow represents the applied magnetic field, and the white arrows indicate the field direction. Color refers to the magnitude of the field strength, with values marked by the legend on the right side. (b) The magnetic field strengths along the axial direction (Z-axis) of the needle were both simulated and measured. The inset shows the direction of data acquisition. The error bars represent the standard deviation (s.d.) from five experiments. (c) The magnetic field gradient along the Y-axis is measured at vertical distances of 5 mm, 10 mm, and 15 mm, and the curves are fitted based on the data points from the simulation.

magnetic field was detected near the iron needle (measured by LakeShore Gaussmeter, model 410). In the simulation, the iron needle had a diameter of 0.6 mm and a length of 60 mm. The precessing field was considered as a static field that made an angle θ (precession angle) with the Z-axis and rotated around it. Therefore, in order to simulate the field distribution around the needle, we studied the case where an iron needle was magnetized by the static field. The applied magnetic field in the simulation was at an angle of 30° to the Z-axis and had a strength of 8 mT. Figure 5.4a illustrates the simulated magnetic field distribution in the vicinity of the needle tip, and Figure 5.4b shows the relationship between the field strength and the distance below the tip. Both the simulated and experimentally measured field strengths decay with an increasing distance from the needle and approach the strength of the applied field (8 mT). The good agreement between the simulated and measured results validates our simulation methods. Field gradient was also induced near the needle. As shown in Figure 5.4c, the relationship between the field gradient along the Y-axis and different vertical distances is plotted. The field gradient had the maximum value of 0.017 T/m, and the minus sign indicates that the direction of the field gradient was opposite to the Y-axis.

5.3.2 Angular Velocity of Droplets

When energized by the precessing magnetic field, microparticle chains are formed due to the attractive magnetic forces between microparticles. The separation distance between chains is determined by the repulsive magnetic forces induced by the out-of-plane component of the field. The rotation of the droplets is caused by the friction force between the particle chains and the inner wall of the droplet. Additionally, the hydrodynamic interaction between droplets depends on the angular velocity of droplets. Thus, before investigating the interactions in an assembled pattern, it is important to analyze the relationship between the applied field and the angular velocity based on the wet friction condition. The friction force exerted from a rotating chain can be expressed as

$$F_f = \mu_k L \tag{5.1}$$

where μ_k and L are the wet friction coefficient and the load force, respectively. In this scenario, we analyze a chain of $2N+1$ microparticles that are labeled from $-N$ to N, with the contact area A located at one end of the chain. The velocity at the end of the chain, which corresponds to the Nth microparticle, can be expressed as $v_N = 2Na\omega\sin\theta$, where a denotes the particle radius, and ω and θ represent the angular velocity and precession angle of the applied field, respectively. The coefficient μ_k is proportional to the rotational velocity of the chain, as [26]

$$\mu_k = (\eta A/hL)v_N \tag{5.2}$$

where h is the gap between the inner surface and the particle chain, and η is the viscosity of the surrounding fluid (DI water). If we define ψ as a constant, *i.e.*, $\psi = \eta A/hL$, the friction force exerted on the droplets by one chain can be expressed as $F_f = \psi v_N L$. Therefore, the total friction torque exerted on a droplet by n microparticle chains becomes

$$\Gamma_f = nF_f \times a_d = n\psi v_N L \times a_d \tag{5.3}$$

where a_d is the radius of a droplet. The Reynolds number, defined as $Re = \rho a_d^2\omega_d/\eta$ with ω_d being the angular velocity of the droplets, is in the range of 0.1–1 during the self-assembly process. This indicates that the self-assembly system is in a low Reynolds number regime. In this regime, the balance between the driven torque and the viscous drag torques results in a steady angular velocity of the droplets. The viscous drag torque on a rotating droplet is reported by Lukerchenko *et al.* [27], as

$$\Gamma_d = -c_d\frac{\rho}{2}\omega_d^2 a_d^5 \tag{5.4}$$

where c_d is the dimensionless drag torque coefficient, ρ is the viscosity of the surrounding fluid (dibenzyl ether). Therefore, the counterbalance relationship between the two torques yields

$$\omega_d = c_e\sqrt{\omega\sin\theta} \tag{5.5}$$

where $c_e = 2\sqrt{n\psi NaL/a_d^4\rho c_d}$ is a constant. Overall, the angular velocity of the droplets can be increased by adjusting the external field to a higher input frequency or a larger precession angle.

5.3.3 Interactions between Droplets

The magnetic interactions between droplets are dominated by the dipole-dipole interaction. Here, we only consider the force of interaction averaged over a field cycle $(2\pi/\omega)$, and the interaction potential is expressed as [28]

$$U(r,\phi,\theta) = -\frac{\mu_o m_d^2}{4\pi}\left(\frac{3\cos^2\phi - 1}{r^3}\right)\left(\frac{3\cos^2\theta - 1}{2}\right) \tag{5.6}$$

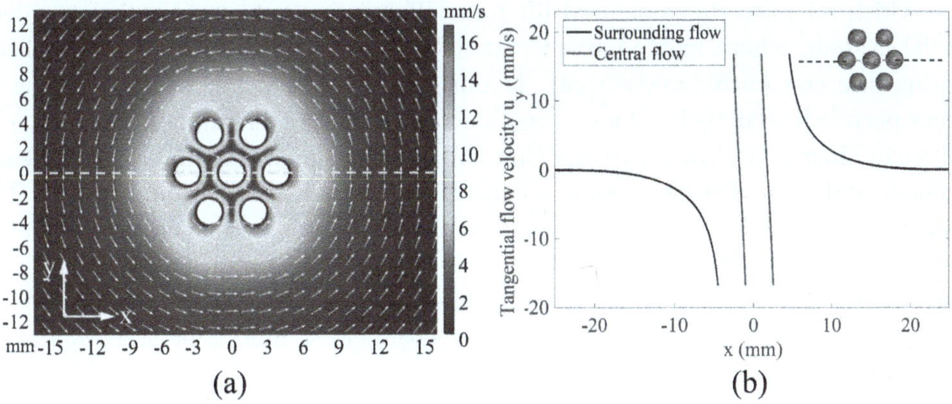

Figure 5.5 (a) Simulated fluid flow induced by the assembled rotating droplets beneath the air-liquid interface. The angular velocity of droplets was set at 6π rad/s. Arrows show the fluid direction, and the color profile denotes the magnitude of the flow velocity (mm/s). (b) Tangential velocity (u_y) of the induced rotational flow along the X-axis (dashed line in (a)). Central flow refers to the induced flow between two droplets, while the surrounding flow refers to the flow outside the pattern. The missing segments in the profile are caused by the presence of three droplets positioned along the X-axis.

where $\boldsymbol{m}_d$ is the magnetic dipole moment of a droplet and is aligned with the external field, ϕ is the angle between the Z-axis and the center vector $\boldsymbol{r}$ of two neighboring droplets. During experiments, all droplets are beneath the air-liquid interface, and the centers of all droplets are coplanar ($\phi = \pi/2$). Therefore, the magnetic force between droplets is obtained by derivation, as

$$F_m = \frac{\partial U}{\partial r}\bigg|_{\phi=\pi/2} = -\frac{3\mu_o m_d^2}{4\pi r^4}\left(\frac{3\cos^2\theta - 1}{2}\right) \tag{5.7}$$

The above analysis indicates that the magnetic interaction can be attractive or repulsive by changing the precession angle θ of the external field, *i.e.*, attractive if $54.74° < \theta < 90°$ and repulsive if $0° < \theta < 54.74°$. The dipolar interaction between droplets averages to zero at a specific precession angle of 54.74°. This adjustable magnetic interaction is distinct from a permanent magnet-based actuation system, where the magnetic interactions between building blocks can only be attractive [19, 29].

When a droplet is energized by the magnetic field, it creates a surrounding rotational flow and moves in a flow created by the other droplets in the assembly. Figure 5.5a shows the simulation results of the induced fluid flow by the assembled pattern, which reveals the presence of two rotational flows: one inside the pattern (central flow) and one outside the pattern (surrounding flow). Figure 5.5b shows the tangential velocity (u_y) of the induced flow along the X-axis, indicating that the flow direction reverses from the central area to the surrounding area. The velocity of the surrounding flow decays while such change becomes almost linear in the central area. The hydrodynamic interactions between droplets are mainly governed by the Magnus effect, which refers to the generated lift force. This is in contrast to rotating objects in a 2D system, where hydrodynamic attraction dominates the Magnus repulsion, resulting in a co-rotating system [30]. In our system, each droplet experiences a repulsion perpendicular to the local direction of flow. However, numerical simulation results by Climent *et al.* demonstrate that two rotating spheres do not experience any repulsion, and their distance remains constant at zero Reynolds number [31]. This simulation is governed by the Stokes equation, and there is no inertia term involved. When finite fluid inertia is included in the system (*e.g.*, $Re = 0.25$), the rotating spheres repel each other. Therefore, the repulsive interaction between droplets arises due to the effect of fluid inertia [32]. The velocity field of fluid generated by the jth droplet can be expressed as

$$\boldsymbol{u}_j(\boldsymbol{x}) = \boldsymbol{\omega}_d \times \boldsymbol{r}_x \left(\frac{a_d}{r_x} \right)^3 \tag{5.8}$$

where $\boldsymbol{r}_x$ represents the position vector defined from the center of the droplet ($r_x = |\boldsymbol{r}_x|$). The hydrodynamic force acting on the ith droplet due to the fluid generated by the jth droplet is given by [33]

$$\mathbf{F}_r = c_f \rho \omega_d^2 \frac{a_d^7 (\mathbf{r}_i - \mathbf{r}_j)}{|\mathbf{r}_i - \mathbf{r}_j|^4} \tag{5.9}$$

where c_f is a constant of proportionality, and $|\mathbf{r}_i - \mathbf{r}_j|$ is the distance between the two droplets. The direction of the vector $|\mathbf{r}_i - \mathbf{r}_j|$ points from the jth to the ith droplet, indicating that the hydrodynamic interaction is repulsive between droplets. Figures 5.6a–c show the hydrodynamic interactions between a pair of rotating droplets. The interaction weakens with an increased separation distance (r, the distance between the center of the two droplets), as seen from the comparison between Figures 5.6a and 5.6b. With an increase in the angular velocity, the interaction between the droplets intensifies, leading to the coupling between induced flows as depicted in Figure 5.6c. The simulated hydrodynamic repulsive forces at various separation distances and angular velocities are shown in Figure 5.6d. Based on Eq. (5.9), the repulsive force has a relationship of $F_r \propto \omega_d^2/r^3$, and the simulation results confirm our analysis. In Eq. (5.9), we have only considered the interactions between two rotating droplets. Since $F_r \propto r^{-3}$, the influence from non-neighboring droplets becomes negligible. Therefore, when calculating the F_r exerted on a droplet, only the forces from neighboring droplets should be considered.

An air-liquid interface around a millimeter-scale floating object deforms and contains either an upward or downward meniscus [34]. The type of meniscus determines the interactions between two floating objects; like menisci attract while unlike menisci repel, which is due to capillarity. The capillary interactions between two droplets in our system are attractive, as they have the same menisci. There are two contributions to the free energy of interaction between the droplets: the surface free energy and the gravitational energy. These energies decrease as the distance between the droplets is reduced [35]. The capillary attraction between two droplets is expressed as [36, 37]

$$F_c = \left(\frac{r}{L_c} \right)^{-\frac{1}{2}} \cdot \frac{\gamma}{2} B^2 C^2 e^{(-r/L_c)} \tag{5.10}$$

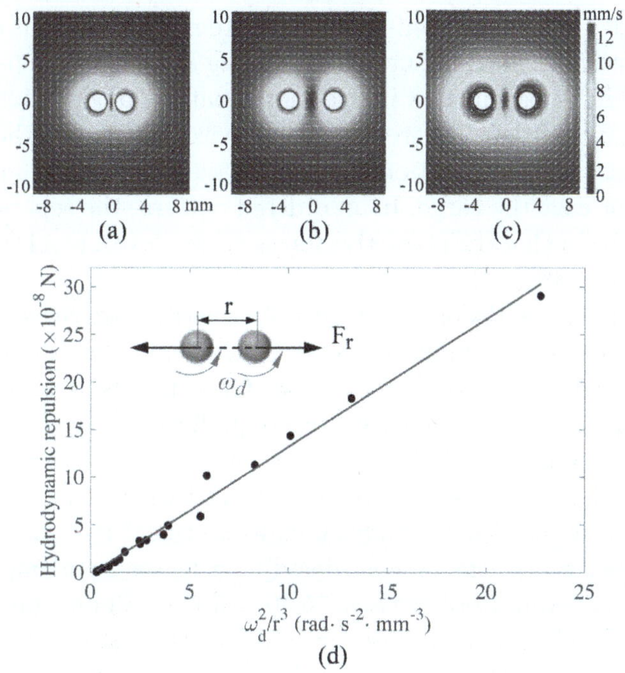

Figure 5.6 Simulation results of the induced fluid flow and hydrodynamic interactions between two rotating droplets beneath the air-fluid interface. (a)–(c) Induced fluid flow with different separation distances (r) and angular velocities (ω_d): (a) $r = 3$ mm, $\omega_d = 4\pi$ rad/s; (b) $r = 5$ mm, $\omega_d = 4\pi$ rad/s; (c) $r = 5$ mm, $\omega_d = 6\pi$ rad/s. (d) Simulated hydrodynamic repulsive forces (F_r) between droplets. The separation distance r was set as 2.5–5 mm, and angular velocities ω_d were set as 2π rad/s, 4π rad/s, and 6π rad/s. Points are data from simulation results, and the line shows the linear fit.

where $\gamma = 1.17 \times 10^{-2} N/m$ is the surface tension of the surrounding liquid (dibenzyl ether), $L_c = \sqrt{\gamma/\rho g}$ is the capillary length and has a value of 1.04 mm. B and C are two dimensionless parameters and are calculated to be 0.85 and 3 [36, 37]. The capillary interaction can be controlled by adjusting the value of γ, which can be achieved by adding surfactants to decrease the surface tension. This will lead to a reduction in the capillary attraction between droplets, resulting in a larger separation distance between droplets. To compensate the attractive forces between droplets, a stronger field gradient is needed to achieve the same pattern. Based on the simulated results shown in Figure 5.4, one way to achieve this is by decreasing the height of the needle. Additionally, a magnetic force induced by the field gradient is exerted on the droplets, pointing toward the center of the pattern, as

$$\mathbf{F}_{\nabla B} = \nabla(\mathbf{m}_d \cdot B) \tag{5.11}$$

where the values of the field gradient are obtained from simulation results (Figure 5.4).

The above simulations and mathematical modeling investigate the different forces acting on the droplets, which is essential for fundamentally understanding the interactions inside the dynamic self-assembly system. This analysis can also guide the tuning of the system's behavior, such as expanding and shrinking patterns. Additionally, by adjusting the parameters in the mathematical model, similar self-assembly systems can be modeled in different fluidic environments. Furthermore, for cargo transportation tasks, the separation distance between droplets should be taken into account to trap or cage the cargo. In an ordered pattern, the separation distance can be estimated by balancing the attractive forces (Eqs. (5.10), (5.11)) and the repulsive forces (Eqs. (5.7), (5.9)).

A dynamically stable droplet pattern is an energy-dissipative structure that requires a continuous energy input (precessing field), and the interactions among the droplets to dominate the pattern formation. Once the external field is turned off, the droplets become a non-dissipative state (equilibrium state), causing the ordered dynamic patterns to be disrupted. In our previous work, we demonstrated that a dynamic pattern with a similar shape could be formed without the use of a needle [38]. In this study, the induced field gradient plays a crucial role in attracting droplets toward the needle, which can be considered as a factor that amplifies the induced attractive forces between droplets (Eqs. (5.10), (5.11)). Similar fundamental interactions among the droplets remain the same, and only the magnitude of the interactions is altered. Consequently, the needle-guided approach enables the formation of a dynamically self-assembled droplet pattern in the dissipative state.

5.4 OPTIMAL SELF-ASSEMBLY AND PATH PLANNING

5.4.1 Optimized Formation of Self-Assembled Pattern

To form an ordered assembled pattern, all droplets require a gathered state to achieve sufficient interactions. The iron needle is manipulated to attract all the droplets using the induced magnetic field gradient around the tip. To ensure an effective gathering process, it is necessary to study the path planning of the needle. The gathering process can be seen as a variant of the Open-Loop Travelling Salesman Problem (OTSP), where the needle attracts all the droplets without revisiting its starting position. The path of the needle is planned based on the hybrid Genetic algorithm [39]. The applied method is based on a parallel implementation of a multi-population steady-state Genetic algorithm involving local search heuristics. It uses a variant of the maximal preservative crossover and the double-bridge move mutation. After conducting iterative calculations, an optimal path is obtained for guiding the needle. The path connects all the droplets and has the shortest length.

Figure 5.7 illustrates the process of droplet gathering and pattern formation, which involves four major procedures:

(1) Acquisition of droplet positions. In Figure 5.7a, the positions of all droplets are obtained using image processing based on color segmentation and threshold. The center of each droplet represents its position.

(2) The droplet positions serve as input for generating a group of random paths, which are compared to obtain an optimized path using the Genetic algorithm.

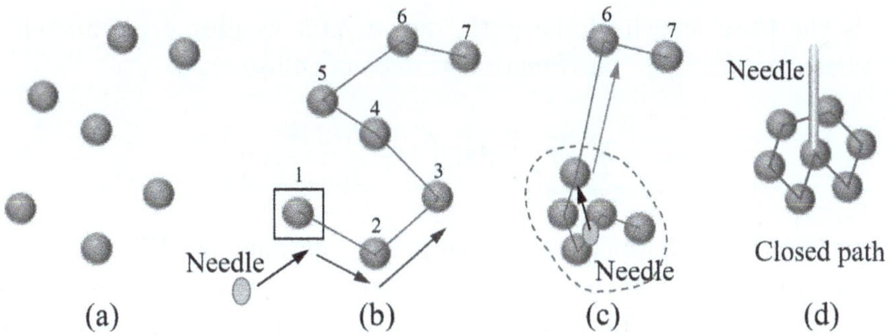

Figure 5.7 Schematic illustration of the gathering and formation of an ordered pattern. (a) The positions of droplets are tracked. (b) The optimal path obtained by iterative calculation. (c) Gathering of droplets by steering the needle along the path. (d) The ordered pattern is formed, and then the path is closed.

The centers of droplets are then connected to form the optimized path, as shown in Figure 5.7b.

(3) The needle is controlled along the optimized path to attract all droplets toward a common point, as depicted in Figure 5.7c. The five droplets enclosed by the dashed circles are moving with the needle toward the sixth droplet.

(4) All droplets are gathered together and the interactions between them are re-balanced to form an ordered pattern gradually. The center of the pattern is defined as the center of all the assembled droplets. The path is closed once the distance between the first and the last droplet falls below a threshold value r_s, as shown in Figure 5.7d.

Following the process of dynamic self-assembly, the resulting ordered pattern is ready to be navigated to perform cargo manipulation tasks.

5.4.2 Optimal Obstacle-Avoidance Path Planning

In intricate surroundings, it is necessary for a mobile object to avoid obstacles during its navigation. We utilize evolutionary algorithms [40] and a path-planning method based on PSO to avoid static obstacles while minimizing the length of the path planned. Our algorithm constructs a smooth third-order spline curve as the path, comprising of n segments and $n+1$ waypoints. The start and the end waypoints (1st and $(n+1)$th) are defined by the position of the assembled pattern and the destination, respectively. The goal of our path planning is to locate M ($M \ll n$) nodes that can interpolate the spline path, minimize the path length, and avoid collisions with obstacles. To simplify this optimization problem, we set the M nodes distribute uniformly along the X-axis between the start and endpoints. Then the y coordinates of the M nodes are determined to minimize the following cost function,

$$Cost = L \times (1 + c_v \times V) \tag{5.12}$$

where L is the total length of the path, and c_v is a weighting parameter used to penalize obstacle collisions. The function V detects collisions, as

$$V = \sum_{j=1}^{N} \sum_{k=1}^{n-1} \left\{ \text{Max} \left(1 - \frac{d(k,j)}{R_c(j)}, 0 \right) \right\} \tag{5.13}$$

where N represents the number of obstacles in the environment, $d(k, j)$ is the distance between the kth waypoint of the path and the jth obstacle. $R_c(j)$ is the radius of the range of the jth obstacle. The function $\text{Max}(a, 0)$ returns the larger value between a and 0. If $\text{Max}(a, 0) > 0$, it indicates that a collision has occurred, and V gives the total level of collisions.

The PSO is employed to solve multi-variable nonlinear optimization problems. The algorithm involves the evolution of a large population of particles to optimize a cost function [41]. The number of particles and generations are denoted as P and G, respectively, where $P \in \mathbb{N}^+$ and $G \in \mathbb{N}^+$. Each particle in the population, denoted as the pth particle at the gth generation, stores its current solution $\mathbf{s}_p^g$, representing the y coordinates of M nodes, as well as its current velocity $\mathbf{v}_p^g$. The best solution obtained by the pth particle until the gth generation is stored in $\hat{\mathbf{s}}_p$. The global best solution found in the swarm population is stored in $\hat{\mathbf{gb}}$, and this optimal solution is updated to all particles. The solution and velocity of each particle are updated using equations below,

$$\begin{cases} \mathbf{v}_p^{g+1} = w\mathbf{v}_p^g + c_1 r_1 (\hat{\mathbf{s}}_p - \mathbf{s}_p^g) + c_2 r_2 (\hat{\mathbf{gb}} - \mathbf{s}_p^g) \\ \mathbf{s}_p^{g+1} = \mathbf{s}_p^g + \mathbf{v}_p^{g+1} \end{cases} \tag{5.14}$$

where w is the inertia weight, c_1, c_2 are the personal and global learning coefficients. To accelerate the convergence speed, we initialize the global best as the straight line from the start point to the endpoint. To reduce the computation time, we set the number of nodes M as 5. We set the number of iterations n as 300 to obtain a smooth path.

5.4.3 Validation of the Path Planning

It is necessary to identify the environment before performing navigation and manipulation tasks. The process of environment registration is shown in Figures 5.8a and 5.8b, where an ordered pattern of five droplets and six pillars are used as the object and obstacles, respectively. The image processing starts with color segmentation. The droplets (red) and obstacles (blue) were separated, and the position of the pattern was tracked. Afterwards, a threshold was utilized to eliminate the background and transform the original image into a binary image, where the obstacles were converted to white regions (Figure 5.8b). Subsequently, the minimum bounding boxes for all obstacles were computed. Before running the navigation algorithm, it's essential to mark the obstacles so that the path planning algorithm can function properly. Because the position of the pattern was determined by the center of five droplets, a safety region with a distance of d_{sa} was added to the bounding boxes to prevent collisions.

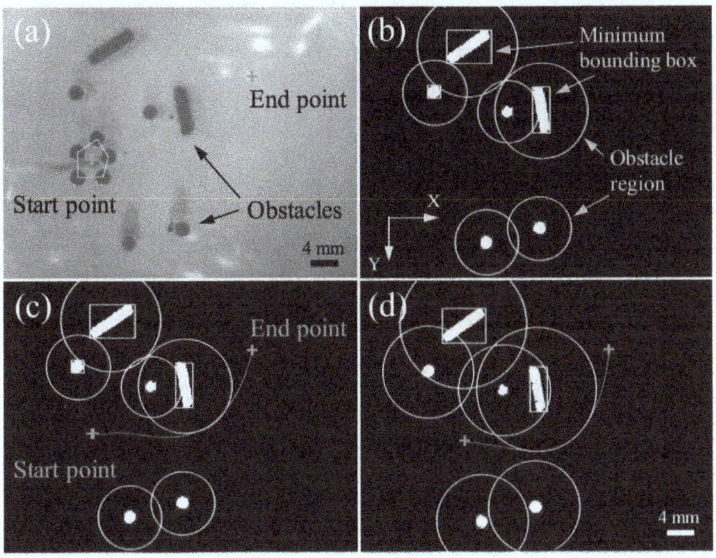

Figure 5.8 Validation of the obstacle-avoidance path planner. (a) The captured experimental scenario. The start point is defined as the center of the pattern. (b) Results of environment registration. (c) and (d) show the two path planning results with different d_{sa}.

The effectiveness of the PSO-based optimal path planning was tested. The parameters of PSO were adjusted because of the trade-off between the computation time and the optimal solution. Increasing the values of P and G leads to a more optimized solution but at the cost of longer computation time [42]. Parameter tuning should be based on specific requirements. In our cases, the minimum requirement is to achieve collision-free navigation of the assembled droplets. After trials with different parameters, the P and G were set as 200 and 50, respectively. As illustrated in Figure 5.8c, the start point was set as the position of the pattern, and the six obstacle regions were calculated. After determining the destination (endpoint), we computed the path while avoiding obstacles. We set d_{sa} to 1.2 times the distance between a droplet and the pattern's center. In order to navigate assembled droplets with a larger pattern, we increased d_{sa} to avoid collisions. As shown in Figure 5.8d, the d_{sa} was increased to 1.5 times the distance, and the optimized path was successfully generated.

To further validate the performance of the PSO-based path planning, a comparison with A* program was conducted (Figure 5.9). A* is a graph traversal and grid-based search algorithm that aims to find the path to a given goal node with the lowest cost [43]. In our system, the feedback image has a resolution of 1600×1200, which corresponds to over 1.92 million pixels. Due to the high resolution, it took more than 10 minutes to complete the A*-based path planning, while the PSO-based calculation only required 20–30 seconds. The computation time can be adjusted by modifying the parameters according to the requirement. In our experiments, the computation time was about 5 s with $P = 200$ and $G = 50$. Additionally, the PSO-based

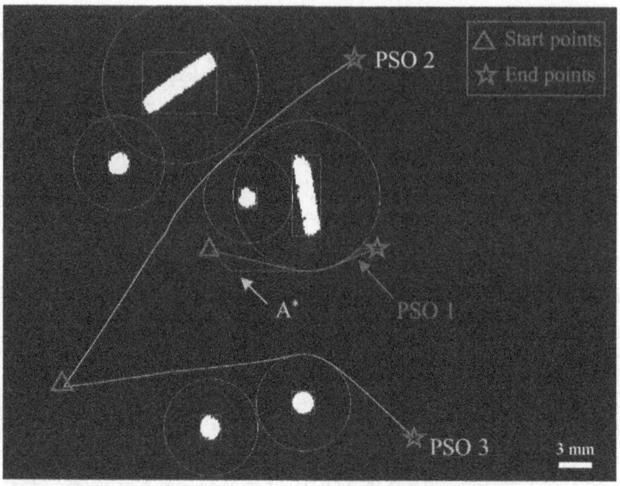

Figure 5.9 The comparison of A*-based and PSO-based path planning.

paths are smoother than those produced by A*, which is beneficial for continuous pattern manipulation.

5.5 EXPERIMENTAL RESULTS AND DISCUSSION

In this section, we demonstrate the optimized process of dynamic self-assembly of droplets, and the ordered pattern was tuned to exhibit reversibly shrinking and expanding. Experimental results for cargo trapping, caging, and transportation using assembled patterns are presented, which has been conducted with integrated obstacle-avoidance capability.

5.5.1 Formation of Self-Assembled Droplets

Each droplet in the acquired images was tracked through mainly three steps of image processing: (1) color segmentation to extract droplets from the background; (2) adding an area threshold to eliminate noise signals; (3) coordinates of the center of all droplets were recognized and tracked using the mean shift tracking algorithm [44]. The input positions for the Genetic algorithm were determined based on the tracked position of the droplets. The path was generated and updated in real-time, and marked with the blue line, as shown in Figure 5.10a. At $t = 8$ s, the needle was controlled to approach the first droplet, which was then attracted and navigated toward the second droplet. Energized by the precessing field, all droplets were rotating and affected by neighboring droplets simultaneously. Meanwhile, the optimized path was updated based on the newly tracked positions. After the gathering process ($t = 32$ s), the needle was stopped, and all interactions between droplets gradually re-balanced.

Here, we set two evaluation criteria to estimate if an ordered, stable pattern is formed: (1) the separation distance between the first and the last droplet (r_{max}) in the optimized path; (2) changes of the center of the pattern (r_c) in a time duration t_s. r_c is

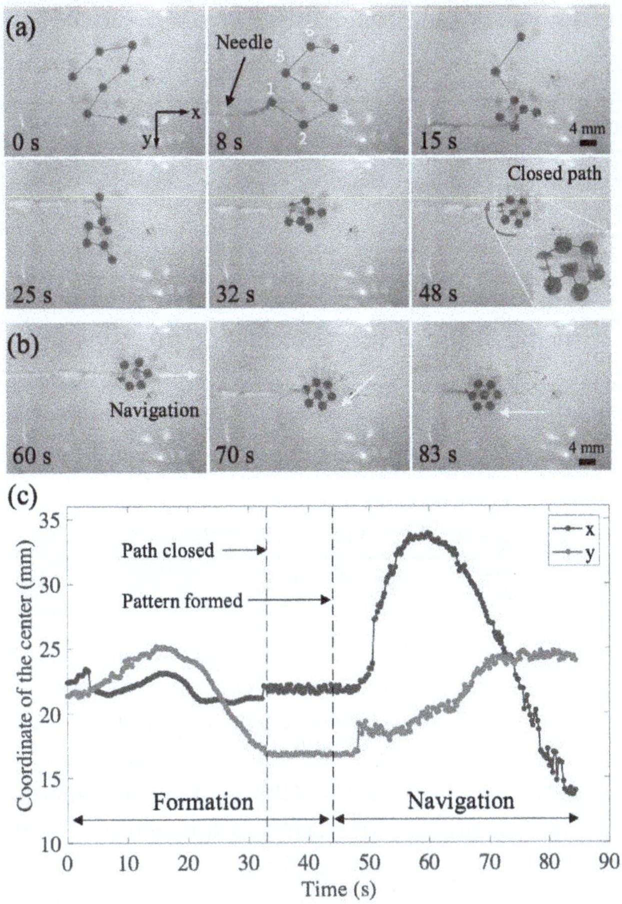

Figure 5.10 (a) Formation process of an ordered pattern guided by the optimized path. The path closed at t = 48 s. (b) Navigation of the assembled droplets. The trajectory is marked by the red line. Applied field parameters: B = 7 mT, f = 4 Hz, $\theta = 30°$. (c) The change of the coordinate of the assembled pattern during the formation and navigation process.

defined as the averaged coordinate of all droplets. In the planned path, the maximum distance occurs between the first and the last droplet. Therefore, the gathering status of droplets can be estimated by monitoring r_{max}. If the value of r_{max} is less than a threshold value r_s, which is defined as several times the diameter of the droplet, the path will be closed, signaling that all the droplets are gathered. As a result of the attraction force from the needle, r_c coincides with the projection of the needle in the XY-plane. Thus, if r_c remains stable without significant disturbances for a time duration longer than t_s, it indicates that successful formation has been achieved. Two criteria are applied to determine the disturbance of r_c: (1) The distance between continuously detected r_c is below a value d_{pf}, as $\sqrt{(x_i - x_{i-1})^2 + (y_i - y_{i-1})^2} < d_{pf}$, then the duration time starts counting; (2) To eliminate accumulated error, the position of latter points must in a range of d_{pf}, compared to all the former points that

TABLE 5.1 Time requirement of forming ordered patterns with/without the assistance of the needle

Number	4	5	6	7	9	13
Times (s) without N	112.8	131.6	128.7	135.7	142	165.5
Time (s) with N	28.5	32.3	34.1	38.5	33.2	42.8
Efficiency improvement	74.73%	75.46%	73.50%	71.62%	76.62%	74.14%

after counting the duration time, as

$$\sum_{j=1}^{i-1} \frac{\sqrt{(x_i - x_j)^2 + (y_i - y_j)^2}}{i-1} < d_{pf} \tag{5.15}$$

where the coordination of the first point is (x_1, y_1). If the coordinate of r_c fails to satisfy either of the two criteria, the duration time stops counting. Once the ordered pattern is formed, the status *SU-AS* (successful assembly) is displayed on the user interface. In this case (Figure 5.10a), we set the $r_s = 4$ mm, *i.e.*, two times the diameter of the droplet, $t_s = 10$ s, and $d_{pf} = 2$ mm. The path generated by the droplets closed at $t = 33$ s, and an ordered pattern was formed at $t = 43$ s. The assembled droplets were then navigated by following the magnetized needle, as shown in Figure 5.10b. Figure 5.10c shows the variation of r_c during the process of pattern formation and navigation. r_c stabilized after the path closed and the pattern was formed after 10 s. Experiments demonstrate the effectiveness of our evaluation criteria during the pattern formation.

By utilizing the magnetized needle, the time required for forming ordered patterns will be reduced. Table 5.1 presents a comparison of the time needed to form various patterns. When the magnetized needle was not used, the assembly process for all patterns took more than 100 s, and the time increased as the number of droplets increased. However, using the needle reduced the formation time by over 70%, to approximately 30–40 s. According to the analysis in Eqs. (5.7)–(5.10), the interactions between droplets decrease significantly as the separation distance increases. Initially, during the self-assembly process, the needle attracts all the droplets, and the interactions between them remain strong, which leads to an acceleration of the process. During the process of pattern formation, the height of the needle was adjusted within a range of 4–14 mm. If the height of the needle exceeded 20 mm, the field gradient became insufficient to collect the droplets effectively, resulting in an extremely low formation efficiency. The applied field strength and input frequency were within the ranges of 5–9 mT and 3–6 Hz, respectively. If a low field strength is combined with a high actuation frequency (*e.g.*, 4 mT, 8 Hz), it can cause the step-out of the droplets, meaning that their rotation becomes asynchronous with the applied field. The back-and-forth motion significantly disrupts the hydrodynamic interaction between droplets, ultimately causing the assembly process to fail.

In our previous study, we showed that comparable patterns could be produced without the use of a magnetized needle [38]. Since weak interactions between droplets lead to the failure of self-assembly, this self-assembly system requires a limited initial distance between droplets (<15 mm, ~8 body lengths of a droplet). In this study, the usage of a needle increased the efficiency of pattern formation by gathering all droplets within a certain range, regardless of their initial positions. The field gradient near the needle provided an attractive force to the droplets. According to the mathematical modeling in Eqs. (5.7) and (5.9)–(5.11), such an attractive force can be treated as a factor to enhance the attractive forces between droplets. The fundamental interactions among droplets did not undergo significant changes. Moreover, the ordered patterns formed due to interactions between droplets, rather than the attractive force from the magnetized needle. The needle was used to gather droplets and improve the time efficiency of the self-assembly process. Therefore, the assembly process was governed by dynamic self-assembly, yielding the self-assembled droplet patterns.

5.5.2 Tuning of an Ordered Pattern

The ordered pattern can be adjusted in a reversible manner by manipulating both the induced field gradient and the interactions between the droplets. According to the simulation presented in Figure 5.4, adjusting the height of the needle can alter the gradient. As shown in Figure 5.11a, the assembly pattern exhibited shrinkage when the distance between the interface and the needle decreased due to the increased field gradient (0–15 s). Conversely, increasing the distance between the interface and the needle causes the pattern to expand (15–27 s). Additionally, the interactions between droplets can significantly impact the pattern. To gain a better estimation of these interactions, we experimentally investigated the relationship between the input parameters of magnetic fields (frequency, precession angle) and the angular velocity of droplets, as shown in Figure 5.11b. The angular velocity increases with increasing input frequency and precession angle, showing good agreement with the analysis of Eqs. (5.1)–(5.5). However, when θ exceeds 60°, the velocity decreases due to the fragmentation of particle chains under high input θ. In a low-Reynolds-number regime, a rotating nanoparticle chain experiences two major torques: magnetic torque and hydrodynamic torque, which counterbalance each other [45, 46]. As the input angle θ increases, the velocity v_N also increases, leading to a corresponding increase in the viscous drag torque until it reaches a critical value where it becomes stronger than the magnetic torque [47]. The particle chains are no longer stable and undergo fragmentation, causing a decrease in both chain length ($(2N + 1) \times 2a$) and the velocity at the end of the chain ($v_N = 2Na\omega \sin\theta$). Based on Eq. (5.2), the decrease in friction force results in a lower angular velocity. In analyzing Eqs. (5.1)–(5.5), we do not consider fragmentation, which resulted in differences between the model and experimental results. Figure 5.11c illustrates the relationship between the height of the needle and the mean separation distance of droplets. The mean separation

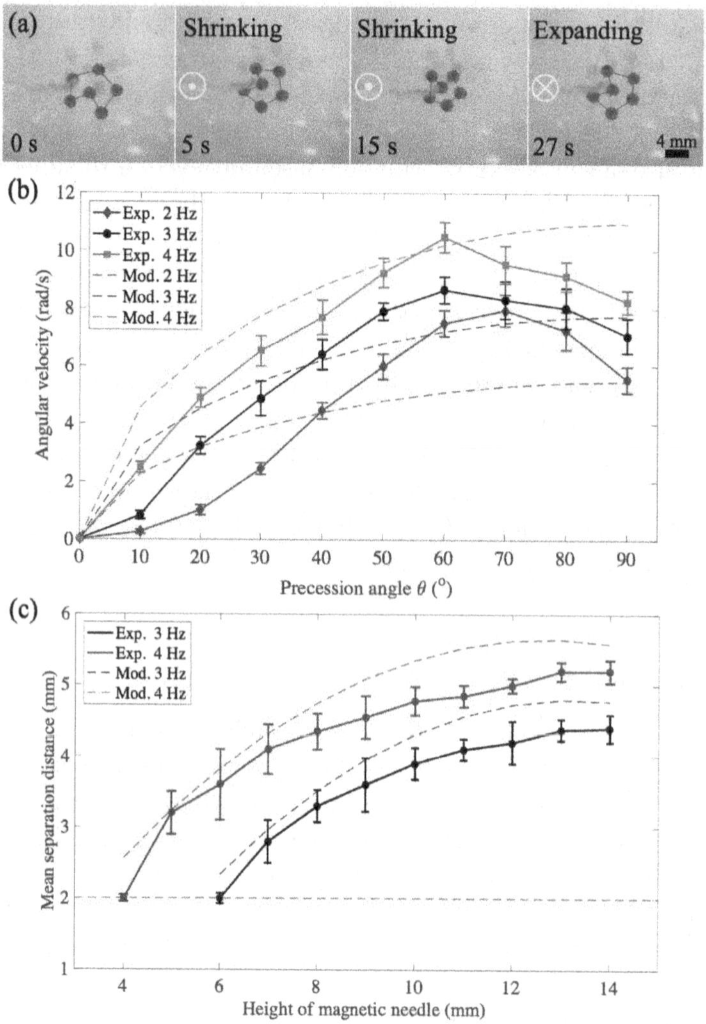

Figure 5.11 (a) Reversible pattern tuned by adjusting the distance between the interface and the magnetized needle. ⊙ and ⊗ indicate the needle's direction of movement, *i.e.*, close to and away from the interface, respectively. The applied field parameters are $f = 3$ Hz and $\theta = 30°$. (b) The angular velocity of droplets (ω_d) versus input precession angles (θ) at frequencies of 2–4 Hz. The results from experiments and the mathematical model are denoted by Exp. and Mod., respectively. (c) The relationship between the mean separation distance ($\overline{r}$) and the height of the magnetized needle (H) at input frequencies of 3 Hz and 4 Hz. All error bars represent the standard deviation obtained from three experiments.

distance, denoted by $\overline{r}$, is the average distance between neighboring droplets. The height, denoted by H, is defined as the distance between the interface and the tip of the needle. Based on Eqs. (5.5) and (5.9), the hydrodynamic repulsive force has a relationship of $F_r \propto \omega \sin(\theta)/r^3$. Hence, increasing the input frequency results in a larger mean separation distance. Moreover, there exists a limit to the minimum mean separation distance, as indicated by the red line in Figure 5.11c, which represents a scenario in which all droplets are in contact with their neighboring droplets. Using the needle improves the efficiency of the reversible pattern expansion in comparison to our previous work. It took approximately 150 s to complete the shrinking-expanding cycle by adjusting the input precession angle ($\overline{r}$ ranges from ~2.5–4.0 mm) [38]. However, by adjusting the height of the needle, the reversible process could be completed in only around 30 s ($\overline{r}$ ranges from ~2.8–5.0 mm).

5.5.3 Cargo Trapping and Transportation

The simulation results in Figure 5.5 demonstrate the occurrence of a localized rotational flow around the ordered pattern. A cargo subjected to the flow experiences a trapping force, which is generated from the inward hydrodynamic force in the flow regions of high vorticity [48]. In addition, the air-liquid interface was influenced by the gravitational force of the droplets: the interface around a droplet was deformed to menisci. A cargo in the menisci experiences a horizontal force and moves toward the droplet [36]. Figure 5.12a illustrates the fluidic trapping and subsequent cargo transportation processes. The polypropylene cargo has dimensions of 2 mm × 2 mm × 1.5 mm. It was situated beneath the air-liquid interface. Four steps were conducted during the process.

(1) The four droplets were gathered and assembled.

(2) The assembled droplets were navigated toward the cargo.

(3) Trapping of the cargo ($t = 78$ s). The induced flow around the pattern caused the cargo to move along the streamlines. The trapping force leads to a decrease in the distance between the cargo and the droplets. Finally, the cargo was trapped and began to orbit around the pattern ($t = 95$ s). To evaluate the trapping status, two criteria were established. The first criterion is the distance between the center of the pattern (r_c) and the cargo. If this distance remains below a predetermined range d_{tr}, a timer starts counting. The timer will stop once the distance exceeds d_{tr}. Since the trapping process is conducted in a static environment, no significant disturbances will affect the process. The second criterion was the time duration. When the timer had a value greater than t_{tr}, the status *SU-TR* (successfully trapped) will be displayed on the user interface. During the experiment, d_{tr} and t_{tr} were set to 8 mm and 15 s, respectively.

(4) The cargo was transported to its destination in a non-contact way. Figure 5.12b illustrates the positions of r_c and the cargo, as well as the distance between them (red line), during different stages of the process, namely trapping, trapped, and transport. The distance between r_c and the cargo decreased gradually during the trapping stage until it reached approximately 5 mm. During transportation, the distance showed slight fluctuations due to drag from the translational motion.

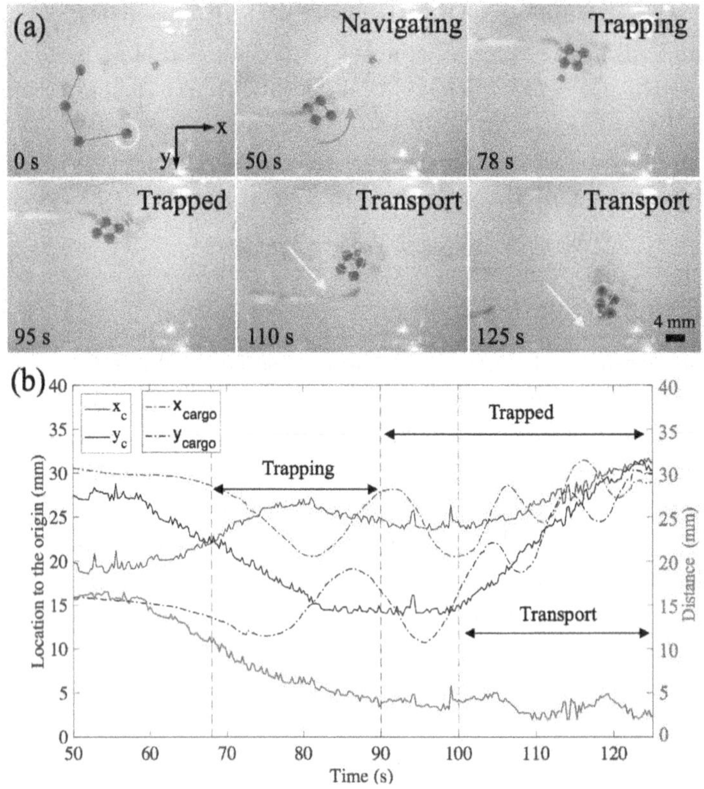

Figure 5.12 Trapping and transportation of cargo. (a) The trapping and transportation process. The green curve represents the trajectory of the cargo, while the yellow arrows indicate the navigation direction of the droplets. Applied field parameters are $B = 7$ mT, $f = 4$ Hz, and $\theta = 30°$. (b) Location of both the assembled droplets and the cargo. The red line plots the distance between the cargo and the center of the pattern.

Cargo transportation can also be achieved by caging the cargo at the center of the pattern. As illustrated in Figure 5.13, where the cargo was successfully trapped at $t = 50$ s. The pattern then expanded to ensure sufficient separation distance between droplets. Based on the characterization results in Figure 5.11, $\overline{r}$ was adjusted to 4.5 mm and cargo was successfully caged at $t = 87.5$ s. The pattern then shrank to prevent releasing of the cargo. Finally, the cargo was transported to the desired location at $t = 103$ s. As observed in simulations shown in Figure 5.5, the rotation direction of the cargo was found to be opposite to that of the rotating droplets due to the induced flow. The two cargo transportation methods have their unique advantages. The trapping method eliminates the need for pattern tuning and offers higher time-efficiency. Additionally, it provides non-contact features that help protect the cargo from surface damage. The caged cargo has a lower risk of accidental release (*e.g.*, excessive drag force), making it a more reliable option for performing tasks in environments with disturbances. In comparison to our previous work [38], the cargo transportation tasks were completed with high time efficiency, due to the effective pattern formation and reversible expansion we showcased in 5.5.1 and 5.5.2.

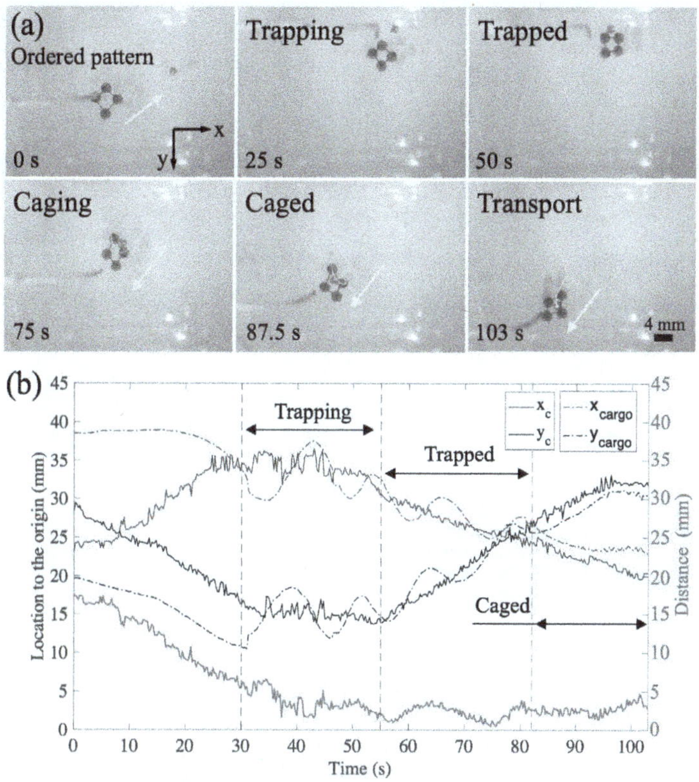

Figure 5.13 Trapping, caging, and transportation of cargo. (a) The green curve illustrates the path of the cargo, while the yellow arrows indicate the navigation direction of the droplets. The applied field parameters are $B = 7$ mT, $f = 5$ Hz, and $\theta = 30°$. (b) The location of the assembled droplets and the cargo. The red line represents the distance between the cargo and the center of the pattern.

In the first scenario, the cargo was primarily trapped by hydrodynamic interactions from the induced fluid and capillary interactions from the menisci. As discussed in Eqs. (5.8)–(5.10), the hydrodynamic interaction has a longer range compared to the capillary attraction between the cargo and droplets [49]. To begin the cargo release process, the first step is to disrupt the induced fluid flow. This can be achieved by setting the input parameter θ to 0. The input field becomes a static field that is perpendicular to the air-liquid interface, and the trapping force of the fluid disappears. The second step involves moving the assembled droplets away from the cargo. By suddenly increasing the distance between the droplets and the cargo, the capillary attraction decayed and the cargo could be released [50]. In the second scenario, a similar approach to our previous work could be utilized to release a caged cargo [38]. By expanding the pattern, the cargo can be released from the central region of the assembled droplets. Following the same two processes of the first trapping case, cargo can be released near the target area. The aforementioned release strategies suggest that the precision of cargo placement is primarily influenced by the induced

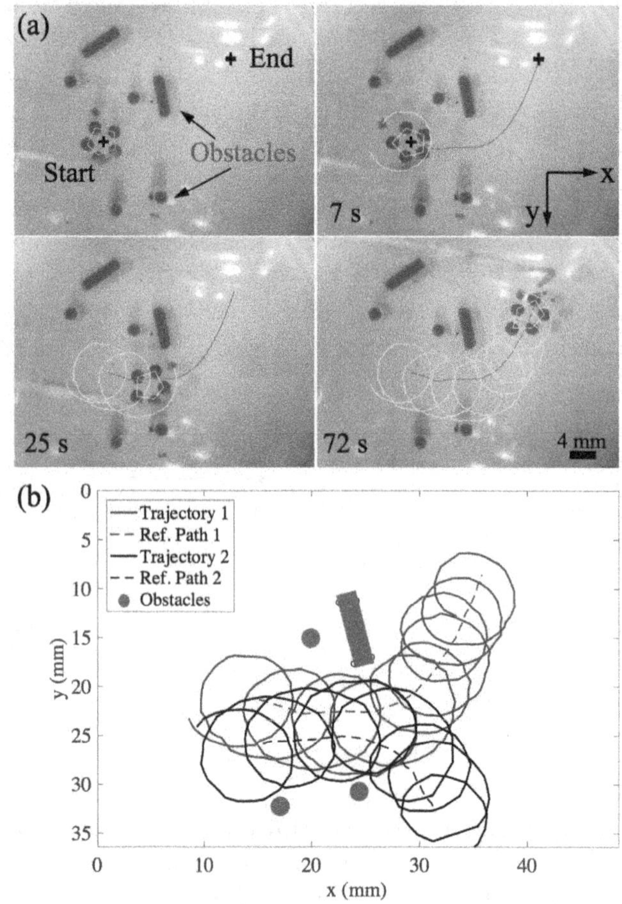

Figure 5.14 Experimental results of the cargo transportation guided by the obstacle-avoidance planned path. (a) Trapping and transportation process. The cargo was successfully trapped and transported to the destination at t = 72 s. The green curve represents the trajectory of the cargo. Applied field parameters in (a) and (b): B = 6 mT, f = 4 Hz, θ = 40°. (b) Obstacle positions and cargo trajectory during the transportation process. The experiment shown in (a) corresponds to the first trajectory.

flow around the pattern. Quickly navigating the droplets away from the cargo can help enhance precision.

5.5.4 Obstacle-Avoidance Cargo Transportation

Experiments were conducted to demonstrate cargo transportation using an obstacle-avoided preplanned path, as shown in Figure 5.14a. The four standing pillars were of the same height as the air-fluid interface, while the two horizontally placed pillars were at the bottom of the fluid. The start point of the path was determined by the cargo's position, while the endpoint was manually selected from the real-time image. The optimized path generated by the PSO-based path planner is shown by the red

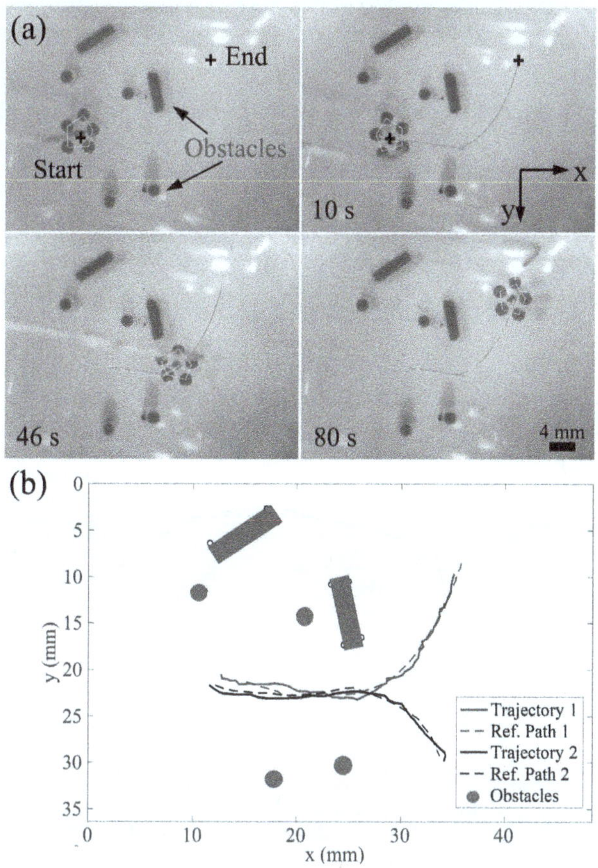

Figure 5.15 (a) Cargo caging and transportation process. The cargo was caged and then transported to the destination at $t = 80$ s. The green curve shows the trajectory of the cargo. (b) Positions of the obstacles and trajectory of the cargo during two cargo transportations. The experiment in (a) denotes the first trajectory.

line. During the computation time (~5 s), the assembled droplets were attracted by the needle, and the position of the pattern was considered unchanged. After successfully trapping the cargo, it was transported and simultaneously orbited the pattern. The pattern followed the needle and transported the cargo to the destination ($t = 72$ s). The trajectory of the cargo was compared to the preplanned path (Ref. path) and the position of the obstacles, as shown in Figure 5.14b. The plot indicates that the cargo was transported without any collision. Figure 5.15a illustrates the process of caging and transporting the cargo. First, the cargo was caged using the same method as shown in Figure 5.13a, and then it was transported along a preplanned path. Figure 5.15b demonstrates that the cargo followed the planned path precisely. We conducted cargo transportation experiments in an environment with more crowded obstacles, where the distance between obstacles was smaller than the two times of d_{sa} (Figure 5.16a). To avoid collisions, the path planner generated a path between the field boundary and the obstacles. Experimental results in Figure 5.16b show that

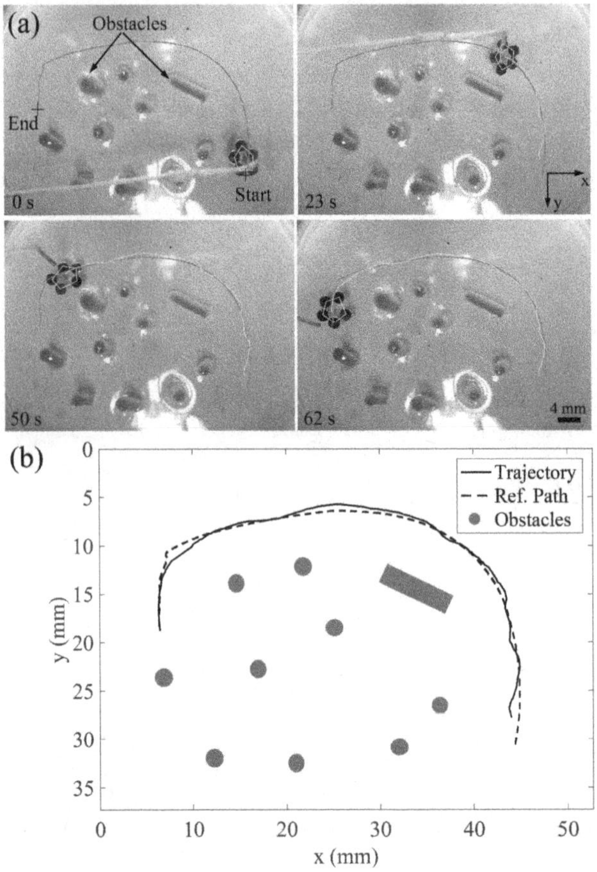

Figure 5.16 (a) Cargo caging and transportation under more crowded obstacle conditions. Applied field parameters: $B = 7$ mT, $f = 4$ Hz, $\theta = 40°$. (b) Positions of the obstacles and trajectory of the cargo during transportation.

the pattern and the transported cargo followed the path and reached the destination without collision. The two cases involved different parameter settings. Since the cargo was orbited during the trapping case, the value of d_{sa} in this case was twice as large as that in the caging case. Disturbances caused by the locomotion of the pattern may affect the trapping stability. Therefore, the number of waypoints n was set as 400 to obtain a sufficient smooth path. In our previous study, we demonstrated the ability to follow a rectangular path with a side length of 10 mm using assembled droplets, which took approximately 400 s [38]. In this work, we significantly improved the time efficiency for transportation. Only 72 s and 80 s were spent for navigating the pattern along the two paths that have the length of 26.4 mm and 29.6 mm, respectively. This represents an improvement in time efficiency of approximately 270% in both cases. Furthermore, the nonlinear attractive force generated by the coil system is difficult to utilize for conducting precise locomotion control. By incorporating a magnetic needle, the droplets can accurately follow the planned path, enhancing their ability for cargo transportation and pattern manipulation within a multi-obstacle environment. The results of our experiments in both cases demonstrate that cargo can be effectively transported using the assembled droplets, which possess the obstacle-avoidance capability. These findings indicate that the assembled droplets can be treated as an effective microrobotic manipulator.

5.6 CONCLUSION

This chapter introduces a control strategy of forming and navigating collective patterns of magnetic droplets at air-liquid interfaces. The collective pattern can be controlled by modulating the inner interactions among droplets, and the navigation and formation efficiency are increased by inducing field gradient near the pattern. The interactions between droplets were studied and mathematically modeled, showing good agreement with experimental results. Dynamic pattern navigation along preplanned paths under precessing magnetic fields was demonstrated by tracking the position of the magnetized needle. By utilizing the reversible pattern expansion and induced fluid flow, cargo can be trapped and further caged before performing transportation tasks. Furthermore, the PSO-based path planner implements the guidance of obstacle-avoidance cargo transportation. The experimental results validate the effectiveness of the proposed strategy in achieving efficient pattern formation, navigation, reversible pattern expansion, and obstacle-avoidance cargo transportation. The proposed method opens new prospects of using self-assembled dynamic pattern as an untethered end-effector for micromanipulation.

Bibliography

[1] Metin Sitti, Hakan Ceylan, Wenqi Hu, Joshua Giltinan, Mehmet Turan, Sehyuk Yim, and Eric Diller. Biomedical applications of untethered mobile milli/microrobots. *Proceedings of the IEEE*, 103(2):205–224, 2015.

[2] Sajad Salmanipour, Omid Youssefi, and Eric Diller. Design of multi-degrees-of-freedom microrobots driven by homogeneous quasi-static magnetic fields. *IEEE Transactions on Robotics*, 37(1):246–256, 2021.

[3] Islam SM Khalil, Anke Klingner, Youssef Hamed, Yehia S Hassan, and Sarthak Misra. Controlled noncontact manipulation of nonmagnetic untethered microbeads orbiting two-tailed soft microrobot. *IEEE Transactions on Robotics*, 36(4):1320–1332, 2020.

[4] Claudio Pacchierotti, Federico Ongaro, Frank Van den Brink, Changkyu Yoon, Domenico Prattichizzo, David H Gracias, and Sarthak Misra. Steering and control of miniaturized untethered soft magnetic grippers with haptic assistance. *IEEE Transactions on Automation Science and Engineering*, 15(1):290–306, 2017.

[5] Yiannis Kantaros, Benjamin V Johnson, Sagar Chowdhury, David J Cappelleri, and Michael M Zavlanos. Control of magnetic microrobot teams for temporal

micromanipulation tasks. *IEEE Transactions on Robotics*, 34(6):1472–1489, 2018.

[6] Wenqi Hu, Guo Zhan Lum, Massimo Mastrangeli, and Metin Sitti. Small-scale soft-bodied robot with multimodal locomotion. *Nature*, 554:81–85, 2018.

[7] Lidong Yang, Qianqian Wang, Chi-Ian Vong, and Li Zhang. A miniature flexible-link magnetic swimming robot with two vibration modes: design, modeling and characterization. *IEEE Robotics and Automation Letters*, 2(4):2024–2031, 2017.

[8] Wuming Jing, Sagar Chowdhury, Maria Guix, Jianxiong Wang, Ze An, Benjamin V Johnson, and David J Cappelleri. A microforce-sensing mobile microrobot for automated micromanipulation tasks. *IEEE Transactions on Automation Science and Engineering*, 16(2):518–530, 2018.

[9] Alper Denasi and Sarthak Misra. Independent and leader–follower control for two magnetic micro-agents. *IEEE Robotics and Automation Letters*, 3(1):218–225, 2018.

[10] Lidong Yang, Qianqian Wang, and Li Zhang. Model-free trajectory tracking control of two-particle magnetic microrobot. *IEEE Transactions on Nanotechnology*, 17(4):697–700, 2018.

[11] Jingjing Bao, Zhan Yang, Masahiro Nakajima, Yajing Shen, Masaru Takeuchi, Qiang Huang, and Toshio Fukuda. Self-actuating asymmetric platinum catalytic mobile nanorobot. *IEEE Transactions on Robotics*, 30(1):33–39, 2013.

[12] Shiva Shahrokhi, Jingang Shi, Benedict Isichei, and Aaron T Becker. Exploiting nonslip wall contacts to position two particles using the same control input. *IEEE Transactions on Robotics*, 35(3):577–588, 2018.

[13] Xiaoguang Dong and Metin Sitti. Controlling two-dimensional collective formation and cooperative behavior of magnetic microrobot swarms. *The International Journal of Robotics Research*, 39(5):617–638, 2020.

[14] Qianqian Wang and Li Zhang. Ultrasound imaging and tracking of micro/nanorobots: From individual to collectives. *IEEE Open Journal of Nanotechnology*, 1:6–17, 2020.

[15] Nahum A Torres and Dan O Popa. Cooperative control of multiple untethered magnetic microrobots using a single magnetic field source. In *Automation Science and Engineering (CASE), 2015 IEEE International Conference on*, pages 1608–1613. IEEE, 2015.

[16] Jiangfan Yu, Ben Wang, Xingzhou Du, Qianqian Wang, and Li Zhang. Ultra-extensible ribbon-like magnetic microswarm. *Nature Communications*, 9, 2018, Art. no. 3260.

[17] Berk Yigit, Yunus Alapan, and Metin Sitti. Programmable collective behavior in dynamically self-assembled mobile microrobotic swarms. *Advanced Science*, 6(6), 2019, Art. no. 1801837.

[18] Jing Yan, Ming Han, Jie Zhang, Cong Xu, Erik Luijten, and Steve Granick. Reconfiguring active particles by electrostatic imbalance. *Nature Materials*, 15(10):1095–1099, 2016.

[19] Wendong Wang, Joshua Giltinan, Svetlana Zakharchenko, and Metin Sitti. Dynamic and programmable self-assembly of micro-rafts at the air-water interface. *Science Advances*, 3(5):e1602522, 2017.

[20] Fernando Martinez-Pedrero, Antonio Ortiz-Ambriz, Ignacio Pagonabarraga, and Pietro Tierno. Colloidal microworms propelling via a cooperative hydrodynamic conveyor belt. *Physical Review Letters*, 115(13), 2015, Art. no. 138301.

[21] Qianqian Wang, Lidong Yang, Jiangfan Yu, Philip Chiu, Y.-P Zheng, and Li Zhang. Real-time magnetic navigation of a rotating colloidal microswarm under ultrasound guidance. *IEEE Transactions on Biomedical Engineering*, 67(12):3403–3412, 2020.

[22] Hong Wang and Martin Pumera. Coordinated behaviors of artificial micro/nanomachines: from mutual interactions to interactions with the environment. *Chemical Society Reviews*, 49:3211–3230, 2020.

[23] Jaakko VI Timonen, Mika Latikka, Ludwik Leibler, Robin HA Ras, and Olli Ikkala. Switchable static and dynamic self-assembly of magnetic droplets on superhydrophobic surfaces. *Science*, 341(6143):253–257, 2013.

[24] Alexey Snezhko and Igor S Aranson. Magnetic manipulation of self-assembled colloidal asters. *Nature Materials*, 10(9):698–703, 2011.

[25] Helena Massana-Cid, Fanlong Meng, Daiki Matsunaga, Ramin Golestanian, and Pietro Tierno. Tunable self-healing of magnetically propelling colloidal carpets. *Nature Communications*, 10(1):2444, 2019.

[26] Andras Z Szeri. *Fluid Film Lubrication.* Cambridge University Press, 2010.

[27] N Lukerchenko, Yu Kvurt, I Keita, Z Chara, and P Vlasak. Drag force, drag torque, and magnus force coefficients of rotating spherical particle moving in fluid. *Particulate Science and Technology*, 30(1):55–67, 2012.

[28] Stefano Giovanazzi, Axel Görlitz, and Tilman Pfau. Tuning the dipolar interaction in quantum gases. *Physical Review Letters*, 89(13):130401, 2002.

[29] Bartosz A Grzybowski, Howard A Stone, and George M Whitesides. Dynamic self-assembly of magnetized, millimetre-sized objects rotating at a liquid–air interface. *Nature*, 405(6790):1033, 2000.

[30] Yusuke Goto and Hajime Tanaka. Purely hydrodynamic ordering of rotating disks at a finite reynolds number. *Nature Communications*, 6:5994, 2015.

[31] Eric Climent, Kyongmin Yeo, Martin R Maxey, and George E Karniadakis. Dynamic self-assembly of spinning particles. *Journal of Fluids Engineering*, 129(4):379–387, 2007.

[32] Jeffrey A Schonberg and EJ Hinch. Inertial migration of a sphere in poiseuille flow. *Journal of Fluid Mechanics*, 203:517–524, 1989.

[33] Bartosz A Grzybowski, Xingyu Jiang, Howard A Stone, and George M Whitesides. Dynamic, self-assembled aggregates of magnetized, millimeter-sized objects rotating at the liquid-air interface: Macroscopic, two-dimensional classical artificial atoms and molecules. *Physical Review E*, 64(1):011603, 2001.

[34] Lorenzo Botto, Eric P Lewandowski, Marcello Cavallaro, and Kathleen J Stebe. Capillary interactions between anisotropic particles. *Soft Matter*, 8(39):9957–9971, 2012.

[35] Bartosz A Grzybowski, Ned Bowden, Francisco Arias, Hong Yang, and George M Whitesides. Modeling of menisci and capillary forces from the millimeter to the micrometer size range. *The Journal of Physical Chemistry B*, 105(2):404–412, 2001.

[36] Dominic Vella and L Mahadevan. The "cheerios effect". *American Journal of Physics*, 73(9):817–825, 2005.

[37] DYC Chan, JD Henry Jr, and LR White. The interaction of colloidal particles collected at fluid interfaces. *Journal of Colloid and Interface Science*, 79(2):410–418, 1981.

[38] Qianqian Wang, Lidong Yang, Ben Wang, Edwin Yu, Jiangfan Yu, and Li Zhang. Collective behavior of reconfigurable magnetic droplets via dynamic self-assembly. *ACS Applied Materials & Interfaces*, 11(1):1630–1637, 2019.

[39] Hung Dinh Nguyen, Ikuo Yoshihara, Kunihito Yamamori, and Moritoshi Yasunaga. Implementation of an effective hybrid ga for large-scale traveling salesman problems. *IEEE Transactions on Systems, Man, and Cybernetics, Part B (Cybernetics)*, 37(1):92–99, 2007.

[40] Ratul Majumdar, Ankur Ghosh, Aveek Kumar Das, Souvik Raha, Koushik Laha, Swagatam Das, and Ajith Abraham. Artificial weed colonies with neighbourhood crowding scheme for multimodal optimization. In *Proceedings of the International Conference on Soft Computing for Problem Solving (SocProS 2011) December 20-22, 2011*, pages 779–787. Springer, 2012.

[41] J Kennedy and R Eberhart. Particle swarm optimization (pso). In *Proc. IEEE International Conference on Neural Networks, Perth, Australia*, pages 1942–1948, 1995.

[42] Lidong Yang, Yabin Zhang, Qianqian Wang, Kai-Fung Chan, and Li Zhang. Automated control of magnetic spore-based microrobot using fluorescence imaging for targeted delivery with cellular resolution. *IEEE Transactions on Automation Science and Engineering*, 17(1):490–501, 2019.

[43] Peter E Hart, Nils J Nilsson, and Bertram Raphael. A formal basis for the heuristic determination of minimum cost paths. *IEEE transactions on Systems Science and Cybernetics*, 4(2):100–107, 1968.

[44] Dorin Comaniciu, Visvanathan Ramesh, and Peter Meer. Kernel-based object tracking. *IEEE Transactions on Pattern Analysis and Machine Intelligence*, 25(5):564–577, 2003.

[45] Qianqian Wang, Jiangfan Yu, Ke Yuan, Lidong Yang, Dongdong Jin, and Li Zhang. Disassembly and spreading of magnetic nanoparticle clusters on uneven surfaces. *Applied Materials Today*, 18, 2020, Art. no. 100489.

[46] Jiangfan Yu, Dongdong Jin, Kai-Fung Chan, Qianqian Wang, Ke Yuan, and Li Zhang. Active generation and magnetic actuation of microrobotic swarms in bio-fluids. *Nature Communications*, 10, 2019, Art. no. 5631.

[47] Sonia Melle, Oscar G Calderón, Miguel A Rubio, and Gerald G Fuller. Microstructure evolution in magnetorheological suspensions governed by mason number. *Physical Review E*, 68(4):041503, 2003.

[48] Kwitae Chong, Scott D Kelly, Stuart Smith, and Jeff D Eldredge. Inertial particle trapping in viscous streaming. *Physics of Fluids*, 25(3), 2013, Art. no. 033602.

[49] Denise Wong, Iris B Liu, Edward B Steager, Kathleen J Stebe, and Vijay Kumar. Directed micro assembly of passive particles at fluid interfaces using magnetic robots. In *2016 International Conference on Manipulation, Automation and Robotics at Small Scales (MARSS)*, pages 1–6. IEEE, 2016.

[50] Tianyi Yao, Nicholas G Chisholm, Edward B Steager, and Kathleen J Stebe. Directed assembly and micro-manipulation of passive particles at fluid interfaces via capillarity using a magnetic micro-robot. *Applied Physics Letters*, 116(4), 2020, Art. no. 043702.

III

Imaging and Localization

CHAPTER 6

Localization of Collective Nanorobots Using Various Imaging Modalities

6.1 INTRODUCTION

Microrobots provide numerous biomedical functions such as targeted delivery [1, 2], biosensing [3], micromanipulation [4, 5, 6], and minimally invasive surgical procedure [7, 8]. Versatile microrobots have been proposed for the usage of a number of actuated techniques (*e.g.*, magnetic fields [9, 10, 11, 12, 13], chemical fuels [14], acoustic waves [15] and biohybrid ways [16, 17]). To realize targeted delivery in a living body, *in vivo* localization of microrobots is an indispensable factor, and their tracked position can be used as the feedback to build a closed-loop control system [18]. Magnetic resonance imaging (MRI) has been applied by Martel *et al.* to locate driven objects and navigate them through a planned path [19, 20]. A group of helical microrobots can also use MRI to image the stomach of rodents [21]. Positron emission tomography (PET) was used to track the position of the catalytic tubular microrobot in the tubular phantom [22]. Recent studies show that the microswarm of artificial bacterial flagella can be imaged in the subcutaneous tissue of mice by infrared fluorescence imaging through the functionalization of fluorophores [23]. Ultrasound imaging is one of the most promising microrobotic imaging tools in medical imaging technology. Compared with MRI, PET/CT, and X-ray imaging, ultrasound imaging technology can provide high spatial and temporal resolution at a lower cost and does not involve ionizing radiation during its use [24, 25, 26, 27, 28]. Taking advantage of its high temporal resolution, that is to say, fast imaging speed, motion control and path planning of a millimeter-scale robotic gripper based on ultrasound feedback are proposed [29]. This feedback is also being used to guide a miniature helical robot to rub blood clots outside the body [30].

Ultrasound imaging relies on acoustic impedance gradients. The scale of microrobots should be larger than the limit of ultrasonic detection, which provides opportunities for localization and control of microrobots *in vivo*. However, the main problem

DOI: 10.1201/9781032665788-6

of microrobot real-time localization is the low signal-to-noise ratio, that is, imaging contrast. One direct way to solve the problem is to use the larger-sized microrobot such as millimeter-scale [31, 30, 29, 32]. However, in a restricted environment, such as bifurcated microvascular systems, key limitations for further application may be encountered. Another way is to use microbubbles. Microbubbles scatter ultrasound waves and obtain enhanced imaging contrast [33, 34]. Bubble-actuated microrobots generate propulsion through catalytic interactions with surrounding chemicals. By tracking the tails of bubbles, these microrobots can be localized indirectly [35]. However, these microrobots need specific catalytic reaction environments such as the stomach, and the reaction rate and time are difficult to control [36]. In order to achieve effective localization and control, the collective behaviors and swarm control of microrobots are worthy of study. A group of microrobots can enhance the contrast of medical imaging, such as MRI [19], PET [22] and fluorescence imaging [23]. Unlike using a millimeter-scale robot, the generated microswarm can be disassembled and reassembled to perform cooperative movements [37]. The building blocks are injected into a restricted environment, navigated to a required location and reassembled again to perform required tasks [38, 39, 40, 41]. Among them, magnetite nanoparticles are regarded as promising candidates, and they have been applied in medical imaging and biosensing [42, 43]. They could be functionalized in a variety of sizes (from a few nanometers to micrometers) and different magnetic properties [44, 45].

In this chapter, firstly we present the localization and real-time navigation of a magnetic nanoparticle-based microswarm guide by ultrasound imagin. Secondly, we present an optimized magnetic driving strategy to enhance the contrast of ultrasonic imaging of colloidal microswarm. Finally, Fluorescence imaging and photoacoustic imaging (PAI) of a rotating microswarm will be introduced.

6.2 REAL-TIME MAGNETIC NAVIGATION OF A ROTATING COLLOIDAL MICROSWARM UNDER ULTRASOUND GUIDANCE

6.2.1 Mathematical Modeling and Simulations

In this section, we use an in-plane rotating magnetic field to generate the microswarm (Figure 6.1a). Microswarms can exhibit motion by adding a small pitch angle (γ) to the rotating field (Figure 6.1b). The motion is achieved by friction asymmetry caused by boundary (substrate) [46]. The generation process is shown in Figure 6.1c. When the external field is turned on, a chain of rotating particles will be formed because of the induced magnetic dipole-dipole gravity between the nanoparticles. At the same time, the fluid interaction between particle chains leads to aggregation behavior, which gradually produces the region of high area density of nanoparticles. The region expands after attracting more particles, resulting in a particle-based microswarm.

The ultrasonic contrast of the microswarm depends on time, that is, the change of the contrast is highly dependent on the direction and lengths of the internal chains. We provide a mathematical model to estimate the chain length changes on the basis of the torque balance. Fe_3O_4@PDA NPs are regarded as spheres with radius a, and they are paramagnetism based on hysteresis loops. The induced dipole moment of a

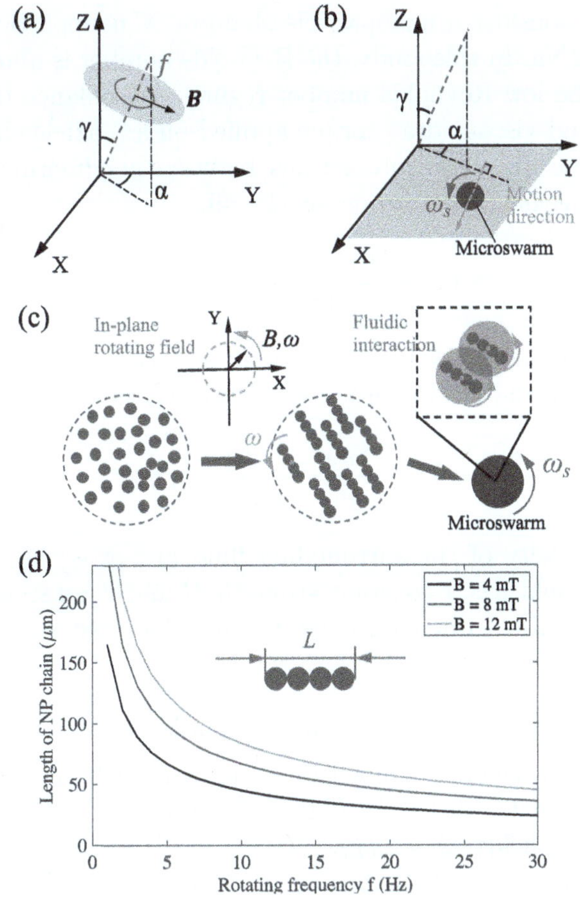

Figure 6.1 (a) Schematic diagram of rotating magnetic fields. The blue line and the arrow represent the normal line and rotation direction of the rotating magnetic field, respectively. The field $\mathbf{B}$ has field strength B and frequency f. α and γ are the yaw angle and pitch angle. (b) Schematic diagram of the microswarm driven by a rotating field on a substrate. ω_s represents the angular velocity of the NP microswarm. (c) Schematic diagram of the generation of an NP microswarm. (d) Relationship between the length of the NP chain and the rotating frequency at different field strengths.

particle in an external magnetic field of a strength B is $\mathbf{m} = \frac{4}{3}\pi a^3 \mu_0 \chi \mathbf{B}$, where μ_o and χ are permeability and vacuum susceptibility, respectively. The induced magnetic force between nanoparticles is expressed as [47]

$$\mathbf{F} = \frac{3m^2}{4\pi\mu_0 r^4}(3\cos^2\beta - 1)\hat{\mathbf{r}} + \frac{3m^2}{4\pi\mu_0 r^4}\sin(2\beta)\hat{\theta} \tag{6.1}$$

where r is the central distance between nanoparticles and β is the phase lag.

Superposition of two sine fields with a 90° phase lag generates an in-plane rotating field, as

$$\mathbf{B}(t) = B\sin(2\pi ft)\hat{\mathbf{x}} + B\cos(2\pi ft)\hat{\mathbf{y}} \tag{6.2}$$

In this section we consider a nanoparticle chain of N nanoparticles, with the chain length being $L = 2Na$. In this study, the Reynolds number is about 1×10^{-3}. Under the condition of the low Reynolds number regime, the balance between the driving magnetic torque and viscous drag torque applied on a particle chain determines the drive. Summing the magnetic interactions between neighboring nanoparticles can calculate the driving magnetic torque, as [48, 49]

$$\Gamma_m = \frac{3\mu_0 m^2(N-1)}{4\pi(2a)^3}\sin(2\beta) \tag{6.3}$$

When the shape factor is taken into account, the viscous resistance moment of a nanoparticle chain in the driving process is expressed as [50]

$$\Gamma_d = \frac{8\pi a^3}{3}\frac{N^3}{\ln(\frac{N}{2}) + \frac{2.4}{N}}\eta\omega \tag{6.4}$$

where η is the viscosity of the surrounding fluid and ω is the angular velocity. A rotating magnetic field has a constant strength B and a rotation frequency f. The defined phase lag is able to be gained by defining the input strength and frequency, that is

$$\sin(2\beta) = \frac{32N\eta\omega}{\mu_0\chi^2 B^2 \ln(N/2)} \tag{6.5}$$

When $\sin(2\beta) < 1$, the chain of nanoparticles rotates synchronously with the external field. In our experiments, all the particle chains show a rotation synchronized with the external rotation fields ($\omega = 2\pi f$).

We can estimate the length of the nanoparticle chain by the balance between the two torques ($\Gamma_d = -\Gamma_m$). Mason number, defined as the ratio of the applied viscous torque divided by the magnetic torque [51]. According to the above definition, the modified Mason number in our scheme is expressed as

$$R_T = 16\frac{\eta\omega\mu_0}{\chi^2 B}\frac{N^3}{(N-1)(\ln(\frac{N}{2}) + \frac{2.4}{N})} \tag{6.6}$$

The critical case is obtained when $R_T = 1$, where the two torques balance each other and nanoparticle chains keep stable. If R_T exceeds unity, the viscous torque becomes greater than the driving magnetic torque, which results in the fragmentation of nanoparticle chains. This may occur by suddenly reducing the field strength or increasing the angular velocity. The change of chain length is calculated by setting $R_T = 1$, and the result is shown in Figure 6.1d. Because of the drag on the chain, the length decreases with increasing frequency. At the same input frequency, increasing the input field strength can result in a longer chain.

In order to understand the fluid interactions between nanoparticle chains, a finite element simulation (COMSOL Multiphysics) is carried out to study the induced fluid flow caused by the rotating nanoparticle chains. As shown in Figure 6.2, the driven nanoparticle chains are modeled as rods with lengths of 60–100 μm. They rotate to their geometric center at frequencies of 6–8 Hz. After more than ten full rotations, the simulation results between Figure 6.2a and 6.2b show that increasing the driving

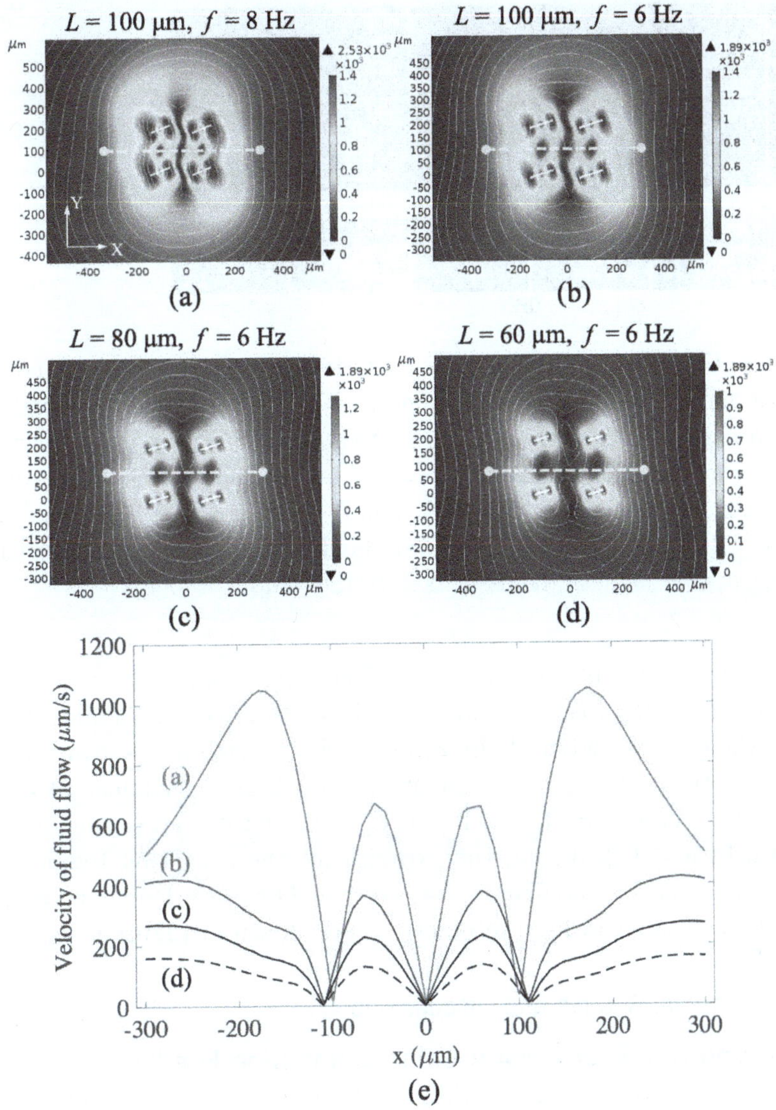

Figure 6.2 Simulation of the fluid interactions between nanoparticle chains. The chain lengths (L) in (a) and (b) are both 100 μm, and in (c) and (d) are 80 μm and 60 μm, respectively. The input rotation frequencies (f) are set to 8 Hz in (a) and 6 Hz in (b-d). The contour lines show the magnitude of the tangential velocity (μm/s), marked by the colored legend on the right. White lines indicate the induced streamlines. (e) Fluid flow induced along the centerline (dashed lines shown in (a–d)) of the pattern under different L and f, as marked from (a) to (d).

frequency can enhance the fluid interaction between chains. However, from Eqs. (6.3)–(6.6), it is known that the chain length decreases with the increase of input frequency. When the chain is short, the fluid interactions between them deceases (Figures 6.2b-d), which leads to an incompact structure of the microswarm (low area density of nanoparticles). Furthermore, if the applied field strength exceeds a critical value, it

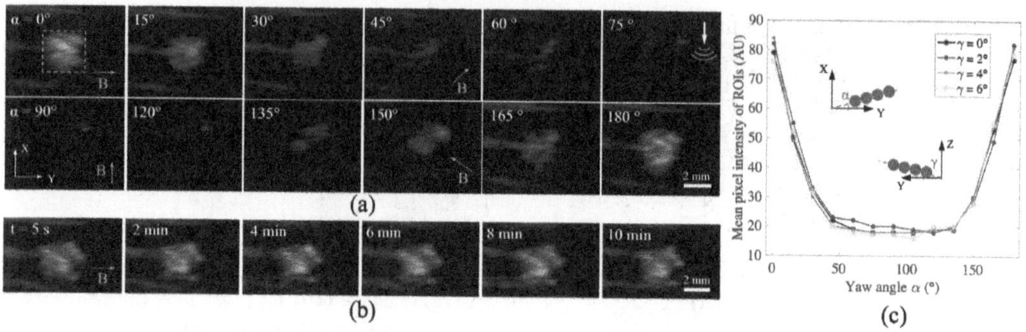

Figure 6.3 (a) Ultrasonic images of nanoparticle chains under the action of an in-plane electrostatic field. The yaw angles change from 0° to 180° at an interval of 15°. The yellow rectangle represents the area of interest (ROI). The white arrows and curves indicate the direction of ultrasonic propagation. All the images are marked with the same ROI. The applied field strength is 7 mT. (b) Ultrasonic images of nanoparticle chains at t = 0–10 mins under the input field $\alpha = 0°$. (c) Mean pixel intensity of ROIs under static magnetic fields at $\alpha = 0–180°$ and $\gamma = 0–6°$.

will lead to aggregation of nanoparticles. Therefore, it is necessary to make a trade-off between the driving frequency and lengths of nanoparticle chains. The fluid flow induced in the central region of the rotating chain pattern is shown in Figure 6.2e, which quantitatively shows the fluid interaction between chains. In order to gain a swarm area of nanoparticles with a high area density, according to the analysis in Figures 6.1d and 6.2, during the experiment, the actuating frequency and field strength are set at 6 Hz and 7 mT, respectively. The chain length is estimated to be 80 μm, and the interchain fluid interactions are shown in Figure 6.2c.

6.2.2 Experimental Results and Discussions

(1) Localization of a Microswarm Using Ultrasound Feedback: Because the microswarm is formed by the aggregation of nanoparticle chains through fluid interactions, we first study the ultrasonic feedback of static nanoparticle chains. Nanoparticle chains assemble along the field direction by applying an in-plane static magnetic field (Figure 6.3a). Change the direction of the chain above by adjusting the yaw angle (α) of the outfield. After the chains reach the static state, the imaging contrast of nanoparticle chains is studied. Ultrasound images are obtained at $\alpha = 0°– 180°$ with an interval of 15°. Where the yaw angles of 0° and 180° are the best imaging contrast, the direction of the chain is perpendicular to the propagation direction of the ultrasonic wave. when the yaw angle increases from 0° to 90° the contrast decreases, then it increases gradually from 90° and reaches the best contrast when $\alpha = 180°$. Figure 6.3b indicates the ultrasound images underneath an in-plane electrostatic field within 10 mins. During experiments, no apparent interference is observed, indicating the influence of ultrasound is negligible. In order to study the relationship between the imaging contrast and the orientation of the nanoparticle chain, the average pixel intensity of the chain region is studied quantitatively. The rectangle area including all the nanoparticle chains is used as the region of interests (ROIs). The average pixel

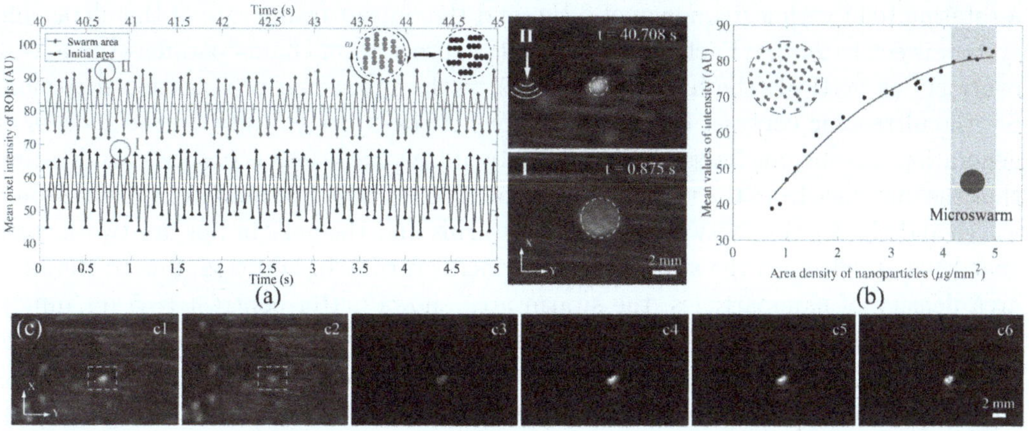

Figure 6.4 Dynamic and enhanced ultrasound imaging contrast. (a) Changes in average pixel intensity for the two ROIs (dashed circles) under a 6 Hz rotating field. The frame rate of the ultrasound imaging system is 24 fps, that is, the continuous 120 frames refer to the Initial area and Swarm area of 0–5 s and 40–45 s, respectively. The dashed lines refer to the mean values of intensity (Swarm area: 81.5, Initial area: 56.4). The white arrow indicates the direction of wave propagation. The applied magnetic field strength is 7 mT. (b) The relationship between the average strength and the area density of nanoparticles. Blue dots come from experimental data and the curve refers to the fitting line of the data. The area density range of a microswarm is marked by the blue area. (c) Image processing. (c1) and (c2) are about the maximum and minimum intensity in a cycle of dynamic contrast. (c3) Image differencing: results of image (c1) subtracted by (c2). (c4) Pixel intensity amplification. The intensity of pixels is multiplied. (c5) Edge extraction. Set a threshold to extract the edges of the microswarm. (c6) Localization. Using the center of the fitted circle can locate the microswarm.

intensity of a ROI is calculated by LabVIEW programs, and the results are plotted in Figure 6.3c. The curve is almost symmetrical amount to $\alpha = 90°$, and the intensity reaches the maximum when $\alpha = 0°$ and 180°. When the chain is perpendicular to the direction of ultrasonic propagation, the scattered ultrasonic wave reaches the maximum. However, if the chain is parallel to the propagation direction of wave ($\alpha = 90°$), only a few sound waves can be scattered. Furthermore, by adding a small pitch angle ($\gamma = 2°– 6°$) to the external field, the chains tilt away from the substrate. Figure 6.3c indicates that adding a small pitch angle will not significantly affect the imaging contrast, which indicates that scattered waves affected by the small tilt of the chain can be ignored.

Then the location of the microswarm under the rotating field is studied. The imaging pairs of the initial region and the swarm region are shown in Figure 6.4a, referring to the regions before (0–5 s) and after (40–45 s) the formation of an effective microswarm, respectively. When t = 0 s, the rotating magnetic field is turned on. We take these two regions as the ROIs and use them to study the changes of ultrasonic contrast when obtaining intensity data frame by frame. The microswarm is driven by a rotating field with a frequency of 6 Hz, and the output frame rate of the ultrasonic system is set to 24 fps. Each data point is the direction of chains parallel (the lowest contrast) or vertical (the highest contrast) to the ultrasonic propagation direction. So, the ultrasonic contrast of the two regions changes periodically. In the process of generation, no obvious interference caused by ultrasonic waves is observed, indicating that the influence from the transducer can be ignored. The low power of the ultrasonic waves and the friction between the microswarms and the gelatin pot are two factors that have an effect on the stability of the microswarms. In addition, due to the high area density of nanoparticles, the swarm area shows better contrast (~5 μg/mm^2). The relationship between imaging contrast and the areal density of nanoparticles is shown in Figure 6.4b. The nanoparticles with different areal densities achieve by controlling the decomposition duration using a dynamic decomposition field [52]. Then a rotating magnetic field with a frequency of 6 Hz is applied to record the imaging contrast at this time. The average pixel intensity is measured from 48 consecutive frames (2 s), and the average intensity represents the average pixel intensity of the 48 frames, which is similar to the methods used in Figure 6.4a. The imaging intensity of the microswarm increases non-linearly with the area density of particles. The average strength of the area with an area density of 4–5 μg/mm^2 is greater than 70. It is also found that even nanoparticles with very low areal density (<1 μg/mm^2) can also contribute to the imaging contrast.

As shown in the image II in Figure 6.4a, the maximum intensity of the swarm area is ~90. When $\alpha = 0°$, this maximum is ~80 in Figure 6.3a, even if the areal density of nanoparticles is only 1.45 μg/mm^2. The length of nanoparticle chains causes the high contrast. Under a static field, the length of nanoparticle chains reaches millimeter scale, increasing the amount of the scattered ultrasound. According to the analysis in Figure 6.1d, the chain length in the swarm region is ~80 μm. However, due to the high area density of nanoparticles, the maximum strength is higher than that in a static field. The analysis above shows that the imaging contrast is affected by the area density of nanoparticles and the length of chains. The averaged pixel intensity of the swarm in Figure 6.4a is 81.5. By using the same calculation method, that is, only the maximum and minimum pixel values in the driving period are calculated, in the case of a static field, the average intensity is about 50 (the maximum of ~80 and the minimum ~20). The areal density of nanoparticles has a more pronounced effect on imaging contrast than chain length.

Making use of the dynamic characteristics and enhanced contrast of the microswarm, the processing method based on image difference is used to locate the microswarm. Figure 6.4c shows the implementation steps of image processing for locating the microswarm. As we discussed in Figure 6.4a, the ultrasonic contrast of the microswarm is time-dependent. By adjusting the frequency at which the rotational field is applied and the display frame rate of the ultrasound system, contrast can be acquired continuously between the highest and lowest values. For example, when the imaging depth is increased from 3 cm to 4 cm, the display frame rate is reduced to 20 fps. By changing the input frequency of the field from 6 Hz to 5 Hz, you can still obtain a continuous change image between the highest and lowest contrast. At the same time, the microswarm remains balanced and maneuverable. As shown in Figure

6.4c3, the signal-to-noise ratio is improved by using the image difference method. After adding a threshold to the image processed by pixel intensity magnification, the microswarm is fitted into a circle. Then the center of the circle is used to represent the position of the microswarm (Figure 6.4c6).

(2) Dose Limitation of Nanoparticle: In order to locate the microswarm effectively, the dose limitation of the nanoparticle should be studied. In clinical application, the recommended therapeutic dose of nanoparticles is usually maintained at low values to avoid dose-related toxicity [53, 54]. There are three main factors that affect the minimum dose required to locate the microswarm. First of all, the coverage of the microswarm. A microswarm with a large coverage area can be gained by using higher doses of nanoparticles, and they can be easily located. However, excessive doses may cause dose-related toxicity to tissues, and some nanoparticles cannot be aggregated into microswarms due to insufficient fluid interaction (Figure 6.5a). In 2 μL aqueous suspension of nanoparticles, the comparison between theoretical and experimental results shows that almost all nanoparticles are clustered into the microswarm. The size of microswarm meets the limit of about 4 mm^2. Second, the imaging depth of the ultrasonic system. The imaging of relatively deep areas requires a low-frequency ultrasound, resulting in a reduction in resolution. In theory, locating the microswarm at a deeper location requires a larger dose. Third, noisy signals can affect the localization of microswarms. This problem can be solved by using dynamic contrast. However, strong noise signals or interference will still affect the positioning.

We study dose limitation at the imaging depth of 5 cm as this depth can reach a variety of human tissues and organs, such as the breast and bladder [55]. Nanoparticles with different doses are used to generate microswarm, and there are 3 cm chicken tissue and 1–2 cm PBS between the ultrasonic transducer and the microswarm (Figure 6.5b). The concentration of Fe_3O_4@PDA nanoparticles aqueous suspension remains the same (5 mg/mL), and the injection volume (0.2–8 μL) controls the dose of the nanoparticles. As shown in Figures 6.5b1 and 6.5b2, the microswarm can be located (red curves) by applying a process based on image difference. However, if the dose is lower than 0.4 μL, the generated microswarm is difficult to locate stably due to the small size and the interference of noise signals. As shown in the case of 0.2 μL (Figure 6.5b3), the locations of the microswarm are marked by dotted circles. The noise signal interferes with the positioning of the microswarm and reports an unwanted tracking position.

(3) *Ex Vivo* Localization of a Microswarm: The microswarm can be located at different depths *in vitro*. The microswarm is produced by using 4 μL nanoparticle aqueous suspension in a gelatin tank with a wall thickness of 5 mm, which is wrapped with chicken tissues. The ultrasound transducer is installed on the surface of chicken tissues with the thickness of 2 cm to 5 cm, and the imaging depth of the ultrasonic system is adjusted to 4 cm to 8 cm to achieve microswarm positioning (Figure 6.6a). However, due to the inverse relationship between ultrasonic length and frequency, the resolution will decrease with the increase of imaging depth. High-frequency ultrasound attenuates with the increase of imaging depth, so the use of low-frequency ultrasound is more reliable for microscanning with relatively deep positioning. When the imagery depth is 4 cm, 5 cm, and 6 cm, the mechanical index (MI) and thermal

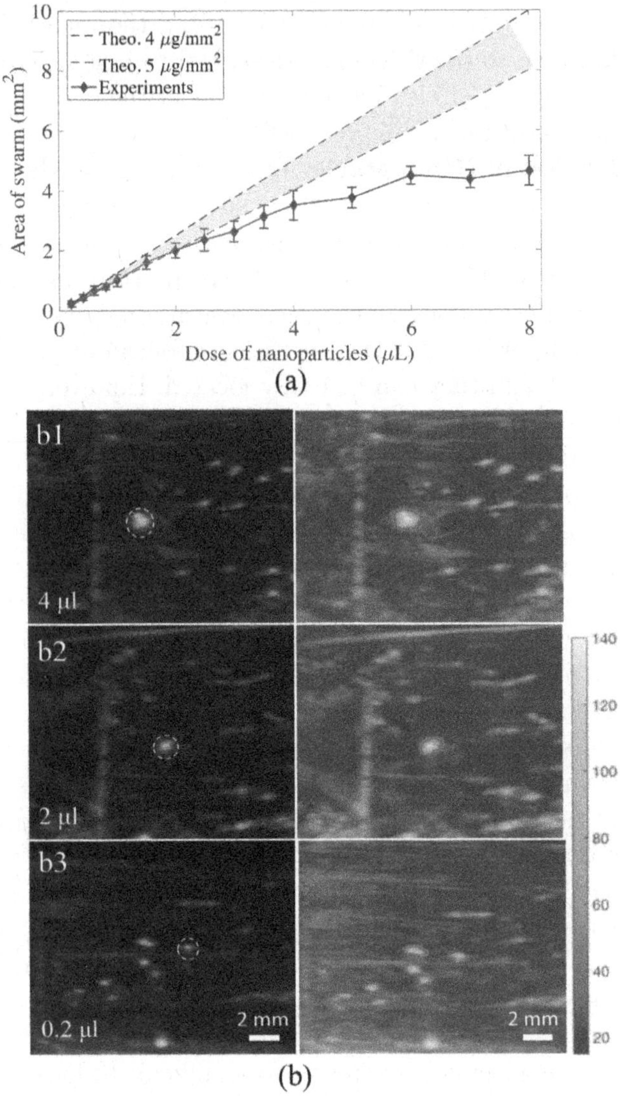

Figure 6.5 (a) The relationship between the microswarm coverage area and the nanoparticle dose. Compare the experimental results with two theoretical estimates: 4 μg/mm^2 and 5 μg/mm^2. All error bars represent the standard deviation (s.d.) of three trials. (b) Ultrasound imaging of microswarm generated by nanoparticles with different doses. The swarm area is marked with a dotted circle. Using MATLAB to draw the pixel intensity distributions, and automatically extract the edge of the microswarm and mark it with red curves.

index score (TIS) are 0.7 and 0.6, respectively. When the image depth increases to 8 cm, both values are 0.4. In all cases, the gain setting (Gn) is 45. When the imaging depth is 4–6 cm (chicken tissue thickness is 2–4 cm), a rotating microswarm is located, as shown in Figures 6.6a1–a3. However, when the image depth is increased to 8 cm, the rotating microswarm cannot be located. This is because the strength of the noise

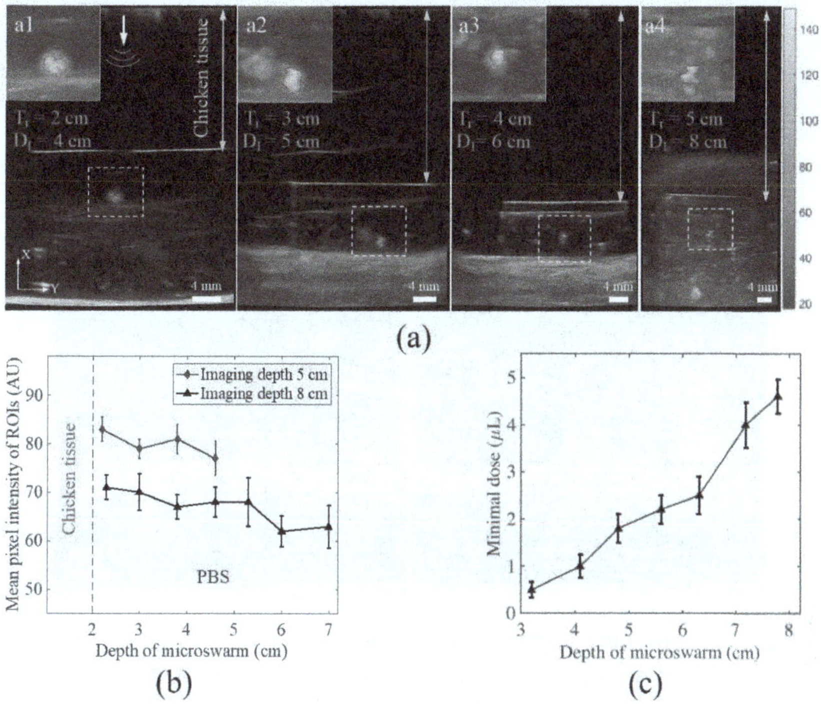

Figure 6.6 (a) Rotating microswarms localized at different depths *in vitro*. Wrap the gelatin jar with chicken tissue with a thickness (T_r) of 2–5 cm and adjust the corresponding imaging depth (D_I) to 4–8 cm. Pixel intensity distributions were plotted with MATLAB (areas marked with dotted rectangles), and the edges of microswarm are marked with red lines. (b) The average pixel intensity of the swarm area at a depth of 5 cm and 8 cm (T_r = 2 cm). All error strips represent the s.d. of three experiments. (c) Minimum dose of nanoparticles used to localize a microswarm at different depths. A gelatin jar is wrapped with chicken tissue to a thickness (T_r) of ~2–7 cm, with the imaging depths setting of 5 cm (T_r: 2–4 cm) and 8 cm (T_r: 5–7 cm). All error bars represent the s.d. of three experiments.

signal is higher than that of the microswarm. Then we increase the dose to 6 μL. Because of the large swarm area, the microswarm can be identified from the noise signal (Figure 6.6a4). Although stronger ultrasound is required at deeper imaging depths, backscattered ultrasound from microswarm is still stronger than ultrasound from the surrounding environments (*i.e.*, tissue, fluid, and gelatin tank). Therefore, larger doses of nanoparticles are required to identify microswarms at deeper depths.

Compared with tissue, there is less attenuation when propagating in liquid (PBS) [56]. We perform *in vitro* experiments using 2 cm thick chicken tissue and increasing the depths of the microswarm in PBS. Figure 6.6b shows the relationship between contrast and depths of a microswarm under the imaging depths of 5 cm and 8 cm. The distance between the microswarm center and the transducer is defined as the microswarm depth. With the increase of microswarm depth in PBS, the contrast decreases slightly. Because of the reduction of resolution, all contrast of 8 cm imaging

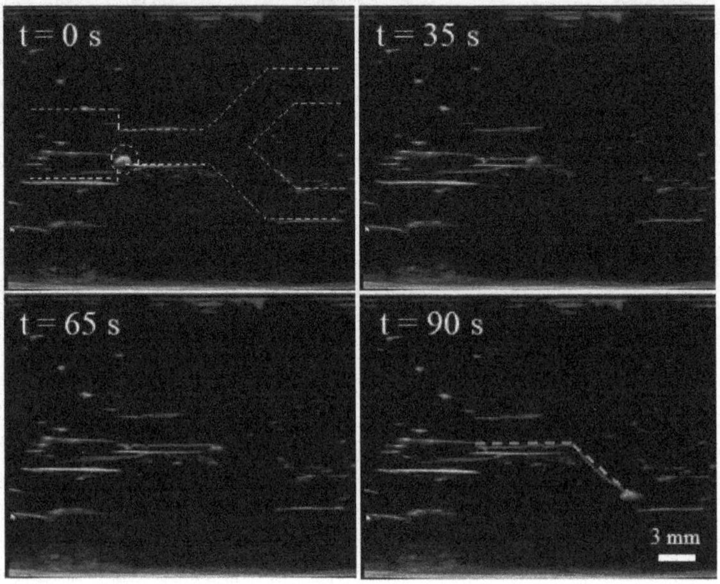

Figure 6.7 Closed-loop control of rotating colloidal microswarms based on ultrasonic feedback. The microswarm navigates along the planned path in the gelatin channel (yellow dashed lines). The red and blue dotted lines represent tracking tracks and planned paths, respectively. The imaging depth is 4 cm. Application field frequency: 6 Hz.

depth is reduced. These results suggest that the microswarms are suitable for use in the lumen of organs, such as the bladder [57]. If a microswarm within a lumen can be localized at shallower depths, it can be localized throughout the lumen (liquid environment). Microswarms can be used in different scenarios, and the corresponding minimum dose needs to be investigated. Figure 6.6c maps the minimum dose of nanoparticles needed to localize microswarms at different depths. During the experiment at the same depth, the dose gradually decreased until the proposed method based on image difference could not locate the microswarm. As the microswarm gets deeper, the minimum dose increases. It takes less than 3 μL to locate the mini-group in the depth of less than 6 cm.

(4) Real-time Closed-Loop Control Using Ultrasound Feedback: We design a PI control scheme, which uses ultrasonic feedback to navigate and rotate in real time along the planned path (Figures 6.7 and 6.8). The microswarm is driven by adding a small pitch angle γ to the application field, and adjusting the yaw angle α controls the direction of motion. The superposition of the field components from the X, Y, and Z axis generates the field. Each shaft is controlled by a pair of the Helmholtz coils. The three field components are expressed as

$$\begin{aligned}B_x &= B\cos\gamma\cdot\cos\alpha\cdot\cos(2\pi ft) - B\sin\alpha\cdot\sin(2\pi ft)\\ B_y &= B\cos\gamma\cdot\sin\alpha\cdot\cos(2\pi ft) + B\cos\alpha\cdot\sin(2\pi ft)\\ B_z &= B\sin\gamma\cdot\cos(2\pi ft)\end{aligned} \tag{6.7}$$

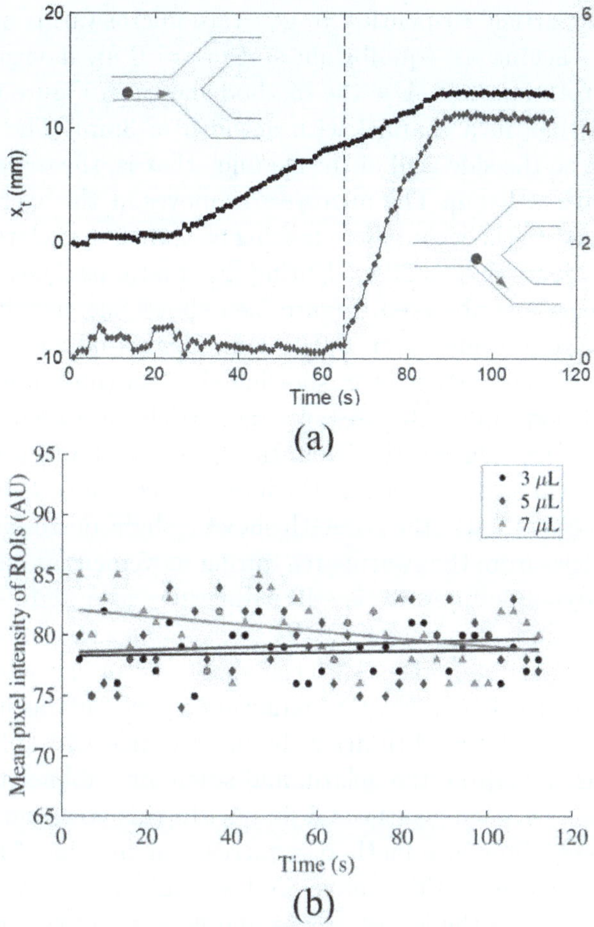

Figure 6.8 Closed-loop control of rotating colloidal microswarms based on ultrasonic feedback. (a) Tracking the position of the microswarm during navigation. Dashed lines indicate changes in the direction of movement toward branches. (b) The change of average pixel intensity in the swarm area during the period driven by different doses of nanoparticles. The average intensity is calculated based on continuous ultrasound images within 2 s. The points are experimental data and the corresponding lines are the linear fitting of the data.

where $\mathbf{B}(t) = B_x\hat{\mathbf{x}} + B_y\hat{\mathbf{y}} + B_z\hat{\mathbf{z}}$. Here, we use static γ during the drive. Therefore, in order to follow a planned path, it is necessary to control the direction of movement of the microswarm, as

$$\alpha(\mathbf{p}(t)) = \mathbf{K}_p(\mathbf{r}(t) - \hat{\mathbf{p}}(t)) + \mathbf{K}_i \int_0^t (\mathbf{r}(\tau) - \hat{\mathbf{p}}(\tau))d\tau \tag{6.8}$$

where α is the yaw angle of the rotating field, $\mathbf{K}_p \in \mathbf{R}^{2\times2}$, $\mathbf{K}_i \in \mathbf{R}^{2\times2}$ are the positive definite gain matrix of the controller, $\mathbf{r}(\mathrm{t}) \in \mathbf{R}^{2\times1}$ is the reference position, and $\hat{\mathbf{p}}(t)$ is the position of the microswarm in the tracking process.

Use 3 μL of nanoparticle suspension to generate microswarms on the left side of the channel. After reaching an equilibrium state (t = 0 s), navigate by adding 4° pitch angles to the rotation field. Use the method shown in Figure 6.4c to track the microswarm in real time in a channel with a width of 3mm. The planned path is calculated according to the side wall of the channel, that is, the distance between the side wall and the path is 1 mm. The microswarm moves at the average speed of 180 μm/s in PBS. Navigate to the right before tasking 65 s, then branch to the bottom and finally reach the destination (t = 90 s). During automatic navigation, no significant ultrasonic disturbances are observed. Figure 6.8a shows the tracking position. The average steady-state positioning error is 0.27 mm. Compared with the body length, the error is ~33.7% of the body length, showing the real-time controllability of the body length. In addition, different doses of nanoparticles are used to automatically navigate the microswarm. During the excitation process, the ultrasonic contrast of the swarm area is kept at a high value and the interference can be ignored, as shown in Figure 6.8b. In the case of 7 μL, the strength shows a slight decrease, which is due to the loss of nanoparticles from the swarm area during movement as discussed in Figure 6.4a. However, the dynamic intensity is still maintained at a high level (the average intensity value > 75) and does not affect the tracking accuracy of the microswarm. According to the analysis of Figure 6.3c, the slight tilt of the nanoparticle chains within the microswarm will not have a significant effect on the imaging contrast. Therefore, different γ can be used to drive the microswarm with different speeds.

The noise signals come from the gelatin and small air bubbles in the side wall of the channel (interface between gelatin and liquid). In this environment with limited interference, the image difference method is carried out in a low frequency manner. All real-time gained images within one second are subtracted by the same image, that is, the first frame with the lowest ultrasound contrast of the microswarm (*e.g.*, Figure 6.4c2). This method can avoid the influence of the frame rate fluctuation and low frequency interference of ultrasonic equipment. In the complex interference environment such as blood vessels, noise signals can be effectively reduced by using high-frequency image differential processing (*e.g.*, Figure 6.4c).

6.3 MAGNETIC ACTUATION OF A DYNAMICALLY RECONFIGURABLE MICROSWARM FOR ENHANCED ULTRASOUND IMAGING CONTRAST

6.3.1 Mathematical Modeling and Simulation

Upon application of an external magnetic field, nanoparticle chains form because of the magnetic attraction force induced between the nanoparticles. In this section, at first, we study the variation of nanoparticle chains within rotational microswarms driven by a nonpolarized rotating field (NRF) or a polarized rotating field (PRF) with different field parameters, and then apply the estimated chain states to build simulations to further study the intraswarm fluid mechanical interaction.

Nanoparticles are regarded as spheres with radius of a_p. The induced dipole moment of paramagnetic particles in the external magnetic field is $\mu = \frac{4}{3}\pi a_p^3 \mu_0 \chi B$, where μ_o and χ are magnetic permeability and susceptibility, respectively, and B is

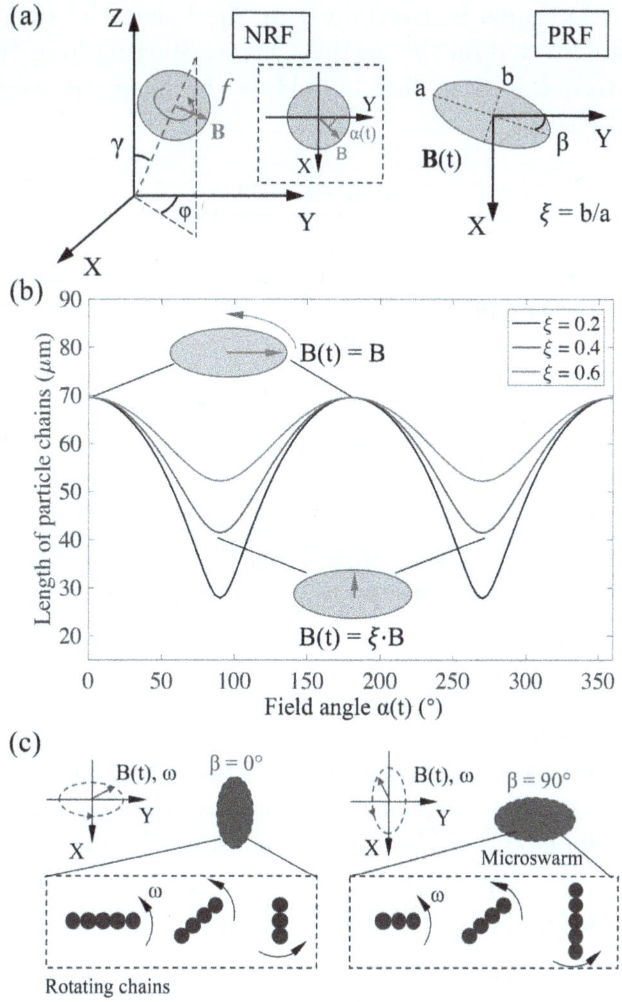

Figure 6.9 The rotating field is used to form and transform the swarm. (a) A schematic diagram of the rotating magnetic field. Left: φ and γ are the yaw and pitch angles of NRF. $\alpha(t)$ represents the field angle that varies with time between the magnetic field and the Y-axis. Right: a and b are the major and minor axes of PRF. β is an elliptical angle, that is, the angle between the major axis and the Y-axis. (b) The relationship between the chain length of PRF and $\alpha(t)$ in a rotation period where ξ is 0.2–0.6. The field parameters are set to $B = 8$ mT and $f = 6$ Hz. (c) Microswarm diagram demonstration of $\beta = 0°$ (left) and $\beta = 90°$ (right) under PRF.

the field strength. The induced magnetic force between nanoparticles is expressed as [47]

$$\mathbf{F}_m = \frac{3\mu^2}{4\pi\mu_0 r^4}(3\cos^2\psi - 1)\hat{\mathbf{r}}_\mathbf{r} + \frac{3\mu^2}{4\pi\mu_0 r^4}\sin(2\psi)\hat{\mathbf{r}}_\theta \tag{6.9}$$

where r is the central distance among the nanoparticles, and ψ is the phase lag. We first think that a microswarm is driven by a non-polarized rotational field (NRF, Figure 6.9a). At a low Reynolds number regime (Re is about 1×10^{-3}), the formation of particle chains is determined by the balance of magnetic torque and viscous drag torque exerted on the particle chains. Starting from the $F_m \propto r^{-4}$, the driven magnetic torque is simplified by adding the magnetic interactions between adjacent nanoparticles, as

[48, 49]

$$\Gamma_m = \frac{3\mu_0\mu^2(N-1)}{4\pi(2a_p)^3}\sin(2\psi) \tag{6.10}$$

For the rotating chain with angular velocity ω, the viscous resistance moment considering the shape factor can be expressed as [50]

$$\Gamma_d = \frac{8\pi a_p^3}{3}\frac{N^3}{\ln(\frac{N}{2})+\frac{2.4}{N}}\eta\omega \tag{6.11}$$

where η is the viscosity of the fluid. Driven by NRF, the equilibrium relationship between the two torques ($\Gamma_d = -\Gamma_m$) gives the value of N, and the length of nanoparticle chain is estimated to be

$$L = 2Na_p \tag{6.12}$$

When a polarized rotating field (PRF, Figure 6.9a) drives the microswarm, the field strength changes with time, as

$$B(t) = B\cos(t)\hat{\mathbf{x}} + \xi \cdot B\sin(t)\hat{\mathbf{y}} \tag{6.13}$$

where B is the maximum intensity in one cycle, and $\xi = b/a$ is the magnetic field ratio. In order to estimate the change in chain length during the drive, we use the Mason number to represent the relationship between the two torques [51]. As known by the definition, the modified Mason number is given by the following formula

$$R_T = \frac{\Gamma_d}{\Gamma_m} = 16\frac{\eta\omega\mu_0}{\chi^2 B(t)}\frac{N^3}{(N-1)(\ln(\frac{N}{2})+\frac{2.4}{N})} \tag{6.14}$$

If $R_T > 1$, the chain breakage of nanoparticles occurs due to the relatively large resistance moment. $R_T = 1$ denotes the critical case where two moments are offset, and the value of $N = N(t)$ is given. Because of the change of magnetic torque, the chain length becomes time-dependent, as $L(t) = 2N(t)a_p$.

Under the action of PRF, the angular velocity remains unchanged, but the field strength changes. Based on the analysis in Eqs. (6.10)–(6.14), the changes of chain lengths in different driving periods of ξ are studied (Figure 6.9b). The calculation parameters are: $\mu_0 = 1.257\times10^{-6}$ V·s/(A·m), $\eta = 1$ mPa·s, $\chi = 0.8$. Due to the decrease of the magnetic driving moment, the chain length decreases with the increase of the magnetic field strength, where fragmentation occurs and the nanoparticle chain breaks down into shorter chains. Figure 6.9c shows the schematic diagram of the internal particle chain state of a PRF-driven microswarm. In the case of $\beta = 0°$, the length of the nanoparticle chain is the longest when $\alpha(t) = 0°$, and the field strength reaches the maximum $B(t) = B$. The vertical relationship between the long axis of the microswarm and the applied PRF is mainly caused by two factors. First of all, when the magnetic field intensity reaches the maximum, the chain is attracted by a relatively strong magnetic linkage-chain interaction, and the particle aggregation effect is enhanced. Secondly, the stronger fluid interaction caused by the longer chain further aggregates the nanoparticle chain. The microswarms shrink along the long axis of the polarization field gradually, and finally they form an elliptical microswarm model. We can change the ellipse angle from 0° to 90°, and the microswarm mode rotates gradually with the PRF and reaches a new direction.

The purpose of simulation is to study the interaction of fluid flow, vorticity, and hydrodynamics caused by particle chains within PRF-driven microswarms. We model each nanoparticle chain as a rod with a length dependent on the field parameter that rotates around its own center to simulate the induced flow around the rotational nanoparticle chain.(Figure 6.10a). In order to simulate the state of the nanoparticle chain when $\alpha(t) = 0°$, here is a particle chain with a length of 70 μm, which rotates at a frequency of 6 Hz (Figure 6.9b, $\xi = 0.6$). Then, to simulate the state of the nanoparticle chain when $\alpha(t) = 90°$ ($\xi = 0.6$), the length of the chain was changed to 43 μm. At this time, the field strength reaches the minimum ($B(t) = \xi \cdot B$), it leads to the shortest chain length. Due to the short chain length, the induced flow rate decreases (Figure 6.10b). Then the vorticity induced by the rotating chain is studied (Figure 6.10c). Hydrodynamic interactions between rotating chains rely on chain-induced vortex mergers [58]. The two eddy currents with higher vorticity are subjected to greater gravity, which is beneficial to the aggregation of nanoparticles [59]. Through the simulation, we can see that when $B(t) = B$, the vortex with larger vorticity will be generated, and the strong hydrodynamic attraction among chains will make the nanoparticles gather in a relatively compact state (Figure 6.10d). Fluid interactions within the PRF-driven swarm mode are simulated (Figures 6.10e and 6.10f), showing that stronger fluid interaction forms when $B(t) = B$. Therefore, from the point of view of chain-chain hydrodynamics and magnetic interaction, the aggregation effect of nanoparticles is enhanced when $B(t) = B$, which explains the vertical relationship between the long axis of the microswarm and the application of PRF.

6.3.2 Estimation of Imaging Contrast of a Rotating Microswarm

We have previously proposed that the angle between the direction of the chain and the direction of ultrasonic propagation determines the imaging contrast of the nanoparticle chains [60]. In this chapter, we define θ_c ($\theta_c \in [0, 90]$) as the angle between the changing direction of the chain and the fixed direction of wave propagation. As shown in Figure 6.11a, under an in-plane NRF, when $\theta_c = 90°$, that is, $\alpha(t) = 0°$, 180°, the best ultrasound imaging contrast of the particle region can be observed, because the backscattered ultrasound reaches the maximum value. The imaging contrast decreases with the decrease of and reaches the minimum value at , that is, the nanoparticle chain is parallel to the direction of wave propagation. With the decrease of θ_c, the imaging contrast decreases and reaches the minimum when $\theta_c = 0°$, when the nanoparticle chain is parallel to the propagation direction of the wave. In order to quantitatively study the relationship between imaging contrast and θ_c of the particle chain, the directional control of particle chain is realized by adjusting the

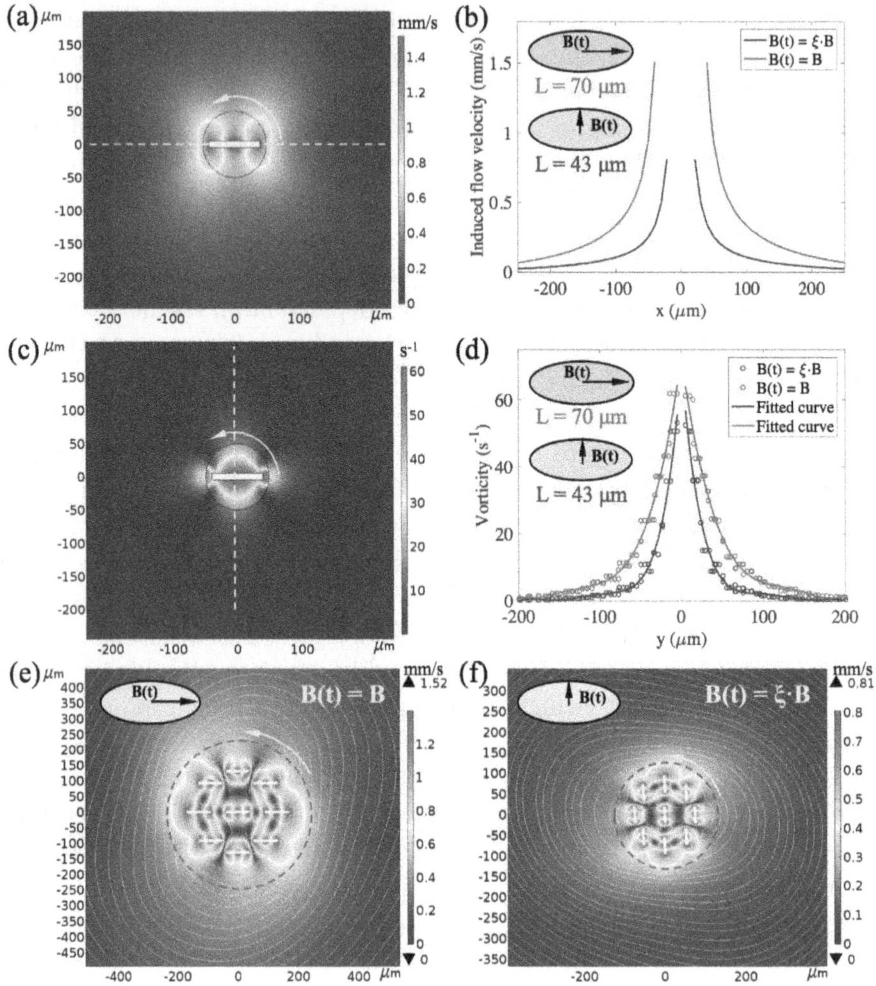

Figure 6.10 Simulation of fluid flow induced by chains of the rotating particles, vorticity, and hydrodynamic interactions between chains. (a) The flow of fluid caused by a rotating chain. The contours represent the magnitude of the velocity of flow (mm/s), marked by the color legend on the right. (b) The speed is drawn along the yellow dashed line in (a). (c) The vorticity caused by the rotating chain. The contours represent the magnitude of the vorticity (s^{-1}). The frequency of NRF in (a) and (c) is 6 Hz. (d) The vorticity is drawn along the yellow dotted line in (c). (e) and (f) show the fluid interactions between the chains within the microswarm when $B(t) = B$ and $B(t) = \xi \cdot B$, respectively. The white line represents the streamlines. The frequency of PRF is 6 Hz and $\xi = 0.6$.

yaw angle $\alpha(t)$ by using in-plane static field (Figure 6.11b). The ultrasonic imaging contrast of the particle chain region is defined by the average pixel intensity (MPI). MPI_{max} is defined as the maximum value of MPI in a rotation period (that is, $\alpha(t)$ = 0°–180° with an interval of 15°). We offer the field strength of 5–8 mT to form different length particle chains. For the field strengths of 5 mT, 6 mT, 7 mT, and

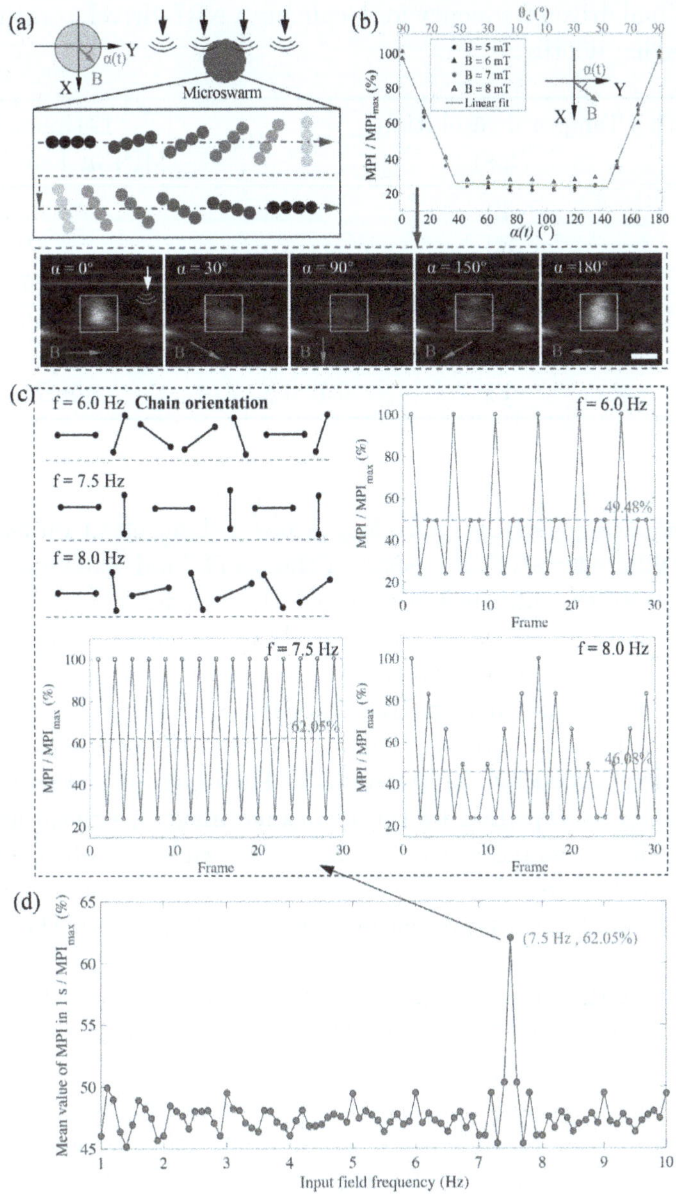

Figure 6.11 Estimation of contrast in rotational microswarm ultrasound imaging. (a) A schematic diagram of the change in the direction of the nanoparticle chain in the microswarm. (b) In a static field in plane, the relationship between the contrast of ultrasound imaging and θ_c. Each data point is the average of the three experiments. The blue rectangles represent the ROIs used to measure the MPI. The scale bar is 2 mm. (c) The change of ultrasonic contrast of microswarms at different input frequencies is estimated. The red dotted line represents the average. The time resolution is set to 30 ft/s. (d) The changes of ultrasound contrast (average MPI within 1 s/ MPI_{max}) of NRF-driven microswarms at different input frequencies is estimated.

TABLE 6.1 Optimal driven frequency for localizing a NRF-driven rotating microswarm at different imaging depths

Imaging depth (cm)	Temporal resolution (fps)	f_{op} (Hz)	Estimated mean MPI in 1 s/ MPI_{max} (%)
2	49	9.8	50.00
3	30	7.5	62.05
4	25	6.2, 6.3	57.28
5	20	5.0 (10.0)	62.05 (100)
6	16	4.0 (8.0)	62.05 (100)
7	14	9.7, 9.8 (7.0)	58.71 (100)

8 mT, the MPI_{max} are 95.2±4.7, 99.2±2.9, 102.7±3.2, and 105.8±3.5 (three trials), respectively, indicating that the chain length has a slight effect on the imaging contrast (contrast difference at 11.1% between the 5 mT- and 8 mT-cases). In order to quantitatively study the influence of θ_c about the imaging contrast and remove the effect of chain length, we use the ratio MPI/MPI_{max}. The study on the relationship between MPI/MPI_{max} and θ_c indicates that the imaging contrast of the particle chain is closely related to θ_c, and there is MPI_{max} when θ_c is 90°.

When the rotating field actuates the microswarms, the periodically varying imaging contrast is determined by the dynamic θ_c. The diagram in Figure 6.11c demonstrates the chain state captured by the ultrasonic imaging system at different field frequencies. So, the estimated θ_c can estimate the changes in ultrasound contrast of the rotating microswarms. For example, the imaging contrast of five continuously generated ultrasonic images representing one cycle varies with the input field frequency of 6.0 Hz (time resolution of the ultrasonic system: 30 fps). The average imaging contrast within 1 s is estimated to be 49.48% of the MPI_{max}. When the input frequency increases to 7.5 Hz and 8.0 Hz, the average value of MPI within 1 s is 62.05% and 46.08% of MPI_{max}, respectively (Figure 6.11c). Therefore, the optimal input frequency needs to be studied to obtain the best ultrasound contrast, that is, the highest average value of MPI. The average MPI within 1 s is calculated by us at the rotation frequency during 1.0–10.0 Hz with an interval of 0.1 Hz. It can be seen from the results that the maximum contrast is acquired when $f = 7.5$ Hz, where the average MPI becomes 62.05% of MPI_{max} (Figure 6.11d). The time resolution of an ultrasonic system varies with imaging depths. Table 6.1 records the optimal input frequencies (f_{op}) for optimal imaging contrast at imaging depths of 2–7 cm. We know that the hydrodynamic interactions between nanoparticle chains are weakened when the driving frequency is less than 4.0 Hz. But when the driving frequency is greater than 10.0 Hz, the length of the chain will be shortened, the aggregation ability of the particles will be weakened, and the stability of the microswarm will be destroyed. So, the f_{op} is estimated in the frequency range of 4.0–10.0 Hz and the interval of 0.1 Hz. Each f_{op} in parentheses represents that the ultrasonic system continuously generates images of $\theta_c = 90°$, that is, all images have the best ultrasonic contrast (MPI_{max}). However, this is difficult to achieve in practical applications for the following reasons.

TABLE 6.2 Magnetic field parameters to form a NRF-driven microswarm with an adjustable chain length

f (Hz)	B (mT)	Chain length (μm)	Area density (μg/mm^2, three trials)
10.0	10.000	59.164	4.63 ± 0.19
8.0	8.054	59.164	4.71 ± 0.24
7.5	7.551	59.164	4.52 ± 0.30
6.0	6.041	59.164	4.50 ± 0.28
5.0	5.034	59.164	4.38 ± 0.41
7.5	6	52.153	4.38 ± 0.30
	7	56.904	4.51 ± 0.29
	8	61.357	4.43 ± 0.32
	9	65.565	4.37 ± 0.36
	10	69.567	4.12 ± 0.15
	12	77.061	3.88 ± 0.47

First of all, in order to make the continuous images of the $\theta_c = 90°$, the time resolution of the ultrasonic system should match the field frequency. But the interference of the time resolution could lead to frame dislocation, or even the interference of one frame could lead to the $\theta_c = 90°$ dislocation. Secondly, the success rate of colony location will be reduced due to the loss of dynamic contrast, especially in noisy environments. Therefore, microswarms positioning at different imaging depths is defined as the alternative optimal frequency (that is, the second highest average MPI).

6.3.3 Experimental Results and Discussions

In this section, ultrasonic imaging is carried out on the microswarm with different driving frequencies and imaging depths to verify the influence of f_{op} on the imaging contrast, and to study the influence of mode transformation on the imaging contrast. Demonstrates *in vitro* swarm localization and microswarms navigation in a limited environment.

(1) Ultrasound contrast under the actuation of NRF: Using NRF with different field strengths and frequencies forms a circular microswarm in 20 seconds. To study the effect of driving frequency on imaging contrast, the length of nanoparticle chains within the micrswarm needs to be controlled. *E.g.*, the estimated length of the chain is 59.164 μm and the NRF of B = 10 mT and f = 10.0 Hz (Eqs. (6.10)–(6.14)). As the driving frequency changes, the field strength also changes accordingly, so that the same chain length can be obtained, as shown in Table 6.2. We define the microswarms area as the region of interest (ROI) used to measure imaging contrast changes. We study the change in ultrasonic contrast of microswarm at different driving frequency, which proves the imaging contrast with periodic changes (Figure 6.12). When the driving frequency is different, the average value of MPI over 3 s shows that the f_{op} is 7.5 Hz when the imaging depth is 3 cm, which is in good agreement with the estimated

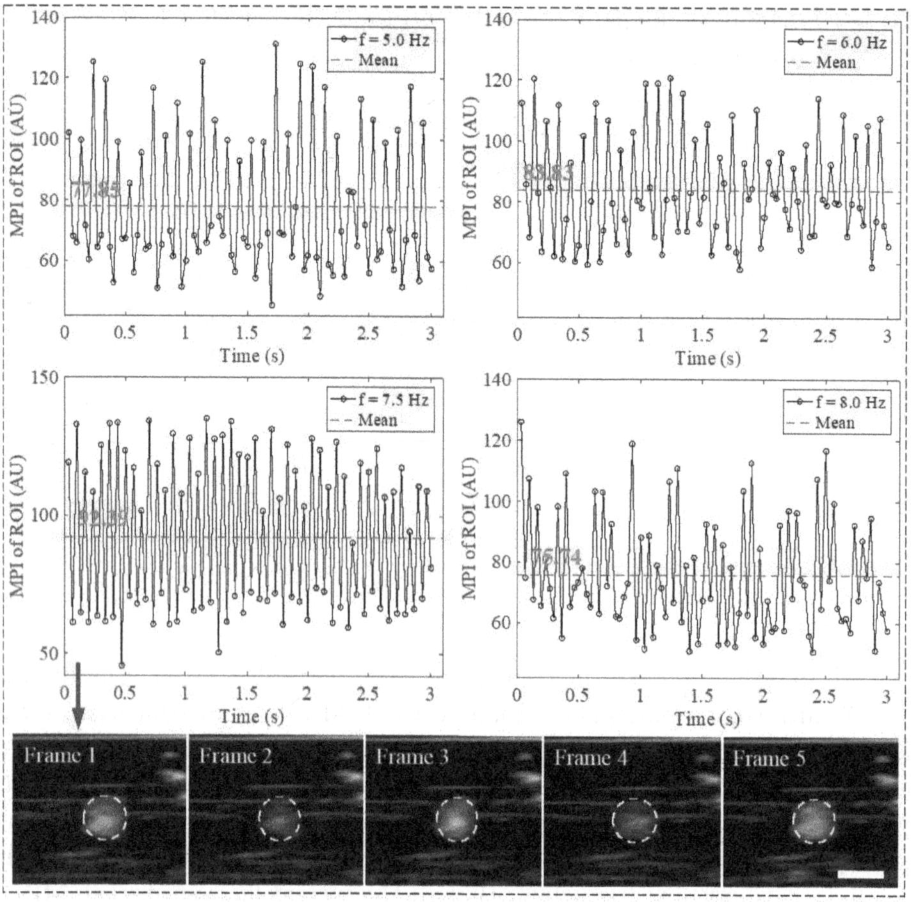

Figure 6.12 The ultrasonic contrast experimental results of the microswarms actuated by NRF. The changes of ultrasonic contrast within 3 seconds (30 feet per second) at different input frequencies. The red dotted line is the average. The scale bar is 2 mm.

value (Figure 6.13a). After the f_{op} was defined, we use different field intensities to investigate the effect of chain length on the imaging contrast ($f = 7.5$ Hz, Figure 6.13b). From the results we can see that the imaging contrast increases when the field strength is 6–9 mT, and decreases when the field strength is greater than 10 mT. Based on Table 6.2, when the strength increases from 6 mT to 9 mT, the chain length increases and the area density is between 4.37–4.51 μg/mm^2. The case of area density of the 9 mT was lower than that of the 7 mT, but we found that better ultrasonic contrast could be observed when $B = 9$ mT. This is due to the relatively strong ultrasonic reflection effect of the longer chain. When $B = 12$ mT is used, the decrease of surface density results in the decrease of MPI; an increase in the chain length to 77.061 μm. The above results show that the length of the chain has an effect on the ultrasonic contrast, and the area density needs to be larger than 4 μg/mm^2 to acquire the enhanced imaging contrast. The field strength should be related to the f_{op}, so that the relatively high regional density and long chain can be maintained.

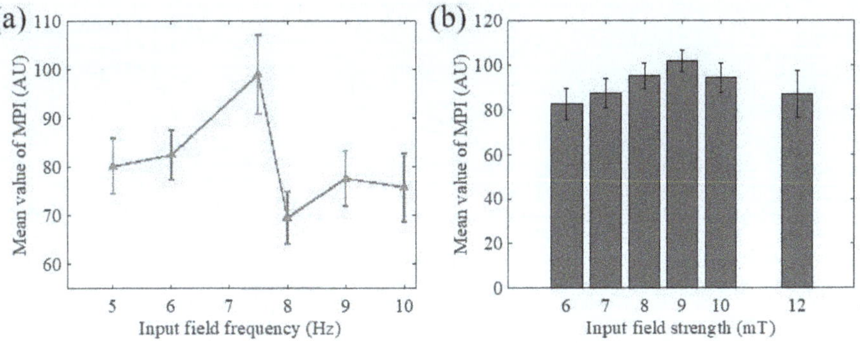

Figure 6.13 (a) The relationship between average MPI within 3 seconds and the frequency of the input field is shown in the figure. Table 6.2 lists the corresponding field strengths in Figure 6.12 and (a). (b) The relationship between average MPI within 3 seconds and the input field strengths. The input field frequency is 7.5 Hz. Each error bar in (a), (b) represents the s.d. of three experiments.

If the drive frequency is higher than the out-of-step frequency, the microswarm exhibits an out-of-step transformation. The magnetic interactions between the out-of-step oscillatory chains become unstable and the weakened hydrodynamic interactions lead to a weakened aggregation capacity; therefore, the microswarms exhibit diffusion behavior as the nanoparticle area density decreases. During the experiment, we actively varied the drive frequency between 5.0 Hz and step-out frequencies (20.0 Hz, 30.0 Hz, 50.0 Hz) at an intensity of 5 mT to study the change in ultrasound contrast (Figure 6.14). The microswarms showed a rotational state ($f = 5.0$ Hz) and an out-of-step state ($f = 20.0$–50.0 Hz) in turn, and the interval was 10 seconds. The average MPI within 2 seconds was used to quantify the change in ultrasonic contrast. It can be seen from the experiment that when a microswarm changes into an out-of-step state, the imaging contrast decreases gradually. By reducing the driving frequency to 5.0 Hz, the imaging contrast gradually recovered with an average MPI of $\sim$90, demonstrating a reversible pattern conversion process. The imaging comparison results of three representative out-of-step microswarms are drawn in Figure 6.15a. In contrast to the imaging comparison of rotating microswarms, MPI does not show a significant time-dependent state because of the irregular motion of the nanoparticle chains. Due to the diffusion behavior, as the frequency increases from 20.0 Hz to 70.0 Hz, the area density of nanoparticles decreases gradually (Figure 6.15b). Therefore, the average MPI and the MPI_{max} of an out-of-step microswarms are lower than the MPI average and the MPI_{max} of a rotating microswarms. From the results, it can be seen that the area density will significantly affect the imaging contrast, for microswarm positioning, microswarms in the out-of-step state should be avoided. In nanoparticle-based therapy, out-of-step microswarms can be used to adjust the coverage area and area density of components, such as magnetothermotherapy [40].

(2) Swarm transformation and ultrasound contrast under the actuation of PRF: The experimental results and analysis of the demonstration mentioned above show that the area density and particle chain can affect the imaging contrast of the

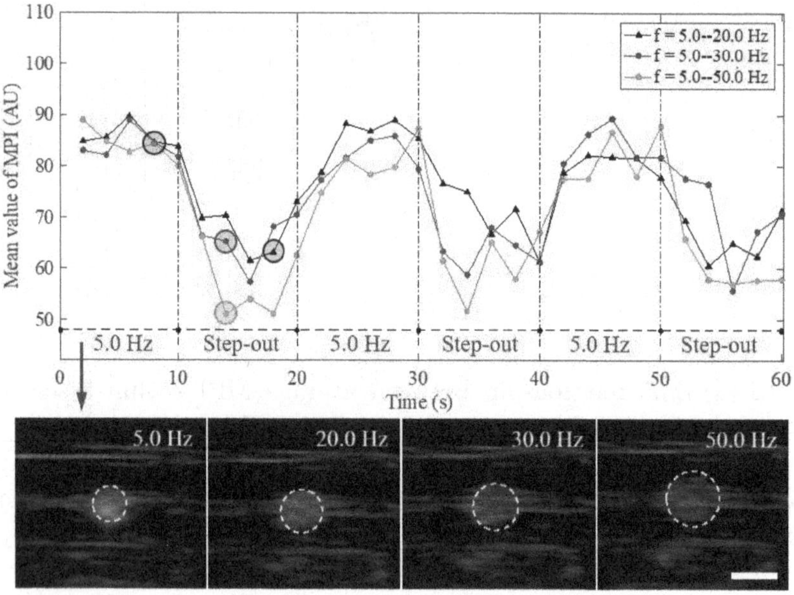

Figure 6.14 Ultrasonic comparison of microswarms driven by NRF with different frequencies. The picture shows taht under the NRF with alternating frequencies, the variation of the average MPI within 2 seconds. When f = 5.0 Hz and out-of-step frequencies are 20.0 Hz, 30.0 Hz, and 50.0 Hz respectively, the time interval between them is 10 seconds. The ultrasonic image shows the corresponding circle-marked swarm areas. The scale bar is 2 mm.

microswarm. In this section, we study the effect of mode conversion on imaging contrast. Driven by PRF, the microswarm can show mode transition. Gradually reducing the field ratio ξ from 1 to 0.2, an elliptical microswarm is formed (Figure 6.16a1). Pattern conversion is a reversible process. By increasing xi to 1, a microswarm of circular patterns is obtained again. (Figure 6.16a2). Elliptic swarms whose major axes are parallel to the direction of wave propagation can also be formed by either directly changing the elliptic angle (*beta*) (*i.e.*, from Figures 6.16a1 to a3) or by changing the elliptic angle to reduce the ratio (from Figures 6.16a2 to a3). We used the latter method to study the change in imaging contrast during image conversion. In the case of $\beta = 0°$ and 90°, the relationship between imaging contrast and field of view ratio is studied (Figure 6.16b). When the angle between the long axis of the microswarm and the propagation direction of the wave is 90°, we find that the contrast increases with the increase of the field ratio. On the contrary, when the field ratio increases from 0.2 to 1 and $\beta = 0°$, the contrast decreases. The changes are analyzed and compared from two aspects: the length of particle chain and the change of pattern shape. As analyzed in Figure 6.11, the imaging contrast is affected by the length and direction of the nanoparticle chain. In the case of $\beta = 0°$, when the external field is perpendicular to the direction of wave propagation, the field strength reaches the maximum value, that is, when $\theta_c = 90°$, $B(t) = B$. Therefore, the maximum length of the nanoparticle chain is beneficial to the imaging contrast. In addition,

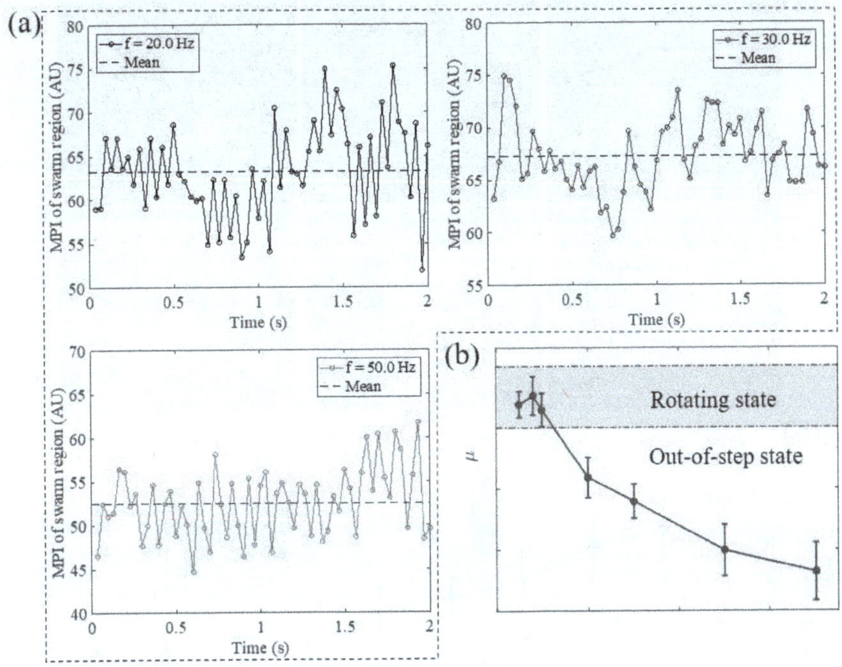

Figure 6.15 (a) When the excitation frequency is higher than the jumping frequency, the MPI in the colony area changes within 2 s. (b) The graph shows the relationship between the areal density of the nanoparticles and the input frequency. Each error bar represents the standard deviation of three tests.

the microswarm is oval in shape and the long axis is parallel to the direction of wave propagation. Compared with the circular microswarm, the imaging contrast is further improved because more nanoparticles in the propagation direction participate in the backscattering of ultrasonic signals. For comparison, when $\beta = 90°$, the length of the chain of nanoparticles is the shortest when it is perpendicular to the direction of wave propagation, that is, when $\theta_c = 90°$, $B(t) = \xi \cdot B$. Reducing the field ratio results in shorter chains, while the swarm pattern shrinks along the direction of wave propagation. Therefore, when ξ decreases from 1 to 0.2, the imaging contrast is lower. In the process of transformation, the change in the region density of nanoparticles can be ignored. The results show that the ultrasonic contrast can be further enhanced by using the mode conversion capability.

(3) Swarm localization *ex vivo*: It is well known that the contrast between dynamic and enhanced ultrasound imaging is very beneficial to microswarm positioning at different depths. Figure 6.17 shows the image processing of positioning and rotating microswarms. Because of the change of θ_c, the microswarm displays dynamic imaging contrasts (Figures 6.17a and 6.17b). An algorithm based on image difference is used to eliminate environmental noise signals, including bubble signals, boundary signals and substrate signals. We subtract the initial image of the microswarm with minimum image contrast from the continuously generated image, and then stack the image to combine the pixel intensity of all the processed images (Figure 6.17c1). The

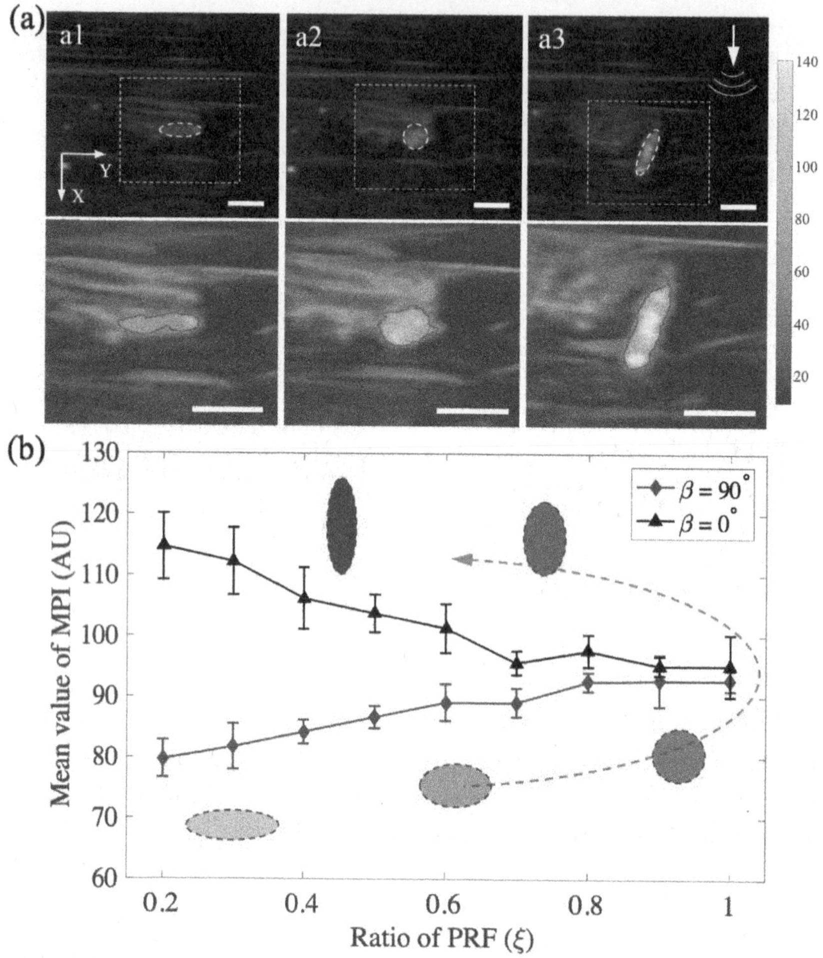

Figure 6.16 Ultrasound imaging of microswarms driven by PRF. (a1)–(a2) The microswarm of circular mode is gained by increasing ξ from 0.2 to 1 in the case of $\beta = 90°$. (a2)–(a3) First, β is adjusted from 90° to 0°, and then ξ is reduced from 1 to 0.2. So that an elliptical microswarms whose long axis is parallel to the direction of wave propagation is gained. Use MATLAB to draw the pixel intensity distributions, and mark the edges of the swarms with a red curve. All scale bars are 3 mm. (b) The change of MPI average value with different ξ in 2 s. The red arrow indicates the mode conversion process. Each error bar represents the s.d. from three trials.

feasibility of this method is tested by using a different number of continuous ultrasonic images (n) (Figure 6.17c2). From the results, it can be seen that 4–10 images are enough to extract ultrasonic signals of the microswarms. The pixel intensities are then multiplied (Figure 6.17d), and apply edge extraction by increasing the threshold. Finally, the microswarm is successfully localized (Figures 6.17e and 6.17f). Furthermore, an electrostatic field parallel to the direction of ultrasound propagation can be applied first to obtain an ultrasound image in which the contrast of the nanoparticle

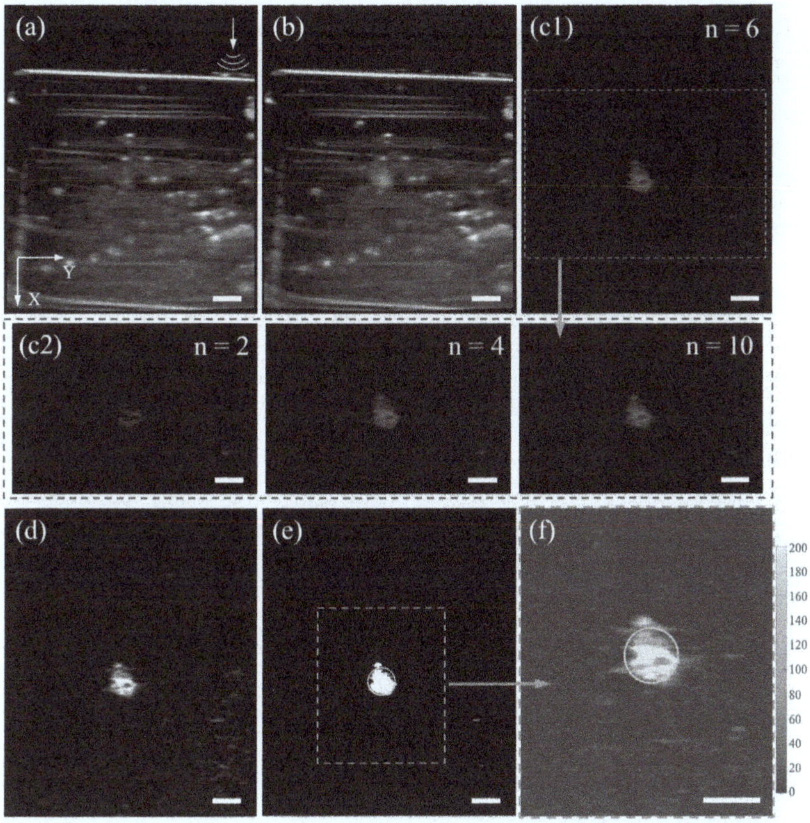

Figure 6.17 Image processing of microswarm positioning. (a) and (b) These two images are typical images of microswarms with minimum and maximum contrast. (c) This figure is a display of the results of image difference and multi-image superposition. (d) In this picture, the pixel intensity is magnified, where the pixel intensity is multiplied by 3. (e) Edge extraction and location. We set a threshold to extract the edge of the microswarm. (f) The pixel intensity distribution of the area is marked by a dotted rectangle in (e). All scale bars are 2 mm.

chains is minimal ($\theta_c = 0°$). The image represents the contrast of the environment and can be applied to the process based on image difference.

In order to further study the feasibility of the proposed method, in order to further study the feasibility of the proposed method, the *in vitro* swarm localization of different depths was carried out. Gelatin jars wrapped in chicken paper towels of varying thickness (Figure 6.18). Microswarms of different depths are formed inside the tank and the imaging depth (d_I) is adjusted according to the depth of the microswarms. Because the ultrasonic frequency is inversely proportional to the wavelength, the greater the imaging depth is, the lower the image resolution is. In order to penetrate the tissue and generate an image with deeper depth information, the ultrasonic length increases and the imaging resolution decreases. Therefore, compared with the relatively shallow imaging (Figure 6.18a1), the ultrasonic image of $d_I = 5$–7 cm is noisier, which poses a challenge to swarm localization (Figures 6.18a2–a4). According

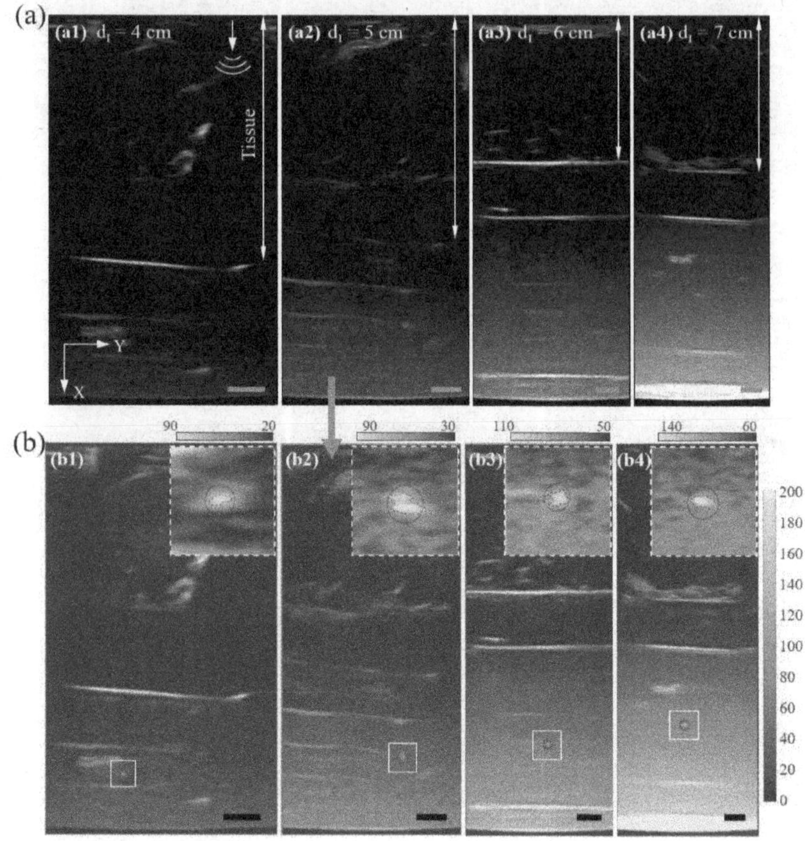

Figure 6.18 Swarm localization *in vitro* with different depths. (a) microswarm ultrasound imaging with different tissue thickness and imaging depth (d_I). Form microswarm in a gelatin jar wrapped with chicken tissue of different thickness. Adjust d according to the depth of the microwave oven. (b) The result of swarm localization after image processing. The color profile represents the pixel intensity, as shown in the color legend on the right. Illustrations are enlarged areas marked by white rectangles.The color legend is located at the top of the illustration. The locations of the colonies are circled in red. All scale bars are 4 mm.

to Table 6.1, the NRF driving frequencies of different imaging depths are adjusted to obtain better contrast of microswarm imaging. Making use of the advantages of dynamic and enhanced imaging contrast, the microswarm is located successfully by using the proposed image processing method (Figure 6.18b). The image superposition of $n = 4$, 4, 6, and 8 were used to obtain the contrast information of the microswarms at $d_I = 4$ cm, 5 cm, 6 cm, and 7 cm, respectively. At the same time, the influence of environmental noise signals on swarm localization can be ignored. In addition, the minimum dose requirement of nanoparticles for swarm localization at different imaging depths is also studied (Figure 6.19). In the course of the experiment, the dose of nanoparticles decreased 1 μg (0.5 μL nanoparticle suspension) each time, until the proposed image processing method could not locate the temperature. Locating the

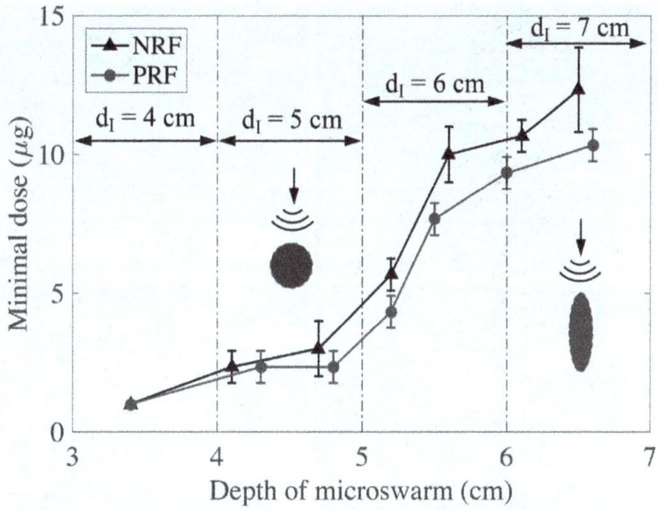

Figure 6.19 Minimum dose requirements for *in vitro* localization of microclusters of nanoparticles at different depths. The imaging depth is adjusted according to the depth of the microswarm. Each error bar represents the s.d. from three tracks. Parameters of the application field of PRF: $\beta = 0°$, $\xi = 0.2$.

microcluster in a deeper position requires a larger dose. The minimum dose requirement is reduced by using mode conversion to enhance the imaging contrast, especially when the depth of the microswarm is more than 6 cm. This real-time image processing method is also suitable for swarm localization during navigation. For example, d_I = 3–5 cm and $n = 6$, image processing requires continuous generation of ultrasonic images within 0.2–0.3 s. Considering that the driving speed of the microswarm is less than one body length (diameter) per second, the positioning accuracy can be kept within half a body length [60].

(4) Swarm navigation and transformation in a confined environment *ex vivo*: Microswarm navigation is carried out in narrow waterways to show morphological adaptation under ultrasonic imaging (Figure 6.20a). Create an *in vitro* environment by wrapping in chicken tissue in the channel. The NRF was first used for microswarm formation, then the microswarm was navigated to a narrow area (t = 25 s). The friction asymmetry near the boundary that is, near the base, by adding a small pitch angle ($\gamma = 4°$) to the rotation field leads to the motion of the microswarm. Then the miniature swarm is converted into an oval pattern by applying PRF and gradually reducing the ξ from 1 to 0.3 to avoid collision with the sidewall (t = 63 s). In the process of navigation, adjusting the yaw angle (φ) of the rotating field controls the direction of motion. Finally, the swram reached its intended destination (tween 90 seconds). Active mode conversion avoids pattern interruption and reduces the impact of pattern-environment interaction, which proves the effectiveness of morphological adaptability.

In the course of the experiment, the change of ultrasound contrast of microswarm was studied (Figure 6.20b). The imaging depth of ultrasonic system is 3 cm. From the analysis of Table 2.1 and the experimental results in Figures 6.12 and 6.13, we can see

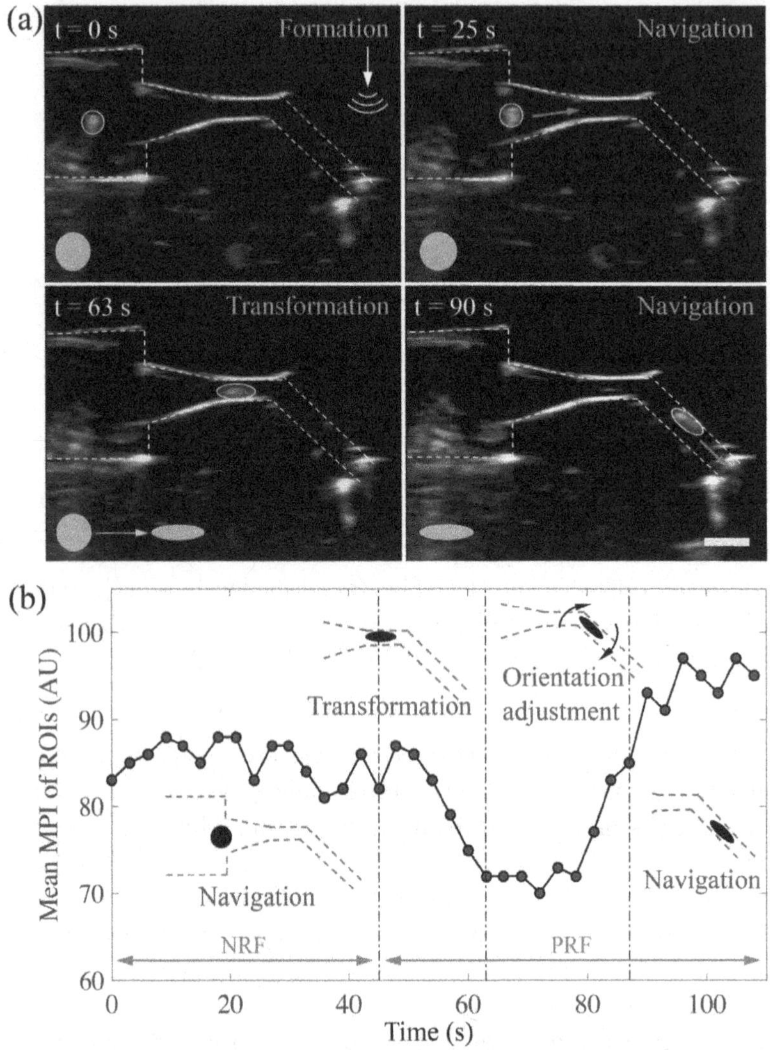

Figure 6.20 Magnetic navigation of microswarms in a narrow environment. (a) Navigation of reconfigurable microswarm under ultrasonic imaging. The yellow dotted line indicates the gelatin channel. Navigate the miniature swarm by adding a 4° pitch angle to the rotation field. The swarm showed a change by adjusting the ξ from 1 to 0.3. The imaging depth is 3 cm. The scale bar is 3 mm. (b) The change of ultrasonic contrast of microswarm in the process of swarm transformation and navigation. As shown in the figure, the process is divided into four steps.

that the best ultrasonic contrast can be obtained when the field parameters of NRF and PRF are set to $f = 7.5$ Hz and $B = 9$ mT. The navigation process can be divided into the following four steps: NRF navigation, PRF conversion, swarm direction adjustment and PRF navigation. The ultrasound contrast of the microswarm shows negligible disturbance driven by NRF and decreases during mode conversion, which is consistent with the discussion in Figure 6.16 (the $\beta = 90°$ case). The direction of the microswarm is adjusted to the alignment channel ($\beta = 45°$); at the same time, the contrast is enhanced due to the increase of microswarm scattering ultrasound. The experimental results show that reversible transformation and controllability can be used to obtain microclusters with environmental adaptability and enhanced ultrasound contrast, which is very important for imaging guidance applications.

(5) Discussion: From the above experimental results, it can be seen that the dynamic comparison of microswarms with different depths is related to the coordination of the frequency of the input field and the time resolution of ultrasonic imaging, which is in good agreement with the theoretical analysis (Section IV). Based on the relationship between θ_c and imaging contrast, the optimal driving frequency f_{op} is calculated, so that the enhanced dynamic ultrasonic contrast can be obtained. From the above experiments, we can also see that the region density of the component and the length of the nanoparticle chain are helpful to the imaging comparison of the microswarm. We also found that to obtain colloidal microswarms with enhanced ultrasonic contrast, the region density should be kept at a relatively high value, and the subunit or subgroup should reach the longest state or elongation state at $\theta_c = 90°$. So we introduce mode conversion and use the polarization of the rotational field of $\xi = 0.2$–0.8 and $\beta = 0°$ to form the longest chain at $\theta_c = 90°$, while maintaining a relatively high region density. The elliptic microswarm with a long axis parallel to the ultrasonic propagation direction was formed, which further enhanced the ultrasonic contrast and the optimal input frequency f_{op}. By utilizing mode conversion to enhance imaging contrast, the minimum dose of nanoparticles can be lowered, thereby reducing the potential toxicity of excess particles. This strategy of enhancing the contrast of colloidal microswarm ultrasound also provides a reference for selecting the position of the imaging probe. As shown in Figure 6.20, the direction of ultrasonic propagation should be kept at a small angle with the long axis of the microswarm. This problem can also be solved by using multiple imaging probes located in different directions [31] or robotic ultrasonic systems [61, 62].

6.4 FLUORESCENCE IMAGING AND PHOTOACOUSTIC IMAGING (PAI) OF A ROTATING MICROSWARM

Synthesis process of the fluorescent nanoparticles is shown in Figure 6.21a. Fluorescence imaging of the swarm formation and spreading of the nanoparticles are demonstrated in Figures 6.21b and 6.21d, respectively. Nanoparticles are suspended in DI water and the fluorescent imaging has a weak imaging feedback because of the low concentration. The nanoparticles are gathered into a relatively smaller region ($t = 6$ s) under a magnetic field gradient, and a rotating magnetic field is then applied for swarm formation (10-16 s). Finally, a microswarm with multiple sub-swarms are formed. The pattern is not an ideal circle because the average diameter of the fluorescent nanoparticles is only 20 nm, resulting in a weak response to the applied magnetic fields. A circular pattern is able to be formed faster using magnetic fields with higher strength. To accurate estimate the coverage area of nanoparticles, imaging binarization, noise removal and connected-body recognition are conducted. The largest area of all the connected bodies is regarded as the coverage area of the major

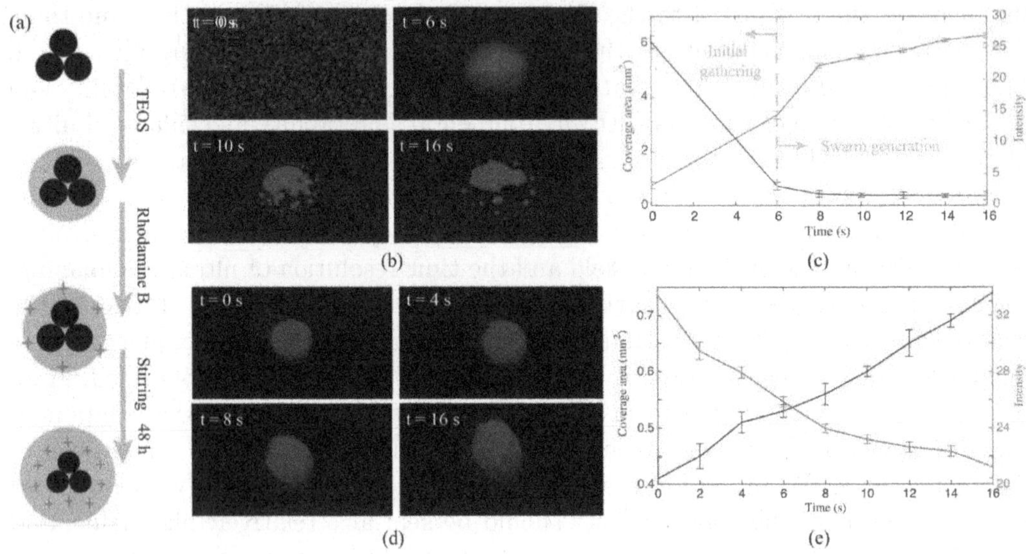

Figure 6.21 Fluorescence imaging for nanoparticles. (a) The synthesis process of fluorescent particles. (b) The real-time imaging of the formation process of a vortex-like nanoparticle swarm. From 0–6 s, the suspended nanoparticles are performed an initial gathering process using a magnetic field gradient. The changes in swarm area and light intensity are shown in (c). (d) The spreading of nanoparticles, and the changes in swarm area and imaging intensity are shown in (e). The error bars indicate the standard deviation from three trials. The imaging intensities are calculated from the coverage regions of the swarms.

swarm. After obtaining the coverage areas at several time points, the data are summarized (Figures 6.21c and 6.21e) and the change in imaging intensity is presented (Figures 6.21c and 6.21e). Figure 6.21c shows weak intensity of the suspended nanoparticles, and the curve of intensity rapidly increases to approximately 14 after the initial gathering. Swarm formation causes a significant effect on the imaging contrast. From 6–8 s, the area of the swarm is shrunk from 0.7 mm^2 to 0.42 mm^2, *i.e.*, the concentration of the particles increases by 67%; meanwhile, the fluorescence intensity increases approximately by 56%. The swarm area continues to decrease when $t = 6$–16 s and finally reaches 0.35 mm^2; whereas the intensity gradually increases to 30. Then the dynamic magnetic field is applied for spreading the concentrated nanoparticles (fluorescence images Figure 6.21d). The swarm is enlarged during the process, while the fluorescence intensity of the nanoparticle swarm becomes lower (Figure 6.21e). From $t = 0$–16 s, the swarm area spreads from 0.42 mm^2 to 0.74 mm^2, showing that the concentration of the nanoparticles and the intensity decrease 43.2% and 36% during the process, respectively. During this short period, the photobleaching effect is negligible. These results show that the particle concentration can significantly influence the fluorescence intensity, and the swarm formation-caused high density of nanoparticles enhances the fluorescent imaging feedback.

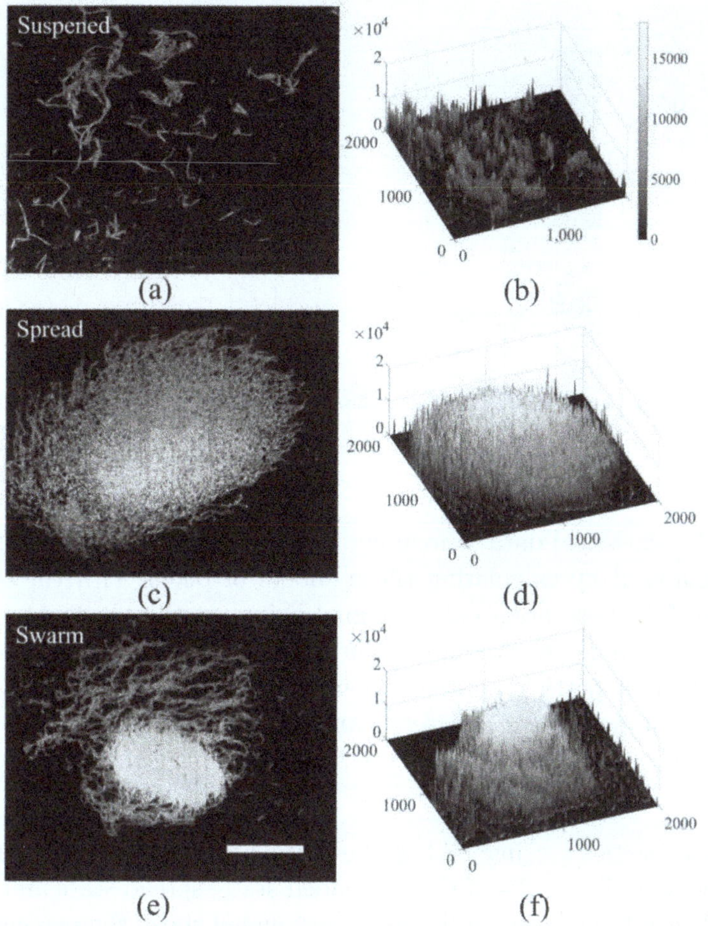

Figure 6.22 Photoacoustic imaging of the nanoparticle swarms with different concentrations, *i.e.* (a) suspended state, (b) spreading state, and (c) swarm state, and the concentrations are 0.7 μg/mm^2, 4.3 μg/mm^2, and 40.5 μg/mm^2, respectively. The color bar indicates the intensity of the imaging feedback. The imaging enhancement of forming a swarm is significant. The scale bar is 1 mm. The color map for (b), (d), and (f) are the same.

Photoacoustic images of nanoparticles with different concentrations are investigated. In Figure 6.22a, the particle suspension is dropped into the tank filled with DI water and the coverage area of the particles reaches 100 mm^2, which leads to a low particle concentration (0.7 μg/mm^2). In this case, the imaging feedback is very weak and most of the nanoparticles are not sufficiently clear. Then most of the particles are attracted into a cluster using a magnetic field gradient, and then the spreading process is conducted under the guidance of photoacoustic imaging (PAI, Figure 6.22b). Compared with Figure 6.22a, the signal is stronger and the contour of the swarm becomes clear. Finally, a concentrated elliptical swarm pattern is formed using rotating magnetic fields. Much concentrated and stronger signals are emitted and shown by the bright yellow ellipsoidal region in Figure 6.22c. The statistical data

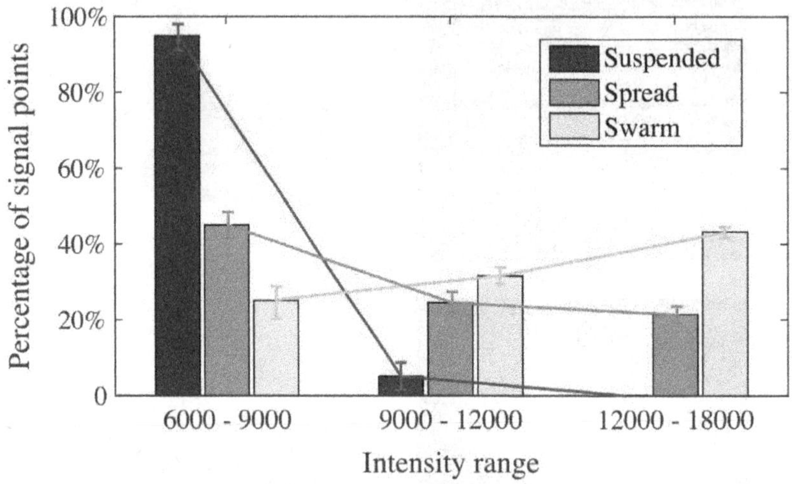

Figure 6.23 The statistical data of imaging feedback intensity. The entire images are statistically analyzed by calculating the numbers of pixels with the corresponding intensity range. The percentages of the signal points on the photoacoustic images in different intensity range are presented. The bars show the relationship between the results with different particle concentrations in the same intensity range, while the curves indicate the percentage difference among the intensity ranges with the same concentration. The error bars indicate the standard deviation from three trials.

of the feedback intensity using PAI is shown in Figure 6.23. The blue, green and yellow bars indicate the results of the suspended state, spread state and swarm state, respectively. When the nanoparticles are in suspended state, the percentage of signal points in the low intensity reaches 95%. The image of the suspended particles has very few signal points in the middle and high ranges of intensity. When the particles are gathered into the spread state, the percentage of signal points gradually decrease with the raising of the intensity range, as shown by the green curve. In this case, the percentage in the middle and high intensity ranges reaches approximately 45%, which are significantly higher compared with the results of suspended state. After the nanoparticle swarm is formed, almost half of the signal points are in high intensity range with another 30% points in the middle range. Therefore, based on the data, it is able to be concluded that the strength of the PAI imaging feedback can be significantly enhanced by inducing swarm formation of nanoparticles.

6.5 CONCLUSION

This chapter firstly introduces a real-time magnetic navigation of rotating colloid microswarms using ultrasonic imaging feedback. Generating magnetite nanoparticle-based microswarms using a rotating magnetic field. The generation process is analyzed, and the internal interaction is simulated. The dynamic ultrasonic contrast of the microswarm is proved by experiments, and the enhanced imaging contrast is obtained because of the high area density of the nanoparticles ($\sim$5 μg/mm^2).

By using dynamic and enhanced ultrasonic contrast media, microswarms are able to locate *in vitro* at depths of 2.2–7.8 cm. The minimum dose of nanoparticles at different depths of microswarms is experimentally studied. In addition, we prove that the microswarm can track the path in real time through closed-loop motion control, and the average steady-state error is 0.27 mm (∼33.7% of the body length). Then, an optimized driving strategy to improve the ultrasound imaging contrast of rotating colloidal microswarms is demonstrated. Because of the angle θ_c which changes with time, dynamic ultrasonic contrast can be seen. Using the relationship between θ_c and imaging contrast, according to the time resolution of ultrasonic imaging with an imaging depth of 2–7 cm, we analyze the optimal driving frequency (f_{op}). It can be seen from the experimental results that the ultrasonic contrast of the microswarm is enhanced at the optimal frequency f_{op}, which is in good agreement with the theoretical estimation. Ultrasonic imaging of the microswarm in the out-of-step state is carried out to verify the influence of θ_c on the imaging contrast and the relationship between regional density and ultrasonic contrast. From the analysis and experimental results, it can be seen that the imaging contrast can be further enhanced by applying PRF-induced mode conversion. In addition, the microswarm is externally located at a depth of 3.4–6.5 cm, and the minimum dose is reduced due to the enhanced imaging contrast of the mode conversion. Finally, paramagnetic nanoparticles as used agents to quantitatively investigate the relationship between the imaging contrast and the areal concentration of the nanoparticles. FI, UI and PAI are applied for observing the nanoparticles with different areal concentrations, which are tuned by two swarm actuation strategies, *i.e.* spreading and vortex-like swarm generation processes. Using all the three imaging modalities, the nanoparticles with lower concentration have relatively weak imaging feedback contrast; while the high-concentrated swarm significantly increases the imaging contrast.

Bibliography

[1] Scott C Lenaghan, Yongzhong Wang, Ning Xi, Toshio Fukuda, Tzyhjong Tarn, William R Hamel, and Mingjun Zhang. Grand challenges in bioengineered nanorobotics for cancer therapy. *IEEE Transactions on Biomedical Engineering*, 60(3):667–673, 2013.

[2] Metin Sitti, Hakan Ceylan, Wenqi Hu, Joshua Giltinan, Mehmet Turan, Sehyuk Yim, and Eric Diller. Biomedical applications of untethered mobile milli/microrobots. *Proceedings of the IEEE*, 103(2):205–224, 2015.

[3] Lidong Yang, Yabin Zhang, Qianqian Wang, and Li Zhang. An automated microrobotic platform for rapid detection of c. diff toxins. *IEEE Transactions on Biomedical Engineering*, 67(5):1517–1527, 2020.

[4] Li Zhang, Jake J Abbott, Lixin Dong, Bradley E Kratochvil, Dominik Bell, and Bradley J Nelson. Artificial bacterial flagella: Fabrication and magnetic control. *Applied Physics Letters*, 94(6), 2009, Art. no. 064107.

[5] Wuming Jing, Sagar Chowdhury, Maria Guix, Jianxiong Wang, Ze An, Benjamin V Johnson, and David J Cappelleri. A microforce-sensing mobile microrobot for automated micromanipulation tasks. *IEEE Transactions on Automation Science and Engineering*, 16(2):518–530, 2018.

[6] Qianqian Wang, Lidong Yang, Ben Wang, Edwin Yu, Jiangfan Yu, and Li Zhang. Collective behavior of reconfigurable magnetic droplets via dynamic self-assembly. *ACS Applied Materials & Interfaces*, 11(1):1630–1637, 2018.

[7] Christos Bergeles and Guang-Zhong Yang. From passive tool holders to microsurgeons: safer, smaller, smarter surgical robots. *IEEE Transactions on Biomedical Engineering*, 61(5):1565–1576, 2013.

[8] Christos Bergeles, Bradley E Kratochvil, and Bradley J Nelson. Visually servoing magnetic intraocular microdevices. *IEEE Transactions on Robotics*, 28(4):798–809, 2012.

[9] Hui Xie, Xinjian Fan, Mengmeng Sun, Zhihua Lin, Qiang He, and Lining Sun. Programmable generation and motion control of a snakelike magnetic microrobot swarm. *IEEE/ASME Transactions on Mechatronics*, 24(3):902–912, 2019.

[10] Shiva Shahrokhi, Jingang Shi, Benedict Isichei, and Aaron T Becker. Exploiting nonslip wall contacts to position two particles using the same control input. *IEEE Transactions on Robotics*, 35(3):577–588, 2019.

[11] Samuel E Wright, Arthur W Mahoney, Katie M Popek, and Jake J Abbott. The spherical-actuator-magnet manipulator: A permanent-magnet robotic end-effector. *IEEE Transactions on Robotics*, 33(5):1013–1024, 2017.

[12] Onder Erin, Hunter B Gilbert, Ahmet Fatih Tabak, and Metin Sitti. Elevation and azimuth rotational actuation of an untethered millirobot by mri gradient coils. *IEEE Transactions on Robotics*, 35(6):1323–1337, 2019.

[13] Lidong Yang, Qianqian Wang, and Li Zhang. Model-free trajectory tracking control of two-particle magnetic microrobot. *IEEE Transactions on Nanotechnology*, 17(4):697–700, 2018.

[14] Islam SM Khalil, Veronika Magdanz, Samuel Sanchez, Oliver G Schmidt, and Sarthak Misra. The control of self-propelled microjets inside a microchannel with time-varying flow rates. *IEEE Transactions on Robotics*, 30(1):49–58, 2014.

[15] Omid Youssefi and Eric Diller. Contactless robotic micromanipulation in air using a magneto-acoustic system. *IEEE Robotics and Automation Letters*, 4(2):1580–1586, 2019.

[16] Mariana Medina-Sánchez, Lukas Schwarz, Anne K Meyer, Franziska Hebenstreit, and Oliver G Schmidt. Cellular cargo delivery: Toward assisted fertilization by sperm-carrying micromotors. *Nano Letters*, 16(1):555–561, 2015.

[17] Chuang Zhang, Jingyi Wang, Wenxue Wang, Ning Xi, Yuechao Wang, and Lianqing Liu. Modeling and analysis of bio-syncretic micro-swimmers for cardiomyocyte-based actuation. *Bioinspiration & Biomimetics*, 11(5), 2016, Art. no. 056006.

[18] Mariana Medina-Sánchez and Oliver G Schmidt. Medical microbots need better imaging and control. *Nature*, 545(7655):406–408, 2017.

[19] Sylvain Martel, Ouajdi Felfoul, Jean-Baptiste Mathieu, Arnaud Chanu, Samer Tamaz, Mahmood Mohammadi, Martin Mankiewicz, and Nasr Tabatabaei. Mri-based medical nanorobotic platform for the control of magnetic nanoparticles and flagellated bacteria for target interventions in human capillaries. *The International Journal of Robotics Research*, 28(9):1169–1182, 2009.

[20] Arash Azizi, Charles C Tremblay, Kévin Gagné, and Sylvain Martel. Using the fringe field of a clinical mri scanner enables robotic navigation of tethered instruments in deeper vascular regions. *Science Robotics*, 4(36), 2019, Art. no. eaax7342.

[21] Xiaohui Yan, Qi Zhou, Melissa Vincent, Yan Deng, Jiangfan Yu, Jianbin Xu, Tiantian Xu, Tao Tang, Liming Bian, Yi-Xiang J Wang, Kostas Kostarelos, and Li Zhang. Multifunctional biohybrid magnetite microrobots for imaging-guided therapy. *Science Robotics*, 2(12, eaaq1155), 2017.

[22] Diana Vilela, Unai Cossío, Jemish Parmar, Vanessa Gómez-Vallejo, Angel Manu Martínez, Jordi Llop, and Samuel Sanchez. Medical imaging for the tracking of micromotors. *ACS Nano*, 12(2):1220–1227, 2018.

[23] Ania Servant, Famin Qiu, Mariarosa Mazza, Kostas Kostarelos, and Bradley J Nelson. Controlled in vivo swimming of a swarm of bacteria-like microrobotic flagella. *Advanced Materials*, 27(19):2981–2988, 2015.

[24] Salvador Pané, Josep Puigmartí-Luis, Christos Bergeles, Xiang-Zhong Chen, Eva Pellicer, Jordi Sort, Vanda Počepcová, Antoine Ferreira, and Bradley J Nelson. Imaging technologies for biomedical micro- and nanoswimmers. *Advanced Materials Technologies*, 4(4), 2019, Art. no. 1800575.

[25] Jin Guo, Chaoyang Shi, and Hongliang Ren. Ultrasound-assisted guidance with force cues for intravascular interventions. *IEEE Transactions on Automation Science and Engineering*, 16(1):253–260, 2018.

[26] Ben Wang, Yabin Zhang, and Li Zhang. Recent progress on micro-and nanorobots: towards in vivo tracking and localization. *Quantitative Imaging in Medicine and Surgery*, 8(5):461–479, 2018.

[27] Guang-Quan Zhou and Yong-Ping Zheng. Automatic fascicle length estimation on muscle ultrasound images with an orientation-sensitive segmentation. *IEEE Transactions on Biomedical Engineering*, 62(12):2828–2836, 2015.

[28] Qianqian Wang and Li Zhang. Ultrasound imaging and tracking of micro/nanorobots: from individual to collectives. *IEEE Open Journal of Nanotechnology*, 2020, accepted.

[29] Stefano Scheggi, Krishna Kumar T Chandrasekar, ChangKyu Yoon, Ben Sawaryn, Gert van de Steeg, David H Gracias, and Sarthak Misra. Magnetic motion control and planning of untethered soft grippers using ultrasound image feedback. In *IEEE International Conference on Robotics and Automation (ICRA)*, pages 6156–6161. IEEE, 2017.

[30] Islam SM Khalil, Dalia Mahdy, Ahmed El Sharkawy, Ramez R Moustafa, Ahmet Fatih Tabak, Mohamed E Mitwally, Sarah Hesham, Nabila Hamdi, Anke Klingner, Abdelrahman Mohamed, et al. Mechanical rubbing of blood clots using helical robots under ultrasound guidance. *IEEE Robotics and Automation Letters*, 3(2):1112–1119, 2018.

[31] Qiyang Chen, Fang-Wei Liu, Zunding Xiao, Nitin Sharma, Sung Kwon Cho, and Kang Kim. Ultrasound tracking of the acoustically actuated microswimmer. *IEEE Transactions on Biomedical Engineering*, 66(11):3231–3237, 2019.

[32] Wenqi Hu, Guo Zhan Lum, Massimo Mastrangeli, and Metin Sitti. Small-scale soft-bodied robot with multimodal locomotion. *Nature*, 554(7690), 2018.

[33] Dimitri Ackermann and Georg Schmitz. Detection and tracking of multiple microbubbles in ultrasound b-mode images. *IEEE Transactions on Ultrasonics, Ferroelectrics, and Frequency Control*, 63(1):72–82, 2016.

[34] Chunxiao Li, Yifan Zhang, Zhiming Li, Enci Mei, Jing Lin, Fan Li, Cunguo Chen, Xialing Qing, Liyue Hou, Lingling Xiong, et al. Light-responsive biodegradable nanorattles for cancer theranostics. *Advanced Materials*, 30(8), 2018, Art. no. 1706150.

[35] Alonso Sánchez, Veronika Magdanz, Oliver G Schmidt, and Sarthak Misra. Magnetic control of self-propelled microjets under ultrasound image guidance. In *IEEE RAS & EMBS International Conference on Biomedical Robotics and Biomechatronics*, pages 169–174. IEEE, 2014.

[36] Emilia S Olson, Jahir Orozco, Zhe Wu, Christopher D Malone, Boemha Yi, Wei Gao, Mohammad Eghtedari, Joseph Wang, and Robert F Mattrey. Toward in vivo detection of hydrogen peroxide with ultrasound molecular imaging. *Biomaterials*, 34(35):8918–8924, 2013.

[37] Jiangfan Yu, Ben Wang, Xingzhou Du, Qianqian Wang, and Li Zhang. Ultra-extensible ribbon-like magnetic microswarm. *Nature Communications*, 9(1), 2018.

[38] Jiangfan Yu, Dongdong Jin, Kai-Fung Chan, Qianqian Wang, Ke Yuan, and Li Zhang. Active generation and magnetic actuation of microrobotic swarms in bio-fluids. *Nature Communications*, 10(5631), 2019.

[39] Zhiguang Wu, Jonas Troll, Hyeon-Ho Jeong, Qiang Wei, Marius Stang, Focke Ziemssen, Zegao Wang, Mingdong Dong, Sven Schnichels, Tian Qiu, et al. A swarm of slippery micropropellers penetrates the vitreous body of the eye. *Science Advances*, 4(11), 2018, Art. no. eaat4388.

[40] Ben Wang, Kai Fung Chan, Jiangfan Yu, Qianqian Wang, Lidong Yang, Philip Wai Yan Chiu, and Li Zhang. Reconfigurable swarms of ferromagnetic colloids for enhanced local hyperthermia. *Advanced Functional Materials*, 28(25), 2018, Art. no. 1705701.

[41] Qianqian Wang, Ben Wang, Jiangfan Yu, Kathrin Schweizer, B. J. Nelson, and Li Zhang. Reconfigurable magnetic microswarm for thrombolysis under ultrasound imaging. In *IEEE International Conference on Robotics and Automation.* IEEE, 2020, accepted.

[42] Zhi Wei Tay, Prashant Chandrasekharan, Andreina Chiu-Lam, Daniel W Hensley, Rohan Dhavalikar, Xinyi Y Zhou, Elaine Y Yu, Patrick W Goodwill, Bo Zheng, Carlos Rinaldi, and Steven M. Conolly. Magnetic particle imaging-guided heating in vivo using gradient fields for arbitrary localization of magnetic hyperthermia therapy. *ACS Nano*, 12(4):3699–3713, 2018.

[43] Kyung Hyun Min, Hyun Su Min, Hong Jae Lee, Dong Jin Park, Ji Young Yhee, Kwangmeyung Kim, Ick Chan Kwon, Seo Young Jeong, Oscar F Silvestre, Xiaoyuan Chen, Yu-Shik Hwang, Eun-Cheol Kim, and Sang Cheon Lee. ph-controlled gas-generating mineralized nanoparticles: a theranostic agent for ultrasound imaging and therapy of cancers. *ACS Nano*, 9(1):134–145, 2015.

[44] Rui Hao, Ruijun Xing, Zhichuan Xu, Yanglong Hou, Song Gao, and Shouheng Sun. Synthesis, functionalization, and biomedical applications of multifunctional magnetic nanoparticles. *Advanced Materials*, 22(25):2729–2742, 2010.

[45] Hongdong Cai, Xiao An, Jun Cui, Jingchao Li, Shihui Wen, Kangan Li, Mingwu Shen, Linfeng Zheng, Guixiang Zhang, and Xiangyang Shi. Facile hydrothermal synthesis and surface functionalization of polyethyleneimine-coated iron oxide nanoparticles for biomedical applications. *ACS Applied Materials & Interfaces*, 5(5):1722–1731, 2013.

[46] Charles E Sing, Lothar Schmid, Matthias F Schneider, Thomas Franke, and Alfredo Alexander-Katz. Controlled surface-induced flows from the motion of self-assembled colloidal walkers. *Proceedings of the National Academy of Sciences*, 107(2):535–540, 2010.

[47] Sibani Lisa Biswal and Alice P Gast. Rotational dynamics of semiflexible paramagnetic particle chains. *Physical Review E*, 69(4), 2004.

[48] H. Singh, P. E. Laibinis, and T. A. Hatton. Rigid, superparamagnetic chains of permanently linked beads coated with magnetic nanoparticles. synthesis and rotational dynamics under applied magnetic fields. *Langmuir*, 21(24):11500–11509, 2005.

[49] Ioannis Petousis, Erik Homburg, Roy Derks, and Andreas Dietzel. Transient behaviour of magnetic micro-bead chains rotating in a fluid by external fields. *Lab on a Chip*, 7(12):1746–1751, 2007.

[50] C Wilhelm, J Browaeys, A Ponton, and J-C Bacri. Rotational magnetic particles microrheology: the maxwellian case. *Physical Review E*, 67(1), 2003, Art. no. 011504.

[51] Sonia Melle, Oscar G Calderón, Miguel A Rubio, and Gerald G Fuller. Microstructure evolution in magnetorheological suspensions governed by mason number. *Physical Review E*, 68(4), 2003, Art. no. 041503.

[52] Qianqian Wang, Jiangfan Yu, Ke Yuan, Lidong Yang, Dongdong Jin, and Li Zhang. Disassembly and spreading of magnetic nanoparticle clusters on uneven surfaces. *Applied Materials Today*, 18, 2020, Art. no. 100489.

[53] Xiaowei Ma, Yuliang Zhao, and Xing-Jie Liang. Theranostic nanoparticles engineered for clinic and pharmaceutics. *Accounts of Chemical Research*, 44(10):1114–1122, 2011.

[54] Aaron C Anselmo and Samir Mitragotri. Nanoparticles in the clinic. *Bioengineering & Translational Medicine*, 1(1):10–29, 2016.

[55] Martin O Culjat, David Goldenberg, Priyamvada Tewari, and Rahul S Singh. A review of tissue substitutes for ultrasound imaging. *Ultrasound in Medicine & Biology*, 36(6):861–873, 2010.

[56] K Zell, JI Sperl, MW Vogel, R Niessner, and C Haisch. Acoustical properties of selected tissue phantom materials for ultrasound imaging. *Physics in Medicine & Biology*, 52(20):N475–N484, 2007.

[57] Carlos Nicolau, Laura Bunesch, Carmen Sebastia, and Rafael Salvador. Diagnosis of bladder cancer: contrast-enhanced ultrasound. *Abdominal Imaging*, 35(4):494–503, 2010.

[58] Jiangfan Yu, Lidong Yang, and Li Zhang. Pattern generation and motion control of a vortex-like paramagnetic nanoparticle swarm. *The International Journal of Robotics Research*, 37(8):912–930, 2018.

[59] MV Melander, NJ Zabusky, and JC McWilliams. Symmetric vortex merger in two dimensions: causes and conditions. *Journal of Fluid Mechanics*, 195:303–340, 1988.

[60] Qianqian Wang, Lidong Yang, Jiangfan Yu, Philip Wai Yan Chiu, Yong-Ping Zheng, and Li Zhang. Real-time magnetic navigation of a rotating colloidal microswarm under ultrasound guidance. *IEEE Transactions on Biomedical Engineering*, 67(12):3403–3412, 2020.

[61] Tianlu Wang, Wenqi Hu, Ziyu Ren, and Metin Sitti. Ultrasound-guided wireless tubular robotic anchoring system. *IEEE Robotics and Automation Letters*, 5(3):4859–4866, 2020.

[62] Christoff M Heunis, Yannik P Wotte, Jakub Sikorski, Guilherme Phillips Furtado, and Sarthak Misra. The ARMM system-autonomous steering of magnetically-actuated catheters: Towards endovascular applications. *IEEE Robotics and Automation Letters*, 5(2):705–712, 2020.

CHAPTER 7

Formation and Navigation of Collective Nanorobots in Dynamic Environments

7.1 INTRODUCTION

Delivery of functionalized nanoparticles in the blood vascular system provides an effective approach to treat vascular-related diseases ranging from vascular occlusion, atherosclerosis, to tumorigenesis. Through intravenous injection, the administered nanoparticles spread passively in the blood circulation system and could reach most of the organs and tissues, providing disease diagnostics and therapy. However, the first-pass metabolism in the liver may cause potential hepatotoxicity and systemic toxicity. The distribution and position of the tiny agents are hard to monitor in real time because of the small size, adding difficulties to the targeted delivery procedure. To overcome these challenges, micro/nanorobots provide a promising approach for active and targeted material delivery [1, 2, 3]. Their on-demand steerability and versatile actuation modes enable the navigation in hard-to-reach and confined environments [4, 5], and various trials have been conducted in cells [6], fluid-filled cavities [7, 8], and blood [9, 10, 11, 12]. However, the drug-loading capacity of an individual micro/nanorobot may meet a critical limitation because of the volume or surface constraint. Their small size challenges real-time imaging and control in a living body, especially in confined, dynamic environments.

To achieve effective delivery, collective behaviors and swarm control of micro/nanorobots are worth investigating. The navigation of microswarms in superficial tissues and relatively stagnant environments is proposed (*e.g.*, eyes and stomach), demonstrating superior performance than the usage of individual small-scale robots [13, 14, 15, 16]. Although swarming micro/nanorobots have shown controllability in the places with negligible flow, the weak interactions between the tiny building blocks challenge the access rate to the target region, especially in dynamic environments. When navigated in the blood vessels, a swarm pattern may be disrupted by complex impacts from bloodstream, such as drag force and blood cells [17]. Two aspects need consideration to stabilize a microswarm before conducting delivery tasks in flowing

DOI: 10.1201/9781032665788-7

environments: introducing strong interactions between building blocks and reducing the impact of bloodstream. The first one can be addressed by inducing attractive interactions between agents. Meanwhile, the swarm should maintain an active status to avoid aggregation. Inspired by the thigmotaxis of sperm, *i.e.*, the tendency of motile sperm to remain close to boundaries, the hydrodynamic drag can be reduced by navigating a microswarm near the boundary of blood vessels, in which the flow velocity is lower than the average velocity. Sperm-hybrid micromotors and their assembled swarm can actively exhibit locomotion near a channel surface to overcome bloodstream and perform multiple cargo or drug delivery [18].

Real-time tracking of micro/nanorobots is crucial when conducting *in vivo* delivery and targeted therapy [19, 20]. Among current medical imaging techniques, ultrasound imaging, as a widely used imaging modality, provides high temporal resolution (*i.e.*, fast imaging speed) with minimum adverse health effects [21]. The typical B-mode ultrasound relies on the gradients of acoustic impedance, and the fast ultrasound feedback enables real-time motion control and path planning of mobile microrobots [22, 23]. However, the low signal-to-noise ratio is a notable issue when tracking tiny agents in dynamic environments. Unlike B-mode ultrasound, Doppler ultrasound (DUS) imaging relies on the Doppler effect, *i.e.*, by measuring frequency shifts in reflected ultrasonic waves that result from the motion of objects. It is originally applied for estimating bloodstream by bouncing high-frequency sound waves from circulating red blood cells (RBCs) [24], and the DUS images are applied to overlay flow data on B-mode ultrasound. It is reasonable to hypothesize that an actuated rotating colloidal microswarm (RCMS) locally disturbs the normal bloodstream and the motion of blood cells, in which the disturbances provide a mechanism for generating DUS signal in situ. Compared to the localization in B-mode ultrasound, both the RCMS itself and the affected region are imaged, and the locally generated DUS signal could be exploited for indirect swarm localization. Therefore, a strategy that integrates swarm control and DUS imaging feedback to perform targeted delivery in dynamic environments is worth investigating.

In this chapter, we introduce the real-time formation and navigation of a RCMS under the guidance of color DUS imaging for active endovascular delivery (Figure 7.1). Driven by rotating magnetic fields, paramagnetic Fe_3O_4 nanoparticles are gathered into a dynamically stable swarm pattern near the boundary of surfaces or vessels. The reduced fluid drag forces and strong interactions between nanoparticles enable the upstream and downstream navigation in flowing environments (mean velocity up to 40.8 mm/s). The access rate of nanoparticles reaches over 90%. The RCMS-induced three-dimensional (3D) bloodstream affects the motion of blood cells and disrupts bloodstream. When emitting ultrasound waves to the RCMS, the Doppler effect is induced by the rotating swarm, which can be detected by DUS imaging modality from multiple viewing configurations. Hence, the 2D planar RCMS can be tracked with ease. The fast DUS feedback enables real-time tracking, navigation, and localized delivery in different flowing environments, *i.e.*, stagnant, flowing, and pulsatile flowing blood, and the swarm-induced DUS signals are able to be detected at a mean velocity up to 50.24 mm/s. Moreover, swarm formation and navigation in the porcine coronary artery are conducted, which validates the delivery strategy in

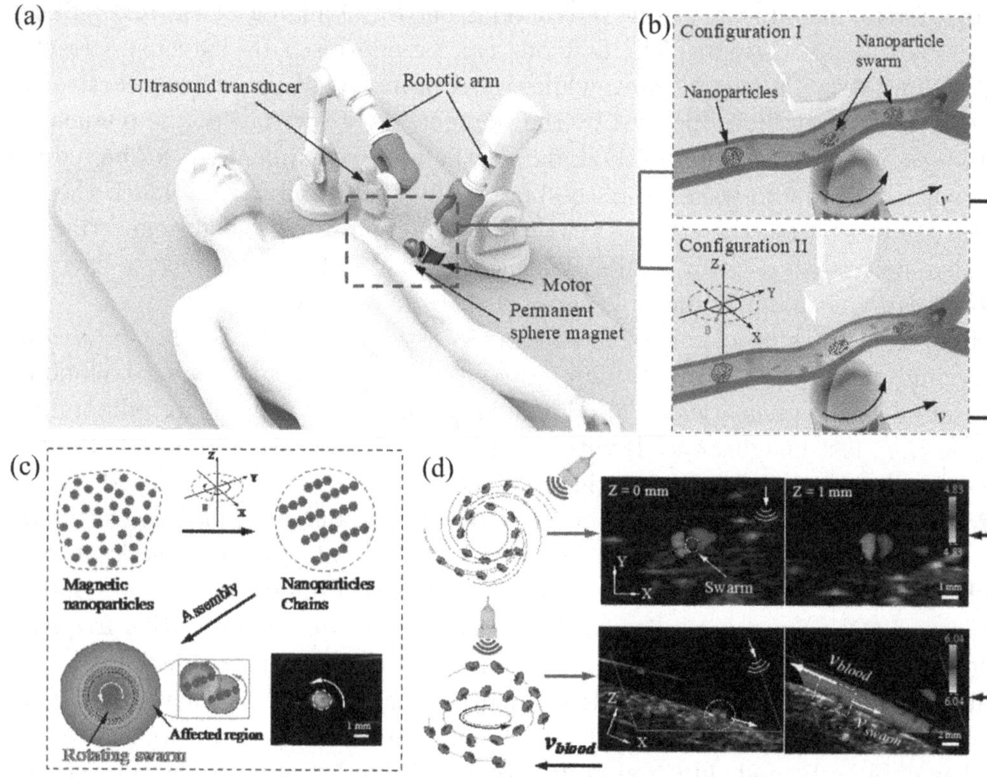

Figure 7.1 Schematic illustration of DUS imaging-guided swarm formation and navigation in blood vessels. (a) The system configurations. (b) Schematic of the swarm navigation in blood vessels. The RCMS is formed, navigated, and tracked in blood vessels with different viewing configurations. (c) The formation process of a RCMS. (d) DUS signal around a RCMS in blood.

ex vivo environments. Moreover, the switchable configurations benefit the formation and tracking of RCMS during the delivery process. The study accomplishes medical imaging-guided swarm navigation and targeted delivery in bloodstream, demonstrating that integrating swarm control and medical imaging techniques holds great promise in active delivery applications.

7.2 FORMATION OF A MAGNETIC NANOPARTICLE MICROSWARM IN WHOLE BLOOD

Formation and navigation of the nanoparticle swarm is conducted by a permanent magnet-based control system. Figure 7.2a shows the simulated magnetic field distribution of the permanent magnet, in which the north and south poles are placed horizontally. The magnetic field is approximately parallel to the XY-plane on the top space of the magnet. The swarm plane (s-plane) is defined as the surface where swarm formation is magnetically controlled, and d_{ms} represents the distance between the s-plane and the top surface of the magnet. The field distribution on the XY-plane

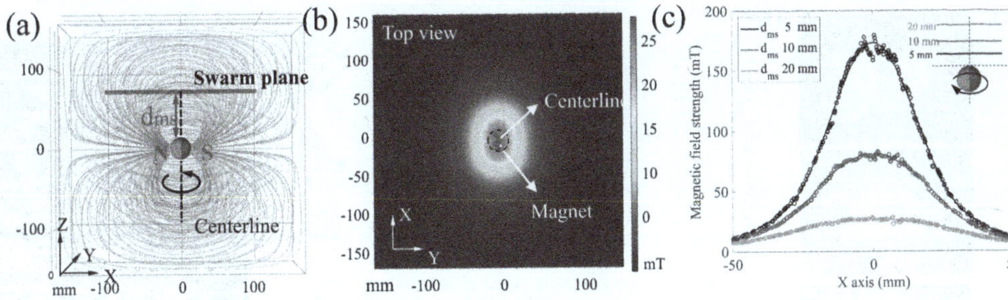

Figure 7.2 (a) Magnetic field distribution of a 25-mm-diameter permanent magnet. The s-plane represents the formation position of a RCMS. (b) A horizontal slice (z = 32.5 mm) of field strength distribution at d_{ms} = 20 mm. (c) Field strength along the X-axis at d_{ms} of 5 to 20 mm. Dots and lines denote simulated data and fitted curves, respectively.

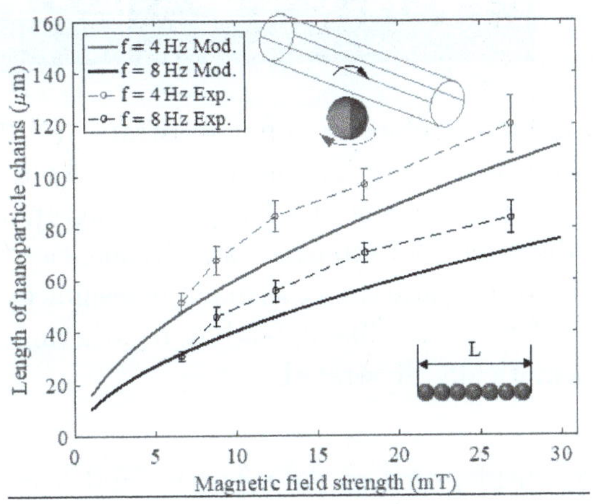

Figure 7.3 The length of nanoparticle chains under different field parameters. Mod. and Exp. denote data from the mathematical model and experiments in glycerol-water solution (viscosity: 4 cp), respectively. Each data point represents the average of three experiments, and each error bar denotes the standard deviation.

at d_{ms} = 20 mm is simulated, and results show that the field strength gradually decreases from the centerline of the magnet (Figure 7.2b). To quantitatively analyze the field distribution, the field strengths along the X-axis with different d_{ms} are plotted. The field strength decreases with both the d_{ms} and in-plane distance to the centerline, as shown in Figure 7.2c. A rotating magnetic field on the s-plane is generated by rotating the magnet. During swarm formation process, rotating nanoparticle chains are first formed due to the induced attractive interaction among nanoparticles. In a low Reynolds number regime (Re: ~0.03), the counterbalanced relationship between magnetic and fluidic drag torques governs the chain formation process [25]. Hence, longer chains are formed by increasing the field strength, whereas fragmentation of chains occurs when increasing the input frequency, because of the enlarged fluidic drag (Figure 7.3). Here, the nanoparticle chains are treated as the basic units. Swarm formations

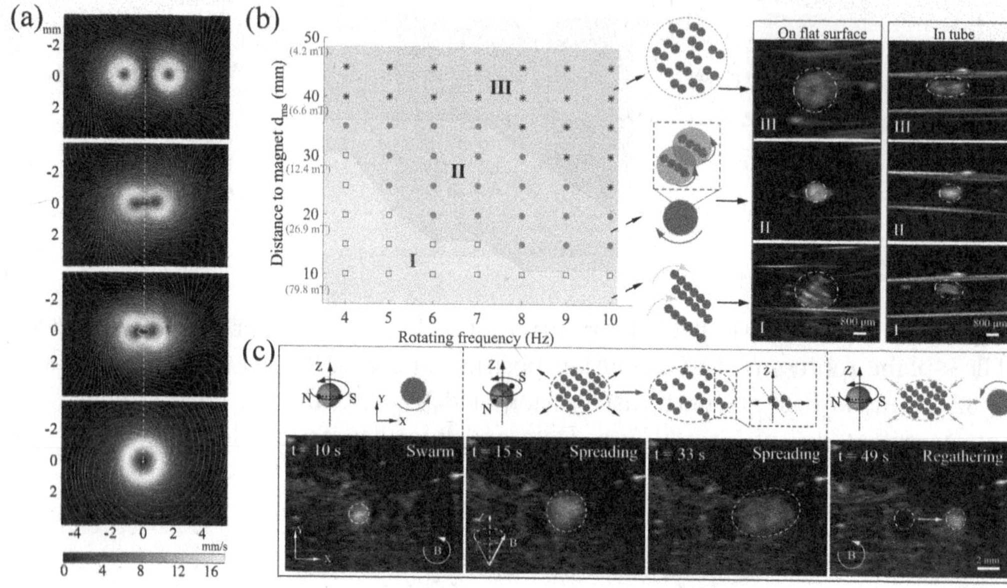

Figure 7.4 Swarm formation in blood on a flat substrate. (a) Simulation of the merging process of two rotational flows. The grayscale and white lines denote the flow velocity and streamlines, respectively. (b) The phase diagram shows the gathering of nanoparticles under different field strengths and frequencies. The right figures correspondingly show the representative experimental results in the three regions. (c) Experimental results of the reversible spreading-regathering of nanoparticles. The applied fields are schematically illustrated.

is analyzed with the consideration of the magnetic and hydrodynamic interactions between chains. During actuation, the induced magnetic interaction between chains changed periodically and averaged to attraction over a cycle. Meanwhile, the magnetic gradient gradually gathers nanoparticle chains into a concentrated region [26]. The locally rotational flow plays an essential role in swarm formation. The long-range attraction between two rotational flows reduced the distance of nanoparticle chains. The two flows tend to merge if the distance reaches a critical value (Figure 7.4a) [27]. After reaching an equilibrium status, a dynamically stable RCMS is obtained.

The magnetic field strength and field frequency significantly regulate the swarm formation process, as experimentally validated in porcine blood (Figure 7.4b). The phase diagram shows that, relatively long nanoparticle chains are formed and tended to repel each other because of the strong hydrodynamic repulsion (region I) [28, 29]. By adjusting the field parameters (d_{ms} and frequency f), longer chains are fragmented into shorter chains, and a dynamic-equilibrium RCMS can be formed (region II). Two criteria are applied to estimate whether swarm formation is completed. First, a dynamic pattern is formed with the area density larger than 4.0 μg/mm^2. Second, the pattern is able to be navigated as an entity, while loosely interacted particle aggregations or short chains cannot be categorized as a stable RCMS. Experiments

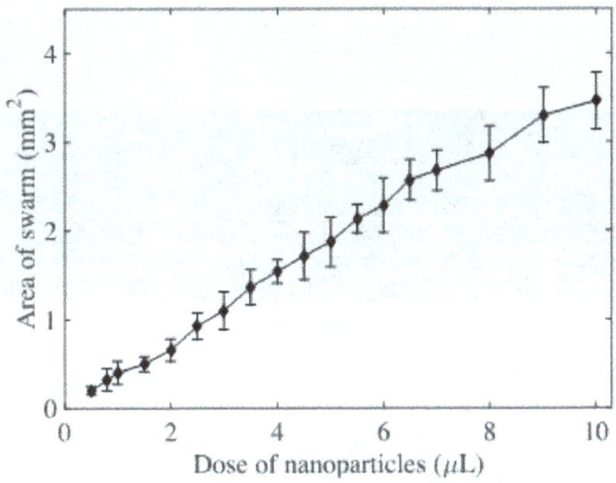

Figure 7.5 Area of RCMSs in blood using different doses of nanoparticles. The area is measured based on B-mode ultrasound images. Each error bar denotes the standard deviation from three experiments.

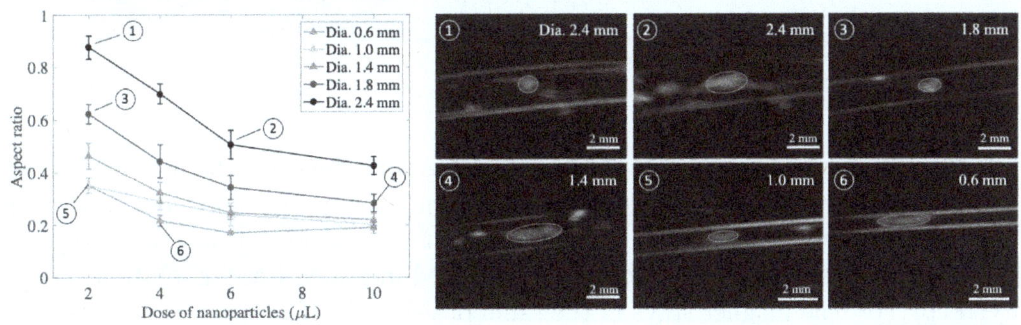

Figure 7.6 Swarm formation tests in different tubes with diameters (Dia.) of 0.6-2.4 mm. The formation tests are conducted in stagnant blood. The aspect ratio represents the length ratio between the short and long axis of a swarm pattern. Each error bar denotes the standard deviation from three trials.

show that the relatively high area density increases the ultrasound contrast of the B-mode imaging [23]. In region III, multiple short chains are formed. Loose-coupled rotating chains with an area density of 1.2–3.8 $\mu g/mm^2$ limit the gathering capability because of the relatively weak magnetic and hydrodynamic interactions. RCMSs with different sizes can be formed using different doses of nanoparticles, as shown in Figure 7.5. Swarm formation on a flat surface and in confined spaces are conducted, where the phase diagrams on both cases maintain the same parameters. RCMS deformed to an ellipse-like pattern with the long axis along with the tube because of the confined formation environments (Figure 7.6).

The RCMS spreads to a larger coverage area under the control of the magnet (Figure 7.4c). By tilting the orientation of N-S poles, the precessing field-induced repulsion between nanoparticle chains enlarges the coverage area of nanoparticles (t = 15–33 s) [30]. A RCMS can be reformed (t = 49 s) after applying a rotating field, demonstrating a reversible spreading-regathering process. During the regathering

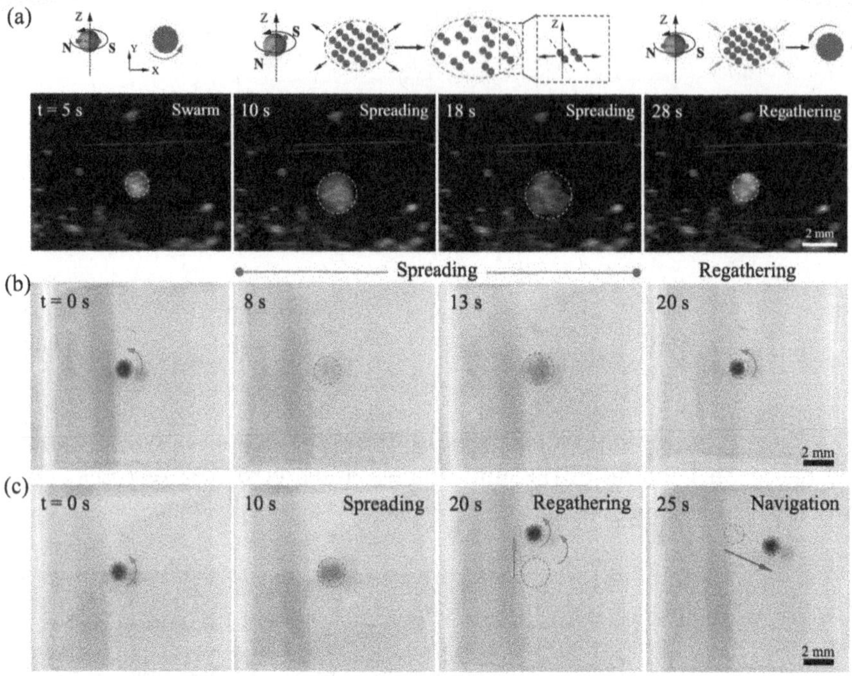

Figure 7.7 Experimental results of the reversible spreading-regathering process. (a) Experimental results of the spreading-regathering process in blood under B-mode ultrasound imaging. The magnet stays in the same position during the gathering-spreading process. (b, c) The process is conducted in glycerol-water solution (viscosity: 4 cp). (b) The magnet stays in the same position. (c) The regathering process is conducted at a new position, followed by swarm navigation.

process, if we move the magnet's position 5 mm along the $+X$-axis, a new RCMS can be formed at the new position that has the distance of around 5 mm to the initial position. If the magnet stays in the same place, a new RCMS can be reformed at the original position (Figure 7.7).

7.3 ROTATING MICROSWARM UNDER DOPPLER ULTRASOUND IMAGING

We investigate the influence of a RCMS on the surrounding environment. Simulation results demonstrate that the rotational flow is locally induced around the RCMS on and above the s-plane (Figures 7.8a and 7.8b). Figure 7.8c show the induced flow velocities at different vertical distances, which quantitatively shows the flow distribution around a rotating microswarm. The flow reaches up to 2.3 mm/s at a 2-mm vertical distance to the RCMS (RCMS radius: 800 μm), which indicates that a rotating swarm can affect the surrounding blood in 3D space. Therefore, detectable Doppler shift could be obtained by the movement of RBCs to the source (ultrasound transducer) by emitting ultrasound waves to the swarm region. To investigate the swarm-induced DUS signal, swarm formation experiments in stagnant blood are conducted

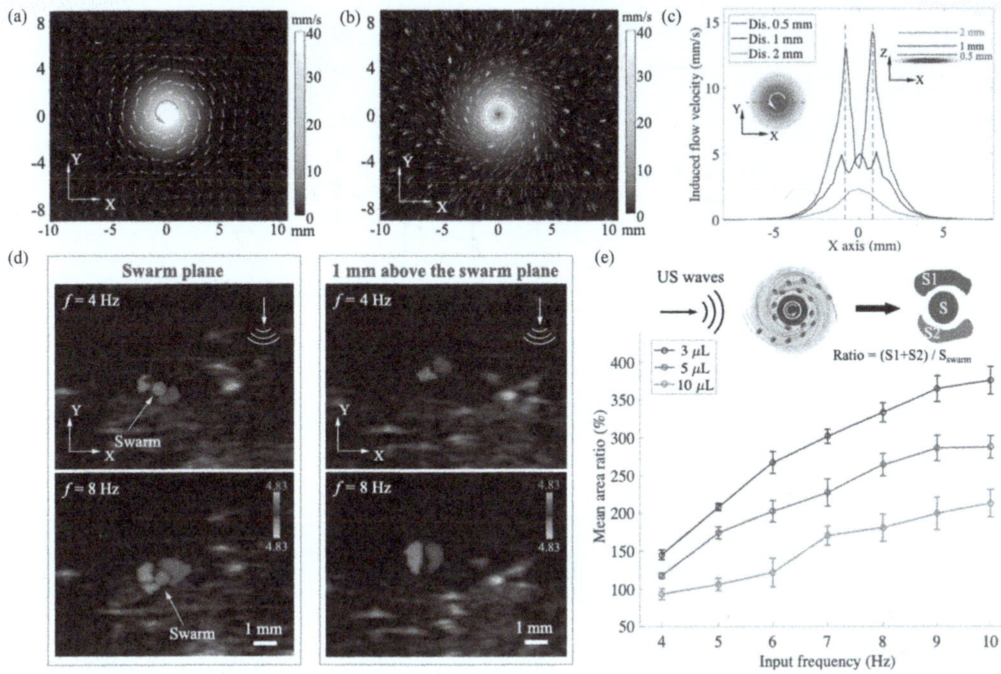

Figure 7.8 Swarm formation and navigation in stagnant blood under DUS imaging. Simulation results of induced flow (a) on the s-plane an (b) 1 mm above the RCMS. The input frequency is 8 Hz. (c) Distribution of induced flow velocity above the s-plane. (d) DUS signals on and above the s-plane. The ultrasound propagation direction is marked on the top right corner. (e) Each error bar denotes the standard deviation from three experiments.

and observed using color DUS mode (Figure 7.8d). Configuration I is used to investigate the DUS signal. The ultrasound propagation direction is parallel to the s-plane. Ultrasound images show both the DUS signal (red and blue colors) and the RCMS (grayscale image) because the DUS signals are overlaid on the B-mode images. Affected by the rotational flow, the blood cells on the left and right sides have opposite moving directions, *i.e.*, moving toward or away from the ultrasound source. Therefore, both red and blue colors can be observed simultaneously. However, the RCMS cannot be directly localized using B-mode signal if the ultrasound waves propagate on the top of the swarm, but the swarm can be indirectly localized based on the swarm-induced DUS signal. In the two cases, the DUS signals are frequency-dependent: a larger affected area and strong DUS signal are obtained by increasing the input frequency from 4 to 8 Hz. To quantitatively investigate the change of Doppler color area at different field parameters, the changes of area ratio with different input frequencies are plotted (Figure 7.8e). Area ratio is defined as the sum of Doppler color area divided by the area of RCMS, and it increases with the input frequency (4–10 Hz). A larger swarm is observed by gathering higher dose of nanoparticles, resulting in an enlarged Doppler color area (Figure 7.9).

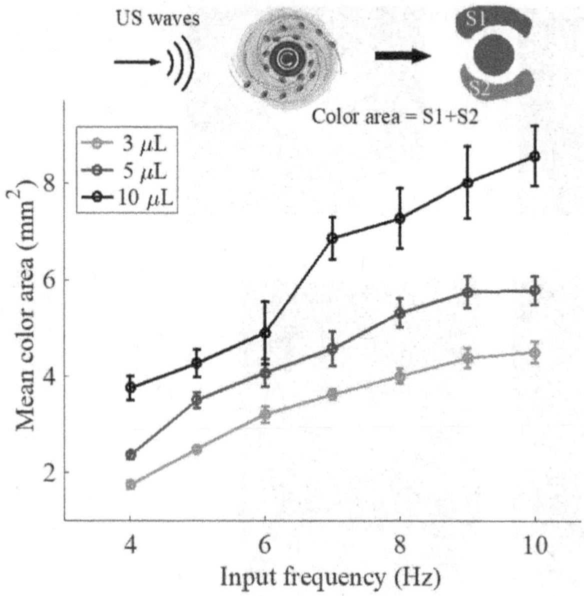

Figure 7.9 The mean area of Doppler colors in stagnant blood in 3 s (14 fps) under input frequencies of 4–10 Hz and doses of 3 μL, 5 μL, and 10 μL. Each error bar denotes the standard deviation from three experiments.

The generation and detection of continuous Doppler signals are essential for conducting DUS-guided navigation. Swarm navigation in stagnant blood is first investigated. The effect on surrounding blood by a moving swarm is simulated in Figure 7.10a, in which the effect on RBCs under different f and swarm locomotion velocity are investigated. The RBCs in the swarm-induced flow experience two main forces: hydrodynamic drag force and trapping force. The latter force is generated from the inward hydrodynamic force in the flow regions of high vorticity [31]. Therefore, in case I, RBCs are trapped and orbiting the moving RCMS. In case II, when increasing the locomotion velocity, RBCs are gradually released from the rotational flow because of the increased drag force. The surrounding RBCs are affected to exhibit rotational motion as well. In case III, an enhanced trapping force is exerted by increasing the input frequency, and more RBCs perform rotational motion that provides the fundamental mechanism for inducing Doppler effect. Besides the field parameters, two ultrasound parameters significantly affect DUS signal: the insonation angle (α) and pulse repetition frequency (PRF). Insonation angle is defined as the angle between the direction of the object motion and ultrasound propagation. The Doppler shift becomes

$$f_d = 2(v/c)f_0 cos\alpha \tag{7.1}$$

where c is the propagation speed of waves in the medium (*e.g.*, tissues and blood), f_0 is the emitted frequency, and v is the speed of reflector (blood cells). A near-90° insonation angle results in a weak signal and the detected velocity of objects (reflectors) close to zero [32]. PRF indicates the number of ultrasound pulses emitted

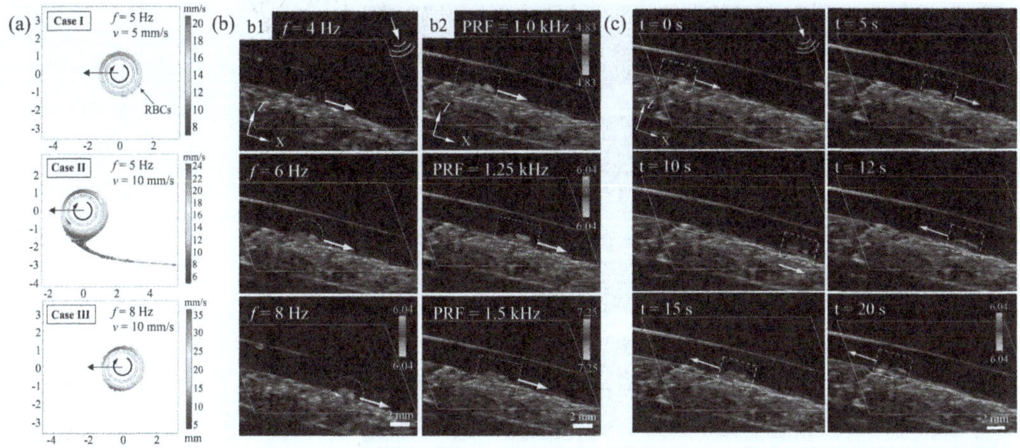

Figure 7.10 (a) Simulation results of the motion trajectories of simulated RBCs (6 μm-diameter microparticles) near a RCMS. The arrows represent the locomotion direction of the RCMS. (b) DUS signal under (b1) different input frequencies and (b2) PRF values. In (b1), PRF = 1.25 kHz; in (b2), $f = 6$ Hz. (c) Navigation of the RCMS under DUS guidance. Parameters: PRF = 1.25 kHz and $f = 6$ Hz.

by the transducer over a designated period of time. When two pulses (pulses 1 and 2) are emitted in a time interval of 1/PRF, a moving reflector (RBCs) moves a short distance between the two pulses, causing the returned pulse 2 to be in a different phase from pulse 1. A new Doppler curve is formed with the frequency equals to f_d by emitting multiple pulses. Therefore, the motion velocity of the reflector is detected, and its moving direction is marked as red or blue color. The DUS signal increases with input frequency under the observation of configuration II (fixed PRF, Figure 7.10b1), showing good agreement with the simulation results (Figure 7.10a). The ultrasound system becomes less sensitive to low blood velocities by increasing PRF (Figure 7.10b2).

Compared to configuration I, configuration II has two advantages. (1) It is hard to keep tracking the s-plane because of the thickness of swarm (<100 μm). The position of a swarm is easier to locate even the imaging plane off the swarm center by applying the configuration II. (2) The DUS signal above the s-plane can be detected along the X and Z directions. Therefore, we apply configuration II during swarm navigation, which is performed by steering the magnet (Figure 7.10c). The swarm navigation is controlled at a mean velocity of 1 mm/s to avoid swarm disruption. The navigation velocity is affected by a more confined space. A high navigation velocity may disrupt the RCMS because of the friction force caused by the boundary and the drag force from blood. The navigation velocity reaches up to 3 to 5.5 mm/s in tubes with diameters of 0.8 to 2.5 mm (Figure 7.11). In addition, continuous DUS signal cannot be observed by directly attracting nanoparticles (no rotation is induced). The nanoparticles gradually stick to the inner wall, and they cannot be actuated as a dynamic pattern, indicating that the interactions inside the rotating swarm play an essential role in swarm formation, navigation, and generation of DUS signal.

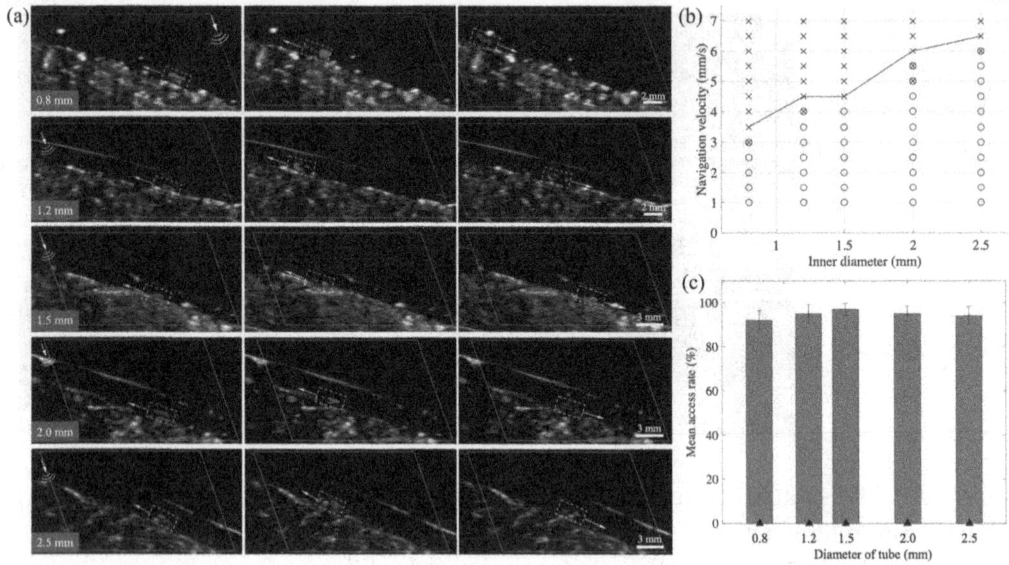

Figure 7.11 (a) Swarm navigation in tubes with different diameters (filled with stagnant porcine whole blood). Yellow arrows denote the navigation directions. (b) Range of navigation velocities in tubes with different diameters. The blue circles and black crosses indicate successful navigation and disruption of swarm, respectively, the overlap between circle and cross indicates successful navigation and disruption of swarm occur in different trials. (c) Access rates of nanoparticles after navigation process in tubes with different diameters. The navigation distance is 40 mm in each trial. Each error bar denotes the standard deviation from five experiments.

7.4 SWARM FORMATION AND NAVIGATION IN FLOWING BLOOD

7.4.1 Pattern Formation and Stability Maintaining of Swarm in Flowing Blood

Due to shear stress, blood velocity near the boundary of a vessel becomes lower than the average velocity, thus, to avoid pattern disruption, the impact of fluidic drag can be reduced by navigating a RCMS near a boundary. Simulations in Figures 7.12a and 7.12b show the flow distribution in a branching pipe, in which the flow velocity along the Z axis is approximately a parabolic profile. The flow stream is significantly reduced near the boundary, compared with the mean flow velocity. As analyzed in Figure 7.2, the field gradient exists along both the horizontal and vertical directions. Therefore, nanoparticles on the s-plane subject to magnetic attraction in parallel and vertical directions, which increases the pattern stability in bloodstream.

Compared to the swarm formation in stagnant blood, the primary influence is the fluidic drag on the RCMS, which affects the hydrodynamic interactions between nanoparticles as well. Experimental results show that such hydrodynamic interactions can be maintained in relatively low-flow rate environments (Table 7.1). The area ratio of swarms in flowing (S_f) and stagnant blood (S_{stag}) environments demonstrates that most nanoparticles can be gathered into the RCMS with an input flow rate of 1–3 mL/min; meanwhile, the control parameters d_{ms} and f affect swarm formation

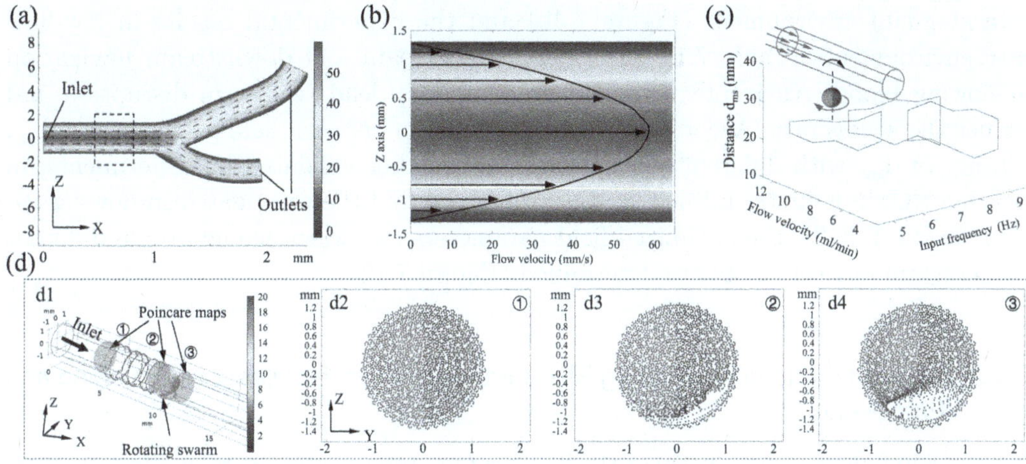

Figure 7.12 Simulation and experimental results of swarm navigation in flowing environments. (a) Simulated bloodstream in a branching pipe (diameter, 2.6 mm). The input velocity is 10 mL/min. (b) Simulated flow distribution along the Z-axis (enlarged region marked by the rectangle in (a)). (c) Range of field parameters (d_{ms} and f) during swarm navigation in flowing environments. (d) Simulation of RBCs flowing through a RCMS. (d2 to d4) Cross sections that have distances of 6 mm (left), 1 mm (left), and 1 mm (right) to the swarm center, corresponding to ①, ②, and ③ in (d1). The input rotating frequency is 6 Hz with a flow rate of 10 mL/min.

TABLE 7.1 Swarm formation tests in flowing blood environments inside a tube (diameter: 2.6 mm)

	Flow rate (mean velocity)	Field parameters (d_{ms})	Formation time	Area ratio (S_f/S_{stag})
Case I	1 mL/min (3.1 mm/s)	30 mm, 6 Hz	10 ± 2 s	94 ± 3%
Case II	2 mL/min (6.3 mm/s)	30 mm, 6 Hz	10 ± 4 s	95 ± 4%
Case III	3 mL/min (9.4 mm/s)	30 mm, 6 Hz	×	×
Case IV	3 mL/min (9.4 mm/s)	20 mm, 6 Hz	16 ± 5 s	87 ± 6%
Case V	3 mL/min (9.4 mm/s)	20 mm, 8 Hz	12 ± 3 s	92 ± 4%
Case VI	4 mL/min (12.6 mm/s)	20 mm, 8 Hz	15 ± 4 s	82 ± 8%

in flowing environments. The comparison between cases III and IV indicates that insufficient magnetic interactions between nanoparticles lead to the failure of formation or pattern disruption. A more stable pattern can be obtained by increasing the input frequency from 6 to 8 Hz (cases IV and V). This is caused by the increased inward trapping force [33]. To effectively form and navigate a RCMS in flowing environments, the field parameters need to be investigated to satisfy the following requirements: (1) Swarm formation in stagnant blood and low-flow rate environments (1–4 mL/min). A reference range of d_{ms} is determined based on the phase diagram of swarm formation in a stagnant environment (Figure 7.4b) and the experimental results in low-flow rate environments (Table 7.1). (2) Effective upstream and downstream navigation in flowing blood. An insufficient field gradient may lead to swarm disruption and reduce the access rate. According to the relationship between field gradient and d_{ms}, a range of d_{ms} with different f is selected and further validated by experiments, in which a RCMS is firstly formed in stagnant blood and then navigated in flowing environments. Finally, the optimized field parameters for swarm navigation in different bloodstream environments are determined (Figure 7.12c).

7.4.2 Swarm Navigation in Flowing Blood Based on Doppler Ultrasound Imaging and Processing

A RCMS in flowing blood disturbs the flow profiles and induces Doppler effect, providing the fundamental mechanism for DUS tracking. We first investigate the influence of a RCMS on flowing RBCs using simulation. Simulated RBCs (6 μm-diameter microparticles) are released from the inlet (Figure 7.12d1). The particles are divided into two groups according to the Y coordinate in the Poincaré map that represents the particle location at its initial position. Under the laminar flow environment, the microparticles remain in the same position before interacting with the RCMS (Figure 7.12d2). After contacting the swarm-induced flow, 6.5% particles change their initial position. After flowing over the RCMS, 12.4% of microparticles are affected by the swarm and move to another half plane (Figures 7.12d3 and 7.12d4), indicating that the normal motion of RBCs are disturbed before contacting the swarm. This disturbance induces Doppler shift by emitting ultrasound pulses to the swarm region. Experimental results demonstrate swarm navigation in flowing blood (Figure 7.13a). The Doppler red and blue colors are dynamically generated around the swarm, therefore, one of the colors can be detected from the background color (bloodstream). Stronger signals can be obtained by increasing the input frequency, as demonstrated in Figure 7.13a1. The swarm can be localized and navigated under the DUS guidance in upstream and downstream manners (Figures 7.13a2 and 7.13a3). Controlled by the magnet-based actuation system, the swarm exhibits locomotion at a mean velocity of 1 mm/s. Because the detectable signal relies on the disruption of normal bloodstream around the swarm, this mechanism may become invalid at a high flow velocity. Moreover, increasing the dose of nanoparticles and the input frequency contributes to stronger signals, which can be applied to applications in relatively high-flow rate environments. The experimental data in Figure 7.13b show the minimal frequency requirements for tracking a RCMS with different flow velocities. The minimal frequency increases with the flow velocity and decreases by using more nanoparticles. However, a 3-μL dose RCMS is hard to be tracked with a mean velocity of 50.2 mm/s because its influence on the bloodstream is too weak to be detected by the DUS imaging. Besides, the increased PRF also weakens the sensitivity of low-velocity flow, failing the real-time swarm localization. The swarm position can be recognized again at an input frequency of 9 Hz by increasing the nanoparticle dose to 5 μL.

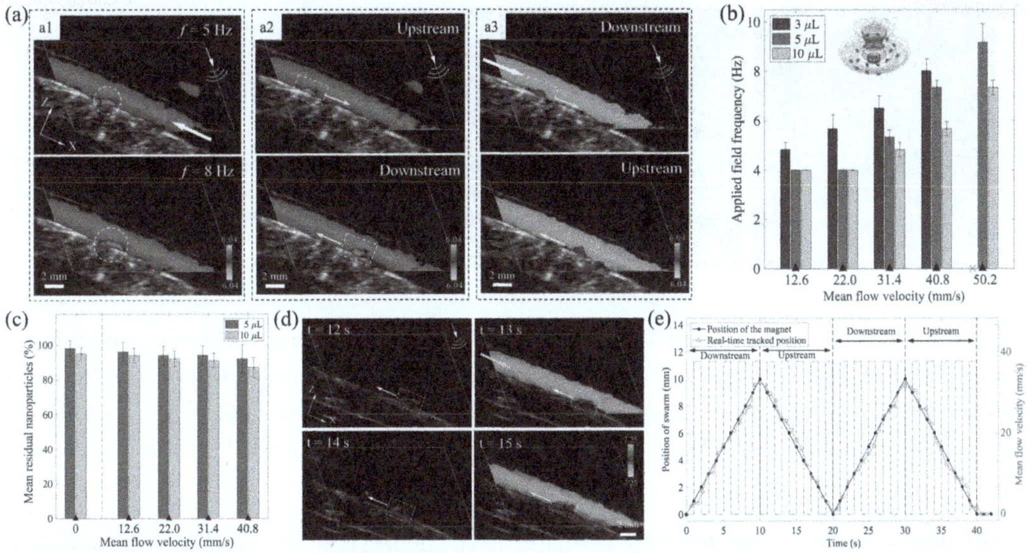

Figure 7.13 (a) Navigation of a swarm in flowing blood at a mean flow velocity of 31.4 mm/s. White and yellow arrows show the flow and swarm navigation directions, respectively. (b) Minimal frequency requirements for tracking a RCMS under different flow velocities. PRF: 1.0 kHz (12.6 mm/s), 1.25 kHz (22.0 to 31.4 mm/s), 1.5 kHz (40.8 mm/s), and 1.75 kHz (50.2 mm/s). Each error bar denotes the standard deviation from three experiments. (c) Recycled residual nanoparticles after navigation under different flow velocities. The zero case represents the control group. Each error bar denotes the standard deviation from five experiments. (d) Navigation of a RCMS in a pulsatile flow environment. The blue and yellow arrows represent the flow direction and the swarm navigation direction, respectively. (e) Comparison between the real-time tracked position and the position of the magnet. The blue dashed line represents the flow profile.

During navigation in flowing blood, the DUS signal dynamically change with no obvious periodicity. The following three steps are designed in the tracking algorithm to improve the tracking effectiveness. First, defining dynamic region of interest (ROI). During the navigation, the swarm followed the magnet's movement. Therefore, the swarm must be located in a confined region near the magnet. The position between the center of the magnet and the end effector of the robotic arm is calibrated before conducting the experiments. A dynamic square ROI centered with the X coordinate of the magnet is defined, which follows the magnet during the navigation process. Second, color extraction and superimposition. The red color areas in ROIs are extracted and the extraction results of n frames are superimposed ($n = 5$–15), avoiding the influence of noise signals and increasing the tracking effectiveness. Third, the superimposed Doppler color's center is calculated, and a Kalman filter is applied to reduce disturbance of the tracking positions. Since the induced DUS signal are distributed around the RCMS on the s-plane and the region above, thus, it is reasonable to treat the center of the superimposed Doppler color as the swarm position. The

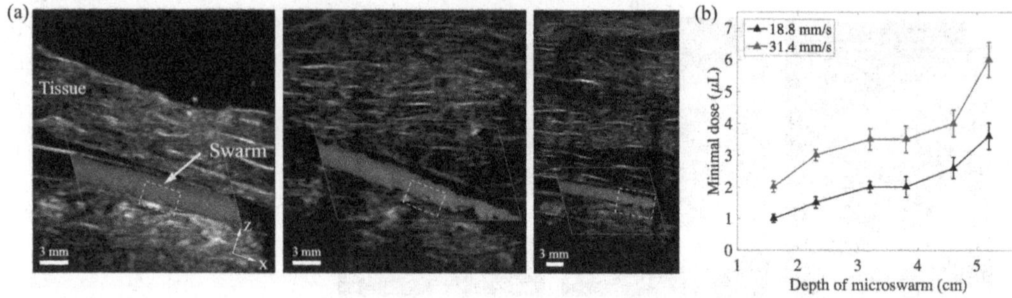

Figure 7.14 (a) Imaging of a RCMS through porcine tissue with different thicknesses (from left to right: 1 cm, 1.8 cm, and 3 cm) under a flowing environment. The mean flow velocity is 31.4 mm/s. Parameters are: $f = 6$ Hz, PRF = 1.25 kHz. (b) Minimal dose requirements for tracking a RCMS at different depths and flow velocities.

comparison between the tracked position and theoretical position is conducted, in which the magnet's position are considered as the theoretical position. The position errors are 0.37 and 0.41 mm during the upstream and downstream navigation, respectively. The overall error 0.34 ± 0.19 mm (three trials), *i.e.*, 21% of the diameter of a RCMS, proving the effectiveness of the tracking approach.

The penetration capability of ultrasound waves can be used for deep tissue imaging. Experiments in Figure 7.14 demonstrated that a RCMS underneath different thicknesses of porcine tissues is successfully tracked. The imaging depth in the ultrasound system is adjusted according to the depth of RCMS. The minimal dose requirements of nanoparticles for localization at different depths are investigated (Figure 7.14), where the dose is reduced gradually until the image process approach failed to localize the swarm. The minimal dose increased when deepening the depth, and around 4 μL is required for localizing a swarm at a 4-cm depth. The nanoparticles are collected, washed, hot air dried, and weighed after finishing the navigation process. Data in Figure 7.13c represent the total weight from 10 trials to reduce the measurement errors. The results in Table 7.1 and Figure 7.13c indicate that the swarm pattern can overcome disruption from flowing blood at a relatively high flow rate, indicating that the interactions between nanoparticles play an essential role in maintaining pattern stability in dynamic environments. Around 90% of nanoparticles are gathered into the RCMS with relatively low flow rates (1–3 mL/min). As a comparison, a RCMS exhibit locomotion in flowing blood with high access rates (~90%) although the flow rate reached over 10 mL/min.

Swarm navigation is implemented in pulsatile flowing environments to investigate the feasibility of our approach. Pulse wave Doppler (PWD) imaging is applied to measure the flow velocity (Figure 7.15) [34]. A mixed tracking algorithm is applied to real-time track the RCMS. In the low-flow region, the DUS signal is extracted and merged using continuous 10 frames, and then the position is determined by analyzing the center of the processed signal. The algorithm in the high-flow region is like that in the constant flow cases. The tracking results are plotted in Figure 7.13e, in which the RCMS is navigated twice in a downstream-upstream cycle. Results show that the overall tracking error in three trials is 0.44 ± 0.21 mm, *i.e.*, 28% of the swarm body

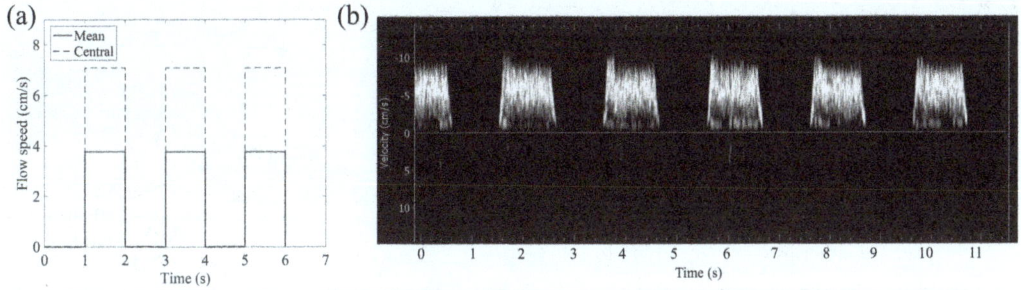

Figure 7.15 Velocity of the pulsatile bloodstream in vitro. (a) Simulation results of the mean flow velocity and the central velocity. Input bloodstream rate: 12 mL/min with a 1 s interval. (b) Measurement of bloodstream in continuous 11 s using pulsed-wave Doppler.

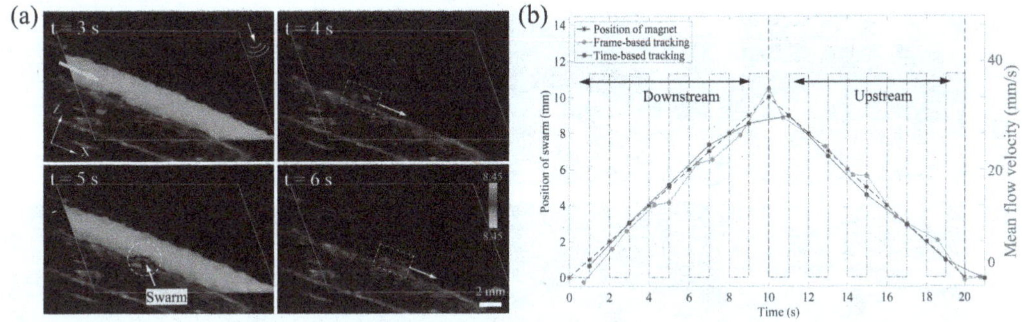

Figure 7.16 Real-time navigation and tracking in a pulsatile flow environment. (a) Navigation of a RCMS in continuous 4 s. Input frequency $f = 8$ Hz, PRF = 1.75 kHz, and the input flow velocity is 14 mL/min. (b) The comparison between time-based and frame-based tracking results.

length. Figure 7.13b indicates that the disturbance from high flow velocity challenges the real-time Doppler tracking. However, the tracking algorithm still effective in the low-velocity region of a pulsatile flow profile. To test the tracking method, we increase flow velocity 14 mL/min and halve the dose of nanoparticles (3 μL; Figure 7.16). The DUS signal in the low-velocity rate region enables the swarm localization, although the swarm cannot be tracked in the high-velocity region. Two tracking algorithms are applied for tracking a swarm: frame-based (n = 10) and time-based tracking approaches (time interval, 1 s). Results show that the overall position errors using frame- and time-based methods are 0.56 ± 0.26 and 0.32 ± 0.22 mm, respectively (Figure 7.16). The RCMS can be localized in this low-dose high–flow rate environment although the tracking frequency became lower, *i.e.*, ∼60% in 12 mL/min-case.

7.5 REAL-TIME SWARM FORMATION AND NAVIGATION IN PORCINE CORONARY ARTERY *EX VIVO*

To validate the feasibility of the delivery strategy, swarm formation and navigation are conducted in porcine coronary artery *ex vivo* (Figure 7.17a). Configuration I is

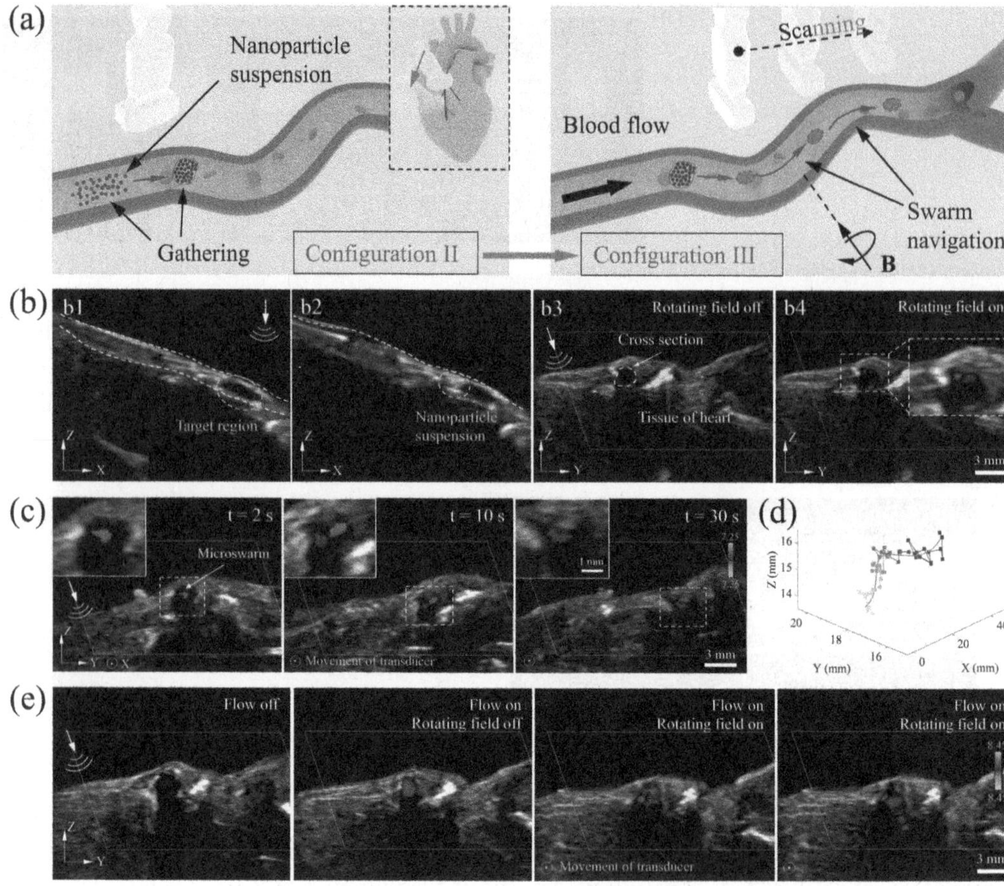

Figure 7.17 Real-time navigation in porcine coronary artery *ex vivo*. (a) Schematic illustration of the nanoparticle release, followed by swarm formation and navigation. The viewing configuration is switched between configurations II and III. (b) The artery is marked by the dashed yellow curves in (b1) and (b2). Blue circles refer to the target region (b1) before and (b2) after releasing nanoparticles into the artery, respectively. (b3 and b4) Ultrasound images before and after applying the rotating magnet. (b1 and b2) and (b3 and b4) are observed with configurations II and III, respectively. (c) Navigation of the RCMS in stagnant blood. The insets show the enlarged images of the region marked by the dashed rectangles. The ultrasound probe is moved along the X-axis. (d) Real-time tracked position of the RCMS. Dots and the red line represent the tracked position and the fitted curve, respectively. (e) Real-time navigation in flowing blood. PRFs are 1.5 kHz in (c, d) and 1.75 kHz in (e).

first applied to observe the artery and choose the target region for releasing nanoparticle. A catheter is used to release nanoparticles inside the artery. Meanwhile, the ultrasound probe is aligned with the catheter for observation of the nanoparticle release, guided by B-mode ultrasound imaging (Figures 7.17b1 and 7.17b2). During swarm formation, system configuration is switched to III because the curved vessel is hard to fully observe using 2D ultrasound images (Figures 7.17b3 and 7.17b4), and the cross section of the vessel is also observed under this configuration. Dynamic DUS signal is detected on the cross section of the vessel after forming a RCMS (Figure 7.17b4). The RCMS is then navigated by controlling the magnet, and the motion of the ultrasound probe is controlled along the X direction and DUS signal on the cross sections (YZ-plane) are recorded simultaneously (Figure 7.17c). The Y, Z and X coordinates of the RCMS are extracted from the ultrasound images and the manipulator, respectively. A frame-merging algorithm is applied to track the RCMS in the vessel (Figure 7.17d). The ultrasound probe enables real-time tracking of the RCMS in the vessel by scanning along the artery. Bloodstream is restored after swarm formation, and the swarm navigation in flowing blood can be conducted by recognizing the induced red DUS signal (Figure 7.17e). Swarm navigation in pulsatile flow environment is performed. During navigation in the low-flow region, the induced DUS signal can be directly applied to swarm localization. The induced red Doppler color can also be recognized from the blue color caused by the bloodstream when navigating the RCMS in the high-flow region. The nanoparticle swarm can be navigated and tracked in stagnant and flowing environments *ex vivo*, showing the effectiveness of our strategy. During experiments, the switchable configurations benefit the swarm formation and navigation process. Configuration II provides a large observation space and is suitable for guiding the nanoparticle release. Considering the relatively large area of DUS signal around a RCMS, the scanning ultrasound probe in configuration III enables the tracking and navigation process in curved blood vessels.

7.6 DISCUSSION AND CONCLUSION

Microrobotic swarms allow simpler building blocks to organize in a coordinated manner to conduct various tasks, such as targeted delivery and micromanipulation [35, 36]. The capability of an individual agent may be affected when scaling down to micro/nanometer scale, whereas their collectives can enhance the functionalities as an entity. For instance, larger delivery capacity of drug and cargo and superior imaging contrast in deep tissue environments can be realized by applying a microrobotic swarm. Although swarm formation in various fluidic environments has been demonstrated, the control of swarm formation and navigation in a dynamic, complex environment requires more fundamental understanding. To fundamentally understand swarm control, we used a permanent magnet–based actuation method to achieve swarm formation, reversible gathering, and navigation in blood with stagnant and dynamic environments. Unlike the navigation of individual microrobots in dynamic environments [11, 37], the swarm control strategy should maintain the pattern stability and against aggregation of the building blocks (*e.g.*, nanoparticles and microrobots) at the same time [18]. The rotating field gathers nanoparticles into a dynamic RCMS, and navigation of the RCMS has been performed (both upstream and downstream) in flowing environments. Moreover, by adjusting the angle between the magnetic dipoles and the s-plane, the swarm can be spread toward an increased coverage area and regathered again. Such a reversible area density of nanoparticles may provide potential applications in magnetic hyperthermia [38]. The swarm formation in Figures 7.4b and 7.4c and Figure 7.8 indicates that a rotating field in the range of ~8 to 30 mT and 4 to 10 Hz is sufficient to form a RCMS in blood. The proposed experiment results provide guidance to the swarm formation process using different magnetic actuation systems, such as the electromagnetic coil system and permanent magnet–based system.

To navigate a microrobotic swarm to a target site, one of the critical challenges is the real-time localization and tracking, which demands high temporal resolution and signal-to-noise ratio [39]. Our study demonstrates the first investigation that uses DUS imaging for real-time tracking a RCMS from multiple viewing angles (Figures 7.1a-c). DUS is originally designed for bloodstream estimation, which is a noninvasive test and is compatible with magnetic fields. Our approach enables real-time tracking of a RCMS in stagnant and flowing blood environments, which is hardly possible using an individual agent in micrometer and sub-micrometer scale. Experimental results indicate that a low dose of nanoparticles is sufficient to generate DUS signal in the dynamic, deep tissue environments. A high flow rate may surpass the locally induced flow and make DUS signal-based tracking ineffective, such as navigation in arteries. Our investigation in a pulsatile-flow environment shows that the induced DUS signal is detectable when the bloodstream reached the relatively low-flow rate region. Although this approach decreases the frequency of position feedback, it showed effectiveness during swarm navigation. Moreover, multiple viewing configurations have been experimentally demonstrated. Configuration I is designed to fundamentally understand the mechanism of RCMS-induced DUS signal in 3D space, in which both the RCMS and the induced DUS signal are observed by adjusting the imaging plane. Configurations II and III could be switched by tuning the probe, as demonstrated in Figure 7.17c. Configuration II is more suitable for swarm navigation in a relatively straight vessel, in which a large region can be imaged and benefits the tracking process. The scanning probe in configuration III enables localized delivery in a more tortuous region. Taking advantage of the 3D DUS signal, the switchable viewing angles provide multiple choices to track a RCMS in different environments. Besides the backscattered wave-based ultrasound imaging approach, recent studies indicate that the light-excited ultrasound waves from microrobots can be applied to real-time localization and tracking, in which the ultrasound waves are generated by light pulse-induced thermoelastic expansion of molecules [40]. This technique may benefit the swarm localization in deep tissue environments by combining the advantages of imaging depth and the high discrimination of microrobotic swarms from the surrounding living tissues.

The passive delivery of nanoparticles through the blood circulation system has the drawbacks of high delivery loss, low specificity, and potential side effects to organs. In this study, we actively navigate nanoparticles in a swarming form, allowing targeted delivery with a high local concentration. After around 20-mm-distance navigation in flowing blood environments, the access rate of nanoparticles could reach over 90%. Long-range navigation of swarms is time-consuming and challenging because of the low access rate. The application of catheter intervention in our study demonstrates a feasible approach in on-demand control of the starting point of swarm navigation. The reduced flow rate realized by the catheter also provides an appropriate environment for releasing nanoparticles and swarm formation. Moreover, it is hard to navigate a medical catheter into the target place through tortuous, small vessels [41]. This issue could be tackled by combing a catheter with a robotic RCMS. After navigating a catheter into a curved region, nanoparticles are released to form a RCMS, and then, the following delivery tasks could be continued by guiding the RCMS (Figure 7.17b). The gathered nanoparticle swarm could reduce adverse effects and delivery loss on other organs and tissues, which is considered a safe, promising approach for targeted therapy. The control parameters in our strategy can be adjusted to deliver various functionalized magnetic micro/nanomachines with real-time feedback control, including nanocarriers of drugs, energy [42, 43], and even imaging contrast agents (*e.g.*, ultrasound [44] and magnetic resonance imaging [45, 46]). To maintain a high access rate of the delivered agents, the interactions between the RCMS and the complex environment inside blood vessels require evaluation before conducting a delivery process, such as the influence from endothelial cells and smoothness of the inner wall of blood vessels.

In summary, we report a DUS imaging–guided approach for real-time navigation and localized delivery of a magnetic nanoparticle microswarm in vascular system. Multiple configurations are realized to conduct delivery tasks in blood vessels, and the position of the RCMS is tracked in real time based on the induced 3D DUS signal. The dynamic Doppler feedback and the fast response of the magnetic control approach enable the targeted navigation in different flowing environments. Moreover, we validate the delivery strategy in the *ex vivo* environment. Our approach shows a promising connection between control and imaging of microrobotic swarms for localized delivery in the blood vascular system, providing a strategy to targeted deliver concentrated agents in flowing environments under medical imaging guidance.

Bibliography

[1] Bradley J Nelson, Ioannis K Kaliakatsos, and Jake J Abbott. Microrobots for minimally invasive medicine. *Annual Review of Biomedical Engineering*, 12:55–85, 2010.

[2] Metin Sitti. *Mobile Microrobotics.* MIT Press, 2017.

[3] Jinxing Li, Berta Esteban-Fernández de Ávila, Wei Gao, Liangfang Zhang, and Joseph Wang. Micro/nanorobots for biomedicine: Delivery, surgery, sensing, and detoxification. *Science Robotics*, 2(4), 2017.

[4] Hakan Ceylan, Immihan C Yasa, Ugur Kilic, Wenqi Hu, and Metin Sitti. Translational prospects of untethered medical microrobots. *Progress in Biomedical Engineering*, 1(1):012002, 2019.

[5] Lukas Schwarz, Mariana Medina-Sánchez, and Oliver G Schmidt. Hybrid biomicromotors. *Applied Physics Reviews*, 4(3):031301, 2017.

[6] Pooyath Lekshmy Venugopalan, Berta Esteban-Fernández de Ávila, Malay Pal, Ambarish Ghosh, and Joseph Wang. Fantastic voyage of nanomotors into the cell. *ACS Nano*, 14(8):9423–9439, 2020.

[7] Zhiguang Wu, Lei Li, Yiran Yang, Peng Hu, Yang Li, So-Yoon Yang, Lihong V Wang, and Wei Gao. A microrobotic system guided by photoacoustic computed tomography for targeted navigation in intestines in vivo. *Science Robotics*, 4(32):eaax0613, 2019.

[8] Xiaohui Yan, Qi Zhou, Melissa Vincent, Yan Deng, Jiangfan Yu, Jianbin Xu, Tiantian Xu, Tao Tang, Liming Bian, Yi-Xiang J Wang, et al. Multifunctional biohybrid magnetite microrobots for imaging-guided therapy. *Science Robotics*, 2(12), 2017.

[9] Rui Cheng, Weijie Huang, Lijie Huang, Bo Yang, Leidong Mao, Kunlin Jin, Qichuan ZhuGe, and Yiping Zhao. Acceleration of tissue plasminogen activator-mediated thrombolysis by magnetically powered nanomotors. *ACS Nano*, 8(8):7746–7754, 2014.

[10] Dengfeng Li, Chao Liu, Yuanyuan Yang, Lidai Wang, and Yajing Shen. Micro-rocket robot with all-optic actuating and tracking in blood. *Light: Science & Applications*, 9:84, 2020.

[11] Yunus Alapan, Ugur Bozuyuk, Pelin Erkoc, Alp Can Karacakol, and Metin Sitti. Multifunctional surface microrollers for targeted cargo delivery in physiological blood flow. *Science Robotics*, 5(42), 2020.

[12] Qianqian Wang, Ben Wang, Jiangfan Yu, Kathrin Schweizer, B. J. Nelson, and Li Zhang. Reconfigurable magnetic microswarm for thrombolysis under ultrasound imaging. In *IEEE International Conference on Robotics and Automation*, pages 10285–10291. IEEE, 2020.

[13] Ania Servant, Famin Qiu, Mariarosa Mazza, Kostas Kostarelos, and Bradley J Nelson. Controlled in vivo swimming of a swarm of bacteria-like microrobotic flagella. *Advanced Materials*, 27(19):2981–2988, 2015.

[14] Ouajdi Felfoul, Mahmood Mohammadi, Samira Taherkhani, Dominic De Lanauze, Yong Zhong Xu, Dumitru Loghin, Sherief Essa, Sylwia Jancik, Daniel Houle, Michel Lafleur, et al. Magneto-aerotactic bacteria deliver drug-containing nanoliposomes to tumour hypoxic regions. *Nature Nanotechnology*, 11(11):941–947, 2016.

[15] Zhiguang Wu, Jonas Troll, Hyeon-Ho Jeong, Qiang Wei, Marius Stang, Focke Ziemssen, Zegao Wang, Mingdong Dong, Sven Schnichels, Tian Qiu, et al. A swarm of slippery micropropellers penetrates the vitreous body of the eye. *Science Advances*, 4(11):eaat4388, 2018.

[16] Jiangfan Yu, Dongdong Jin, Kai-Fung Chan, Qianqian Wang, Ke Yuan, and Li Zhang. Active generation and magnetic actuation of microrobotic swarms in bio-fluids. *Nature Communications*, 10:5631, 2019.

[17] Yongzhi Qiu, David R Myers, and Wilbur A Lam. The biophysics and mechanics of blood from a materials perspective. *Nature Reviews Materials*, 4(5):294–311, 2019.

[18] Haifeng Xu, Mariana Medina-Sánchez, Manfred F Maitz, Carsten Werner, and Oliver G Schmidt. Sperm micromotors for cargo delivery through flowing blood. *ACS Nano*, 14(3):2982–2993, 2020.

[19] Mariana Medina-Sánchez and Oliver G Schmidt. Medical microbots need better imaging and control. *Nature*, 545(7655):406, 2017.

[20] Xuanhe Zhao and Yoonho Kim. Soft microbots programmed by nanomagnets. *Nature*, 575:57–59, 2019.

[21] Azaam Aziz, Stefano Pane, Veronica Iacovacci, Nektarios Koukourakis, Jürgen Czarske, Arianna Menciassi, Mariana Medina-Sánchez, and Oliver G Schmidt. Medical imaging of microrobots: toward in vivo applications. *ACS Nano*, 14(9):10865–10893, 2020.

[22] Wenqi Hu, Guo Zhan Lum, Massimo Mastrangeli, and Metin Sitti. Small-scale soft-bodied robot with multimodal locomotion. *Nature*, 554(7690):81–85, 2018.

[23] Qianqian Wang, Lidong Yang, Jiangfan Yu, Philip Wai Yan Chiu, Yong-Ping Zheng, and Li Zhang. Real-time magnetic navigation of a rotating colloidal microswarm under ultrasound guidance. *IEEE Transactions on Biomedical Engineering*, 67(12):3403–3412, 2020.

[24] Ammar A Oglat, MZ Matjafri, Nursakinah Suardi, Mohammad A Oqlat, Mostafa A Abdelrahman, and Ahmad A Oqlat. A review of medical doppler ultrasonography of blood flow in general and especially in common carotid artery. *Journal of Medical Ultrasound*, 26(1):3, 2018.

[25] Harpreet Singh, Paul E Laibinis, and T Alan Hatton. Rigid, superparamagnetic chains of permanently linked beads coated with magnetic nanoparticles. synthesis and rotational dynamics under applied magnetic fields. *Langmuir*, 21(24):11500–11509, 2005.

[26] Stefano Giovanazzi, Axel Görlitz, and Tilman Pfau. Tuning the dipolar interaction in quantum gases. *Physical Review Letters*, 89(13):130401, 2002.

[27] Ch Josserand and M Rossi. The merging of two co-rotating vortices: a numerical study. *European Journal of Mechanics-B/Fluids*, 26(6):779–794, 2007.

[28] Alexey Snezhko and Igor S Aranson. Magnetic manipulation of self-assembled colloidal asters. *Nature Materials*, 10(9):698–703, 2011.

[29] Koohee Han, Gašper Kokot, Shibananda Das, Roland G Winkler, Gerhard Gompper, and Alexey Snezhko. Reconfigurable structure and tunable transport in synchronized active spinner materials. *Science Advances*, 6(12):eaaz8535, 2020.

[30] Qianqian Wang, Jiangfan Yu, Ke Yuan, Lidong Yang, Dongdong Jin, and Li Zhang. Disassembly and spreading of magnetic nanoparticle clusters on uneven surfaces. *Applied Materials Today*, 18:100489, 2020.

[31] Kwitae Chong, Scott D Kelly, Stuart Smith, and Jeff D Eldredge. Inertial particle trapping in viscous streaming. *Physics of Fluids*, 25(3):033602, 2013.

[32] Mitchell Cassin and Ann Quinton. What is the more common method of obtaining velocity measurements in carotid artery studies: a 60° insonation angle versus a convenient insonation angle? *Sonography*, 6(1):5–9, 2019.

[33] A Lecuona, U Ruiz-Rivas, and J Nogueira. Simulation of particle trajectories in a vortex-induced flow: application to seed-dependent flow measurement techniques. *Measurement Science and Technology*, 13(7):1020–1028, 2002.

[34] Haroon Zafar, Faisal Sharif, and Martin J Leahy. Measurement of the blood flow rate and velocity in coronary artery stenosis using intracoronary frequency domain optical coherence tomography: Validation against fractional flow reserve. *IJC Heart & Vasculature*, 5:68–71, 2014.

[35] Daniel Ahmed, Thierry Baasch, Nicolas Blondel, Nino Läubli, Jürg Dual, and Bradley J Nelson. Neutrophil-inspired propulsion in a combined acoustic and magnetic field. *Nature Communications*, 8:770, 2017.

[36] Gašper Kokot and Alexey Snezhko. Manipulation of emergent vortices in swarms of magnetic rollers. *Nature Communications*, 9:2344, 2018.

[37] Semi Jeong, Hyunchul Choi, Gwangjun Go, Cheong Lee, Kyung Seob Lim, Doo Sun Sim, Myung Ho Jeong, Seong Young Ko, Jong-Oh Park, and Sukho Park. Penetration of an artificial arterial thromboembolism in a live animal using an intravascular therapeutic microrobot system. *Medical Engineering & Physics*, 38(4):403–410, 2016.

[38] Elio Alberto Perigo, Gauvin Hemery, Olivier Sandre, Daniel Ortega, Eneko Garaio, Fernando Plazaola, and Francisco Jose Teran. Fundamentals and advances in magnetic hyperthermia. *Applied Physics Reviews*, 2(4):041302, 2015.

[39] Guang-Zhong Yang, Jim Bellingham, Pierre E Dupont, Peer Fischer, Luciano Floridi, Robert Full, Neil Jacobstein, Vijay Kumar, Marcia McNutt, Robert Merrifield, et al. The grand challenges of science robotics. *Science Robotics*, 3(14), 2018.

[40] Azaam Aziz, Mariana Medina-Sánchez, Jing Claussen, and Oliver G Schmidt. Real-time optoacoustic tracking of single moving micro-objects in deep phantom and ex vivo tissues. *Nano Letters*, 19(9):6612–6620, 2019.

[41] Yoonho Kim, German A Parada, Shengduo Liu, and Xuanhe Zhao. Ferromagnetic soft continuum robots. *Science Robotics*, 4(33):eaax7329, 2019.

[42] Mahdi Karimi, Amir Ghasemi, Parham Sahandi Zangabad, Reza Rahighi, S Masoud Moosavi Basri, H Mirshekari, M Amiri, Z Shafaei Pishabad, A Aslani, M Bozorgomid, et al. Smart micro/nanoparticles in stimulus-responsive drug/gene delivery systems. *Chemical Society Reviews*, 45(5):1457–1501, 2016.

[43] Ben Wang, Kai Fung Chan, Jiangfan Yu, Qianqian Wang, Lidong Yang, Philip Wai Yan Chiu, and Li Zhang. Reconfigurable swarms of ferromagnetic colloids for enhanced local hyperthermia. *Advanced Functional Materials*, 28(25):1705701, 2018.

[44] Kyung Hyun Min, Hyun Su Min, Hong Jae Lee, Dong Jin Park, Ji Young Yhee, Kwangmeyung Kim, Ick Chan Kwon, Seo Young Jeong, Oscar F Silvestre, Xiaoyuan Chen, Yu-Shik Hwang, Eun-Cheol Kim, and Sang Cheon Lee. ph-controlled gas-generating mineralized nanoparticles: a theranostic agent for ultrasound imaging and therapy of cancers. *ACS Nano*, 9(1):134–145, 2015.

[45] Tae-Hyun Shin, Youngseon Choi, Soojin Kim, and Jinwoo Cheon. Recent advances in magnetic nanoparticle-based multi-modal imaging. *Chemical Society Reviews*, 44(14):4501–4516, 2015.

[46] George J Lu, Arash Farhadi, Jerzy O Szablowski, Audrey Lee-Gosselin, Samuel R Barnes, Anupama Lakshmanan, Raymond W Bourdeau, and Mikhail G Shapiro. Acoustically modulated magnetic resonance imaging of gas-filled protein nanostructures. *Nature Materials*, 17(5):456–463, 2018.

CHAPTER 8

Magnetic Navigation of Collective Cell Microrobots in Blood

8.1 INTRODUCTION

In micromanipulation, biosensing, targeted delivery, and minimally invasive surgery, untethered microrobots offer promising capabilities [1, 2, 3, 4, 5]. Under external fields, these remotely controlled micromachines are able to be navigated in complex media to perform challenging tasks, such as active delivery in bovine vitreous humour, blood, peritoneal cavity, and gastrointestinal tract [6, 7, 8, 9]. However, the tiny size and volume of a single microrobot are limitations for the delivery capability. Thus, it is required to repeat delivery procedures. Recently, introducing collective behaviors of microrobots holds great potential in tackling these challenges [10, 11]. In comparison with the application of individual microrobot, collective microrobots can be utilized to achieve controlled delivery in a batch (*e.g.*, materials, drugs, energy) [12, 13, 14], and can be gathered to enhance the contrast of medical imaging [15]. However, there are challenges in the navigation of collective microrobots in dynamic environments (*e.g.*, blood vessels), mainly due to the impact of fluid flow and the heterogeneous fluidic environment [16]. The fluidic drag may disrupt the collective pattern and challenge navigation efficiency and access rate.

In order to perform navigation tasks *in vivo*, medical imaging systems must be utilized to provide imaging feedback for tracking microrobots [17, 18]. Among current medical imaging techniques, ultrasound imaging is particularly advantageous due to its high temporal resolution and lack of ionizing radiation, making it a safe and effective means of localizing mobile microrobots [19, 20, 21]. Ultrasound images are generated through the reflection of ultrasound waves from the target. The amplitude of the reflected sound waves, as well as the time it takes for them to travel, provide information for producing the image. Typically, a medical ultrasound imaging system can penetrate up to a depth of approximately 10 cm. To localize a microrobot, the imaging plane must be adjusted to interact with the microrobot. However, due to the

DOI: 10.1201/9781032665788-8

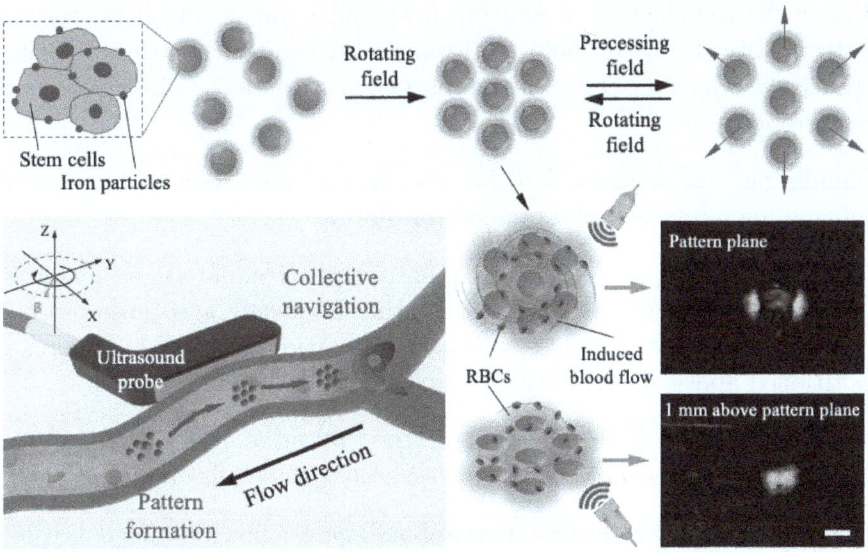

Figure 8.1 Schematic illustration of collective pattern formation and navigation of rotating cell microrobots under ultrasound Doppler imaging. Using a rotating magnetic field to form the pattern and using a precessing field to adjust it reversibly. The pattern-induced blood flow causes the generation of Doppler signals on and above the pattern plane. The collective microrobots are navigated upstream against blood flow near a boundary while simultaneously localized using the ultrasound Doppler feedback. The scale bar is 2 mm.

size limitation, it can be difficult to locate a mobile microrobot using a typical two-dimensional ultrasound imaging system. Unlike B-mode ultrasound imaging, which relies on the gradients of acoustic impedance, ultrasound Doppler imaging is designed based on the Doppler effect. This involves measuring frequency shifts in reflected ultrasonic waves resulting from the motion of objects. Doppler ultrasound has been widely used in clinics to measure blood flow by bouncing high-frequency sound waves from red blood cells (RBCs). During actuation, a mobile microrobot can influence the surrounding fluids, which has been utilized for tasks such as manipulating cargo or acting as a fluidic tweezer [22]. It is possible to speculate that an actuated microrobot may disrupt the normal blood flow and the motion of RBCs, which could be detected using ultrasound Doppler imaging [23]. Furthermore, an assembled pattern of microrobots could intensify the disturbances, resulting in an enhanced Doppler effect. Compared to B-mode imaging, the use of Doppler imaging allows for both the microrobots and the affected regions to be localized, and the induced Doppler signals can be utilized to indirectly localize the microrobots.

In this chapter, we propose ultrasound Doppler imaging and navigation of collective cell microrobots in blood (Figure 8.1). Stem cell microrobot is treated as a biocompatible agent or bio-hybrid carrier for cell delivery and regenerative medicine [24]. It is actuated and exhibits locomotion under magnetic fields. We achieve the following aspects:

(1) Under the influence of a rotating field and a precessing field, the collective patterns of cell microrobots are formed and reversibly gathered in blood, respectively, which agrees with the mathematical model of interactions between microrobots.

(2) Simulations are conducted to investigate the blood flow induced around the moving microrobots and its impact on RBCs.

(3) The induced Doppler signals are quantitatively compared and analyzed under various input parameters such as rotating frequency and pulse repetition frequency of ultrasound waves, including scenarios where the imaging plane is positioned above the collective pattern.

(4) The navigation and localization of the collective microrobots using power Doppler ultrasound imaging are carried out on both flat and uneven surfaces.

(5) The navigation of collective microrobots against flowing and pulsatile flowing blood with different flow rates is experimentally investigated and analyzed.

8.2 MATHEMATICAL MODELING

8.2.1 Actuation of Cell Microrobots in Stagnant and Flowing Blood

In a low-Reynolds-number regime, the motion velocity of a rolling object is slower than the circumferential velocity due to the fluid layer between the object and boundary. To analyze the relationship between input frequency and locomotion velocity of cell microrobots, a wet friction condition is applied. We consider a rotating cell microrobot, which has a mass of m and a radius of R and is exposed in a rotating magnetic field with the input frequency f and pitch angle γ to the Z-axis, as depicted in Figure 8.2a. In the vertical direction, the load force F_L acting on the substrate is equal to the sum of gravitational force and buoyancy of the microrobot, which can be expressed as $F_L = mg - \rho V g$, where V is the volume of the microrobot, which can be calculated as $V = 4\pi R^3/3$. In the horizontal direction, the drag force F_d balances the friction force F_f, so we have $F_f = -F_d$. The friction force is proportional to the load on the substrate, as

$$F_f = \mu_f F_L \tag{8.1}$$

where μ_f is the wet friction coefficient, which is proportional to the rotational velocity (v_e) of the cell microrobot [25], as $\mu_f = \psi v_e$. We assume that ψ is a constant, and the frictional torque becomes

$$\Gamma_f = F_f \cdot R = \psi v_e F_L R. \tag{8.2}$$

Under the wet condition, the fluid shear stress is estimated as $\tau = \eta(\partial u/\partial z)$ and approximates to $\eta(v_e/h)$, where u is the velocity vector, η is the dynamic viscosity of the fluid, and h is the distance between the cell microrobot and substrate [26]. Therefore, the drag torque caused by the shear stress is expressed as

$$\Gamma_d = \tau A \cdot R = \frac{\eta A}{h} v_e R \tag{8.3}$$

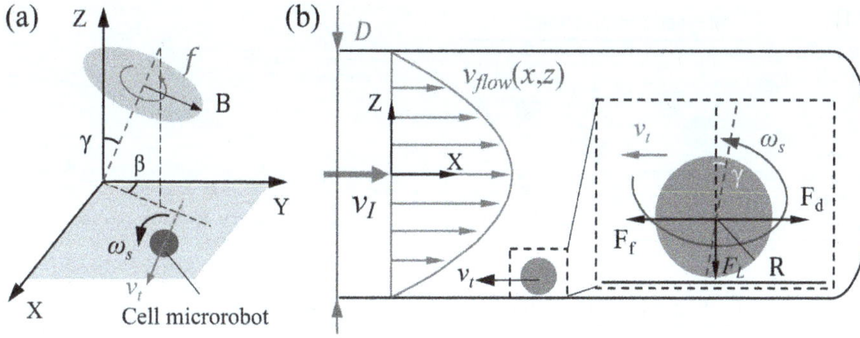

Figure 8.2 Schematic illustrations of (a) the rotating magnetic field and (b) the forces exerted on a rotating cell microrobot in a flowing condition. The input flow rate is denoted by v_I, while $v_{flow}(x, z)$ represents the distribution of the flow velocity.

where A is the contact area that fluid shear stress works on. Given the balance of the two torques yields $\mu_f = (\eta A/hF_L)v_e$. During experiments, the term $\psi = \eta A/hF_L$ maintains constant, which validates our assumption in Eq. (8.2). Under a rotating magnetic field, the rotational velocity in the XZ-plane becomes $v_e = 2\pi fR \cdot \sin\gamma$. The rotational component in the XY-plane does not contribute to the rotation-to-translation transition. Defining $A = 2\pi R$, we can further derive the friction force in Eq. (8.1) as

$$F_f = \mu_f F_L = \psi F_L \cdot 2\pi fR \cdot \sin\gamma. \tag{8.4}$$

At low Reynolds numbers, the drag force on a sphere moving with a translational velocity v_t is estimated as $F_d = 32\eta R v_t/3$ [27]. Therefore, the balance between the friction force and the drag force yields

$$v_t = \frac{3\pi\psi F_L}{16\eta} \cdot f\sin\gamma. \tag{8.5}$$

When driven below the step-out frequency, the above equation indicates that the locomotion velocity is proportional to the input field parameters (f and γ).

Driven in the flowing environment, the increased fluidic drag will affect the locomotion of the microrobot. In the case of a microrobot moving upstream in a blood vessel with the diameter D and flow rate v_I. Velocity v_{flow} varies along the Z-axis due to the boundary effect, as illustrated in Figure 8.2b. The velocity distribution can be approximated by a parabolic profile, as $v_{flow}(x, z) = 2[1-2(x^2+z^2)/D]v_{mean}$, where $v_{mean} = v_I/(\pi D^2/4)$ is the mean flow velocity. The drag force on a cell microrobot is affected by the equivalent mean flow velocity, which can be calculated as $\overline{v} = \int_{-D/2}^{-D/2+2R} v_{flow}dz/2R$. Thus, we can determine the drag force exerted on the microrobot as $F_d = 32\eta R(v_t + \overline{v})/3$, and the Eq. (8.5) changes to

$$v_t = \frac{3\pi\psi F_L}{16\eta} \cdot f\sin\gamma - \overline{v}. \tag{8.6}$$

Based on this analysis, indicating that if the input flow rate exceeds a threshold value, the actuation velocity will become zero or even negative, which will result in downstream passive motion, *i.e.*, $\int_{-D/2}^{-D/2+2R} v_{flow}dz = 2R(3\pi\psi F_L/16\eta) \cdot f\sin\gamma$.

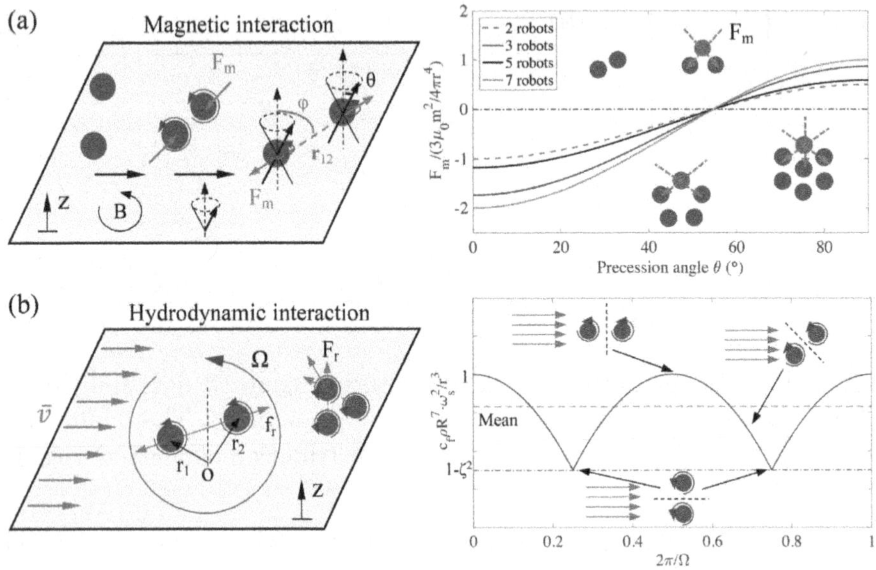

Figure 8.3 Schematic illustrations of the interactions between cell microrobots. (a) The left figure depicts the magnetic interaction between cell microrobots under an in-plane rotating field and a precessing field with $\theta < 54.7°$. The right figure shows how the magnetic interaction varies with θ for different patterns of cell microrobots. (b) The left figure illustrates the hydrodynamic interaction between cell microrobots. The right figure shows the change in hydrodynamic interaction during one precession cycle ($2\pi/\Omega$) with an input flow rate of $\overline{v}$.

8.2.2 Interactions between Cell Microrobots in Stagnant and Flowing Blood

The induced magnetic dipolar interactions between two cell microrobots, with magnetic moments $\mathbf{m}_1$ and $\mathbf{m}_2$, actuated under a magnetic field, can be described by [28]

$$U_{m1,2} = \frac{\mu_0}{4\pi}\left[\frac{\mathbf{m}_1 \cdot \mathbf{m}_2}{r_{12}^3} - 3\frac{(\mathbf{m}_1 \cdot \mathbf{r}_{12})(\mathbf{m}_2 \cdot \mathbf{r}_{12})}{r_{12}^5}\right] \tag{8.7}$$

where μ_0 is the magnetic permeability of free space, and $r_{12} = |\mathbf{r}_1 - \mathbf{r}_2|$ represents the separation distance between the two microrobots. There is no net force exerted on the microrobots due to the uniformity of the exerted rotating magnetic fields. Therefore, the magnetic interaction between the microrobots is due to the induced magnetic dipole-dipole interaction. Driven by a precessing magnetic field, as $\mathbf{B}(t) = B\{\sin\theta[\cos(2\pi ft)\hat{\mathbf{x}} - \sin(2\pi ft)\hat{\mathbf{y}}] + \cos\theta\hat{\mathbf{z}}\}$, where θ is the precession angle to the Z-axis, f is the input frequency, and $\hat{\mathbf{x}}$, $\hat{\mathbf{y}}$, $\hat{\mathbf{z}}$ are the unit vectors, the average magnetic interaction between cell microrobots over a field cycle is given by [29]

$$U(\varphi, \theta, r_{12}) = -\frac{\mu_0 \mathbf{m}_1 \cdot \mathbf{m}_2}{4\pi}\left(\frac{3\cos^2\varphi - 1}{r_{12}^3}\right)\left(\frac{3\cos^2\theta - 1}{r_{12}^3}\right) \tag{8.8}$$

where φ is the angle between $\mathbf{r}_{12}$ and the Z-axis (Figure 8.3a). During actuation, microrobots are coplanar on the substrate ($\varphi = \pi/2$). Therefore, the magnetic force between cell microrobots is calculated as

$$\mathbf{F}_m(\theta, r_{12}) = \frac{\partial U}{\partial r_{12}} = -\frac{3\mu_0 \mathbf{m}_1 \cdot \mathbf{m}_2}{4\pi \mathbf{r}_{12}^4}\left(\frac{3\cos^2\theta - 1}{2}\right). \tag{8.9}$$

The magnetic interaction between cell microrobots can be controlled to switch between repulsion ($0° < \theta < 54.7°$) and attraction ($54.7° < \theta < 90°$), as indicated by Eq. (8.9). At the magic angle $\theta = 54.7°$, the magnetic interaction becomes zero. Under a rotating magnetic field with $\theta = 90°$, such as $\mathbf{B}(t) = B[\cos(2\pi ft)\hat{\mathbf{x}} - \sin(2\pi ft)\hat{\mathbf{y}}]$, the magnetic attraction gathers microrobots together. However, when using a precessing magnetic field with $\theta < 54.7°$ (Figure 8.3a), the magnetic interaction among the gathered microrobots becomes repulsive.

Each rotating cell microrobot in a collective pattern is driven by a rotating magnetic field and induces a rotational flow, causing it to move within the flow created by the other microrobots. The Magnus effect, which generates a lift force, governs the hydrodynamic interactions between these microrobots. As a result, the interaction between them is influenced by the effect of fluid inertia [30, 31]. Here, we examine the hydrodynamic interaction between two cell microrobots that rotate with an angular velocity of ω_s, as illustrated in Figure 8.3b. The lift force acting on robot 1 from robot 2 is proportional to the induced flow $u_1 = \omega_s R$ and the fluid viscosity η. The inertia term involves the Reynolds number $Re = \rho R^2 w_2/\eta$, where ρ denotes fluid density and w_2 represents the shear rate induced by robot 2 in the vicinity of robot 1. w_2 is proportional to $\omega_s R^3/r_{12}^3$. Therefore, the hydrodynamic interaction between two rotating cell microrobots is expressed as [32]

$$\mathbf{F}_r = c_f \rho \omega_s^2 R^7 \frac{(\mathbf{r}_1 - \mathbf{r}_2)}{|\mathbf{r}_1 - \mathbf{r}_2|^4} \tag{8.10}$$

where c_f is a constant of proportionality. The direction of the hydrodynamic force $\mathbf{F}_r$ points from the second to the first robot, indicating that the interaction between the cell microrobots is repulsive. Since $F_r \propto \omega_s^2/r_{12}^3$, the separation distance could be enlarged by increasing f. In a dynamic environment, hydrodynamic interaction is influenced by the flow rate and the angle between the vector $\mathbf{r}_{12}$ and the flow direction $\overline{\mathbf{v}}$. The induced flow of robot 1 becomes $u_1 = \omega_s R + (\mathbf{M}(-\pi/2)\mathbf{r}_{12}) \cdot \overline{\mathbf{v}}$, where $\mathbf{M}(-\pi/2)$ represents the rotation matrix. The shear rate changes to $w_2 \propto [\omega_s R - (\mathbf{M}(-\pi/2)\mathbf{r}_{12}) \cdot \overline{\mathbf{v}}]R^2/r_{12}^3$. The precession angular velocity (Ω) of the collective microrobots affects the angle ζ between $\mathbf{r}_{12}$ and $\overline{\mathbf{v}}$. For a co-rotation system of two microrobots, the induced velocity by robot 2 near robot 1 is $u'_{1,2} = \omega_s R^3/r_{12}^2$. The precession angular velocity is defined as $\Omega = u'_{1,2}/(r_{12}/2)$, and we have

$$\Omega = 2\omega_s \frac{R^3}{r_{12}^3}. \tag{8.11}$$

Therefore, the separation distance and the driven frequency determine the change of the angle between $\mathbf{r}_{12}$ and $\overline{\mathbf{v}}$, so as the hydrodynamic interaction F_r. To illustrate the force value over an actuation cycle, we can express Eq. (8.10) as

$$\mathbf{F}_r(t) = \frac{c_f \rho R^5}{|\mathbf{r}_1 - \mathbf{r}_2|^3} u_1 u_2 \hat{\mathbf{r}}_{12} \tag{8.12}$$

where $\hat{\mathbf{r}}_{12}$ represents the unit vector of $\mathbf{r}_{12}$. Figure 8.3b illustrates how the force F_r acting on a microrobot changes over one precession cycle ($2\pi/\Omega$), with a mean flow velocity set as $\overline{v} = \zeta\omega_s R$. The maximum interaction occurs when the vector $\mathbf{r}_{12}$ becomes parallel to $\overline{\mathbf{v}}$.

In the low-Reynolds-number regime, the interaction between magnetic and hydrodynamic forces is counterbalanced and governs pattern formation, as

$$\mathbf{F}_m = -\mathbf{F}_r. \tag{8.13}$$

By adjusting the input field strength B, rotating frequency f, and precession angle θ, the separation distance between cell microrobots in a collective pattern can be controlled. Among patterns of two, three, five, and seven-cell microrobots, the analysis above shows that each microrobot in the seven-robot pattern experiences a relatively stronger magnetic interaction from neighboring microrobots due to the presence of the center microrobot, as schematically illustrated in Figure 8.3a. The seven-microrobot pattern exhibits better stability under the same input field and flow disturbance (*e.g.*, blood flow), making it the primary object of investigation.

8.3 SIMULATIONS OF INDUCED BLOOD FLOW AND MOTION OF RBCS

Simulations are conducted to investigate how a rotating cell microrobot affects the surrounding blood (Figure 8.4). The microrobot is treated as a 500 μm diameter sphere, and a fluid viscosity of $\eta = 4$ mPa · s is used to simulate whole blood viscosity. Following 5 seconds of continuous rotation, the induced flow profile was obtained (Figure 8.4a). The Reynolds number is calculated as $Re = \rho R^2\omega_s/\eta$, where $\rho = 1.04 \times 10^3$ kg/m^3 represents the fluid density, and Re is calculated in the range of 0.1–0.59. In this low-Reynolds-number regime, the induced flow velocity can be described by $\mathbf{u}(x) = \omega_\mathbf{s} \times \mathbf{r}_x(R/r_x)^3$, where $\mathbf{r}_x$ is a position vector defined from the center of the microrobot. The results of the simulated and theoretical flow velocity along the X-axis (u_y) are shown in Figure 8.4b, where the observed difference in velocity is due to the presence of fluid inertia [33]. As a microrobot rotates, it generates flow in three-dimensional space. The simulated flow in the plane located one body length above the microrobot's center (z = 0.5 mm) is shown in Figure 8.4c, and the velocity distribution on planes at various heights is also investigated (Figure 8.4d). As the distance from the cell microrobot increases, the velocity of the flow decreases. At a plane of z = 1 mm (*i.e.*, two body lengths above the microrobot's center), a flow velocity of ~0.2 mm/s is obtained. Simulations are also performed in a tubular environment to replicate the pattern-induced flow in blood vessels (Figures 8.4e and 8.4f). Compared to the induced flow generated by a cell microrobot, the pattern-induced flow has a larger area of interaction with the environment. This enhanced disturbance to the blood and RBCs inside the vessel can improve the generation of Doppler signals, which are critical for real-time pattern localization.

Ultrasound Doppler imaging relies on the Doppler effect, with the mobile RBCs serving as the ultrasound reflectors. Simulations of particle trajectory were conducted to investigate the impact of mobile collective microrobots on RBCs. We take a collective pattern of seven-cell microrobots as our study object (Figure 8.5 - Figure 8.8).

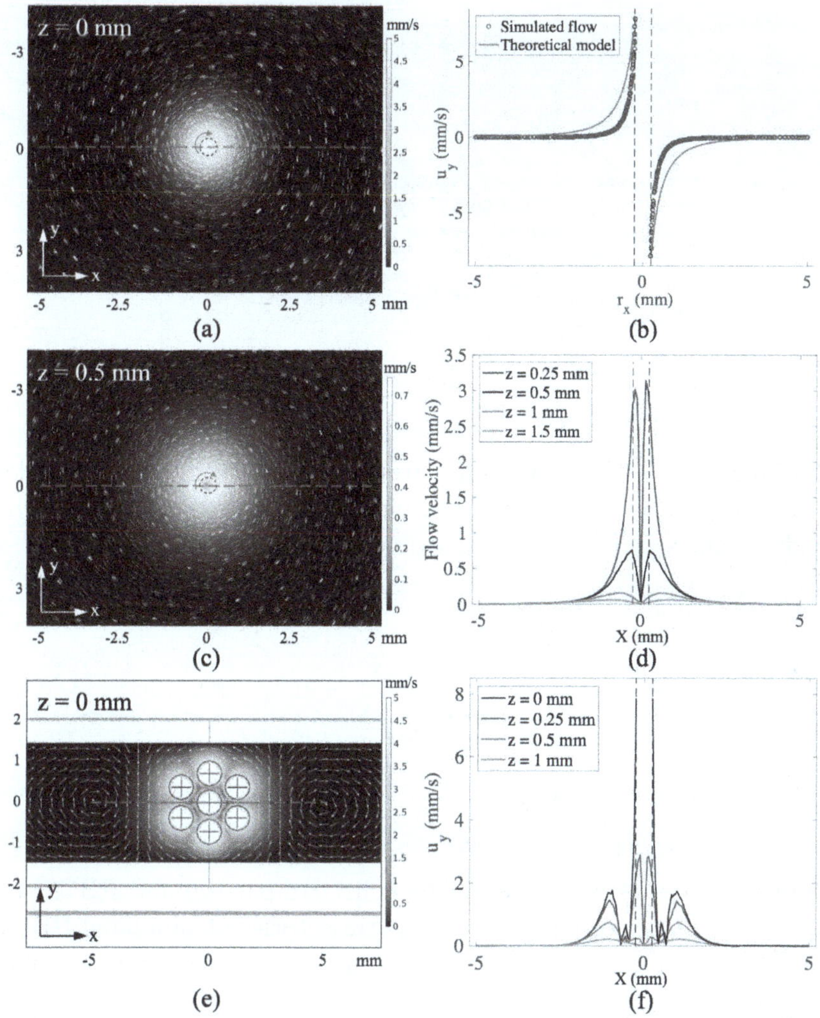

Figure 8.4 Simulations of the induced blood flow by a single cell microrobot and a collective of microrobots. (a) The induced fluid flow distribution at z = 0 is displayed, with arrows indicating the flow direction and the color profile showing the magnitude of the flow velocity (mm/s). (b) The simulated and theoretical tangential flow velocity (u_y) along the X-axis (dashed line in (a)). The missing segment of the curve is caused by the presence of the cell microrobot located at the origin. (c) The induced fluid flow distribution at z = 0.5 mm. (d) The simulated tangential flow velocity at different heights along the X-axis (dashed line in (c)). (e) The induced fluid flow distribution of a seven-microrobot pattern at z = 0 in a 4 mm-diameter tube. (f) The simulated tangential flow velocity along the X-axis (dashed line in (e)). The input frequency in simulations in (a), (c), and (e) is 5 Hz.

To simulate collective motion in the opposite direction, a laminar flow is introduced from the left-hand side of the X-axis and flows toward the right-hand side (Figure 8.6a). Each microrobot rotates around its own center at the same frequency, and the

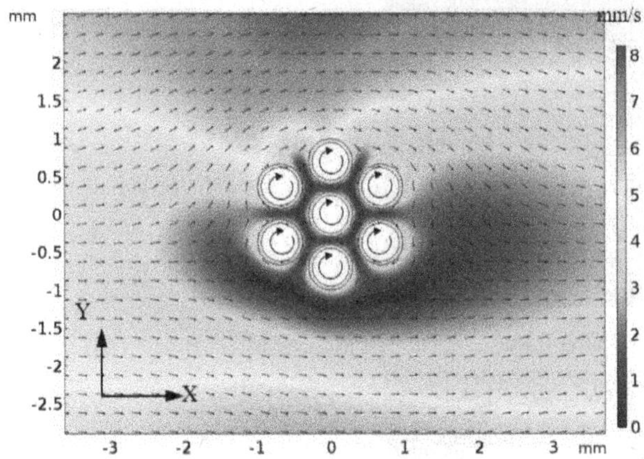

Figure 8.5 Simulation of the flow profile around the pattern. The flow velocity is 5 mm/s as indicated by the arrow, and the input frequency is 3 Hz. The unit for the color legends is mm/s.

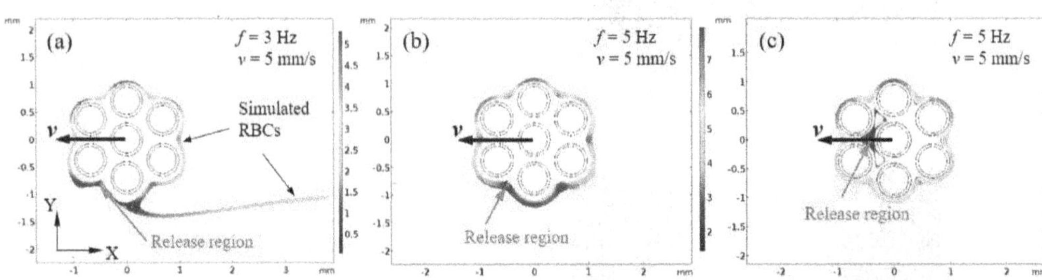

Figure 8.6 Interactions between the mobile collective pattern and RBCs at different input frequencies. The color curves show the trajectories of simulated RBCs ($t = 15$ s), and the release region is marked by the red arrows. The unit for the color legends is mm/s.

pattern disturbs the laminar flow. To simulate the movement of RBCs, a group of microparticles with a diameter of 6 μm (according to the diameter of pig RBC, and this size is also similar to human RBC [34]) is released at $t = 5$ s. The induced flow affects the simulated RBCs (SRBCs), causing them to exhibit a circular-like motion trajectory near the microrobots (Figure 8.6). Two primary forces act on the SRBCs: the drag force from the viscous fluid and the trapping force from the inward hydrodynamic force in the areas of high vorticity [35]. As a result, the SRBCs exhibit a drag force-dominated rotational motion and become trapped by the pattern. Some of the SRBCs are released from the pattern at $f = 3$ Hz due to the suppressed trapping force by the relatively larger drag force (Figure 8.6a). Figures 8.6a and 8.6b suggest that the trapping force increases with increasing rotating frequency. The motion of SRBCs between microrobots is also trapped in a circular-like trajectory around the pattern (Figure 8.6c). The simulation results suggest that the Doppler effect generated by the induced blood flow around a collective pattern can be detected using ultrasound Doppler imaging.

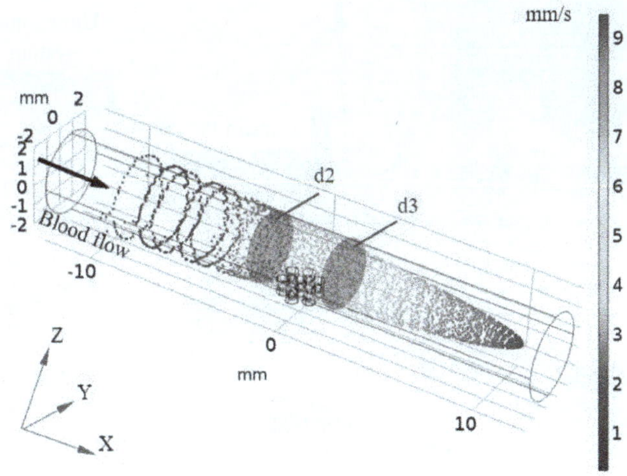

Figure 8.7 Simulation of RBCs flowing through collective microrobots with a rotating frequency of 5 Hz. The unit for the color legends is mm/s. The unit for the color legends is mm/s.

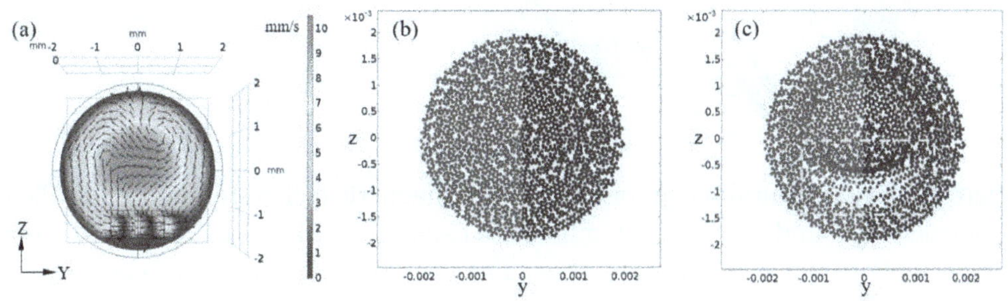

Figure 8.8 The induced flow profile at YZ-plane (x = 0.3 mm, (a)). (b) and (c) show the distribution of RBCs on cross-sections positioned at x = -1 mm and x = 1 mm to the pattern center, respectively, as marked in (a). The unit for the color legend is mm/s.

To further investigate the underlying mechanism of the Doppler signal induced by collective microrobots in flowing blood conditions, a group of SRBCs was released from the inlet of a 4 mm-diameter tube with a mean flow velocity of 5 mm/s (Figure 8.7). Figure 8.8a illustrates the disturbance of the pattern to the normal blood flow on the YZ-plane. To visualize the motion of SRBCs, they are classified into two groups based on their initial Y coordinate in the Poincaré map: red if Y < 0 and blue if Y > 0. Under the laminar flow condition, the microparticles remain stationary on the YZ-plane before approaching the pattern (Figure 8.8b). However, after flowing over the pattern, some of the particles change their position due to the pattern-induced distortion of the flow profile (Figure 8.8c). The results suggest that ultrasound pulses emitted toward the collective pattern can generate Doppler shift, leading to Doppler signal generation in a flowing condition.

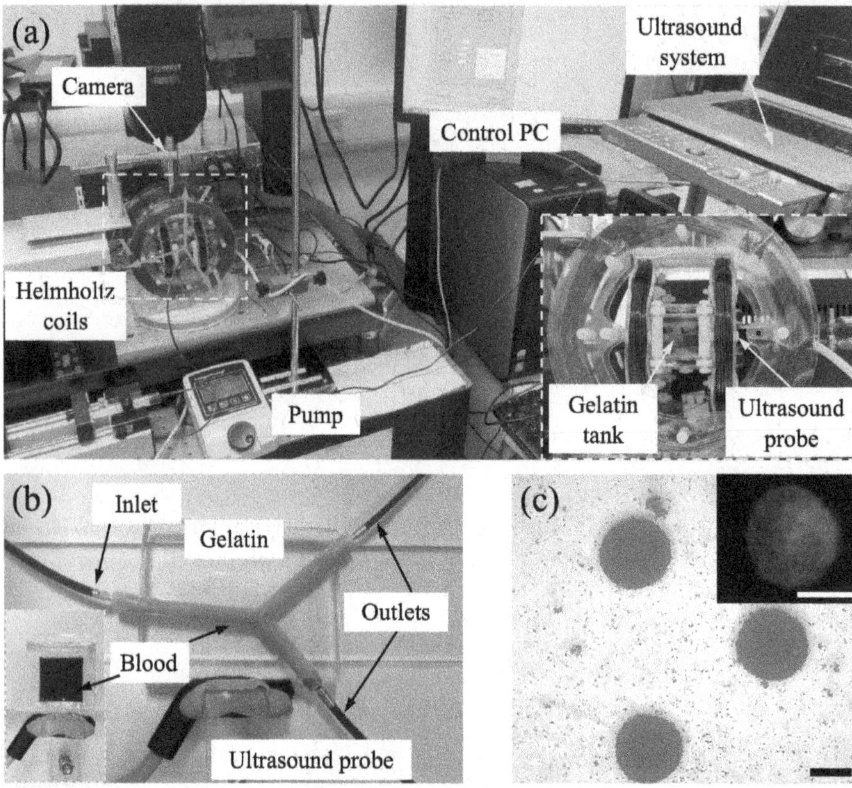

Figure 8.9 Experimental setup. (a) The electromagnetic coil system was controlled by a controller box and a lab PC. A miniature camera was mounted on top to monitor the assembly of the tank and the probe. The tank was placed at the central working region. (b) Experimental validation using gelatin tanks. The tank and tube were filled with porcine whole blood. Blood flow was controlled by a programmable pump. (c) Live stem cell microrobots under fluorescence microscopy. The image shows the morphology of the microrobots and the distribution of magnetic iron particles. The scale bars are 500 μm.

8.4 EXPERIMENTAL SETUP AND CELL MICROROBOTS

The experimental setup includes a three-axis Helmholtz coil system, an ultrasound imaging system, and gelatin tanks. The coil pairs were driven by three servoamplifiers (ADS 50/5 4-Q-DC, Maxon Inc.), and the field parameters were controlled by a LabVIEW program running on a lab PC. An ultrasound system (Terason t3200, Teratech Corporation, USA) with an ultrasound probe (16HL7, Teratech Corporation, USA) was integrated with the magnetic actuation system for imaging cell microrobots (Figure 8.9a). During experiments, the imaging depth was set to 3 cm, and results were recorded at 14 fps using power Doppler mode. For stagnant blood environments, a gelatin tank containing porcine whole blood and cell microrobots was used and placed in the central working area of the coil system. Experiments in flowing blood were conducted inside a 4 mm inner diameter tube (Figure 8.9b), with the flow rate controlled by a programmable pump (TJP–3A, LongerPump, China).

Carbonyl iron microparticles, which were 2–3 μm in diameter, were coated with a polydopamine (PDA) layer under alkaline conditions. 100 mg of carbonyl iron were ultrasonically dispersed in 30 mL of Tris(hydroxymethyl)aminomethane solution. The pH of the solution was adjusted to 8.5 using hydrochloric acid prior to the addition of 20 mg dopamine hydrochloride. The suspension was mechanically stirred for 240 min in a 4°C ice bath. The resulting magnetic particles were then harvested using a magnet and washed three times with ethanol and DI water.

Rat mesenchymal stem cells expressing green fluorescent protein (MSC-GFP) were cultured in Dulbecco's modified Eagle's medium (DMEM) containing 10% fetal bovine serum (FBS) until they reached 80% confluency in a 150 mm dish. The cells were then washed with phosphate-buffered saline (PBS) and treated with Trypsin to form a cell suspension. The suspension was collected and centrifuged at 1000 rpm for 5 min to remove metabolic waste and cell debris. The cells were then diluted with DMEM to a cell density of 10^6 ml^{-1}. The resulting cell suspension was well mixed with magnetic particles and cultured in a 96-well non-adhesive plate for 2 days to form a 3D spherical structure (Figure 8.9c). The volume percentage of living stem cells in a typical cell microrobot was calculated to be 92.4% based on the volume of a cell microrobot and the dose of magnetic particles (the diameter of a mature cell robot was ∼600 μm, the initial cell number was 10^6 cells/mL, and the particle amount was 40 μg). These results demonstrate the high percentage of stem cells inside the cell robot.

8.5 EXPERIMENTAL RESULTS AND DISCUSSION

8.5.1 Ultrasound Doppler Imaging of a Cell Microrobot in Blood

We first used power Doppler mode to investigate the Doppler signals induced by a rotating cell microrobot. As shown in Figure 8.10a, no significant Doppler signal was detected at an input frequency of 1 Hz. However, when the frequency was increased to 3 Hz, the color area of Doppler signals around the cell microrobot was displayed and further enlarged by adjusting the frequency to 5 Hz. We superimposed the Doppler color area onto the B-mode grayscale image in our ultrasound system, enabling us to observe both the microrobot and the Doppler signals. Simulation result in Figure 8.4 demonstrates that the fluid above a rotating microrobot ($z > 0$ mm) is also affected. Figure 8.10b shows imaging results with the imaging plane positioned 1 mm above the microrobot's center. Doppler signals are detected with $f > 2$ Hz, and increase as the input frequency is increased. We investigated the relationship between the color area ratio and the input frequency at $z = 0$ mm and $z = 1$ mm (Figure 8.10c). The color area ratio is defined as the ratio of the Doppler signal area to the area of the microrobot in the B-mode image. The decrease in the color area at $f > 5$ Hz, indicating that the actuation was above the step-out frequency. This suggests that the microrobot's rotation was not synchronized with the field due to the increased drag torque. In addition to the field parameters, pulse repetition frequency (PRF) can also have a significant impact on Doppler signals. PRF refers to the number

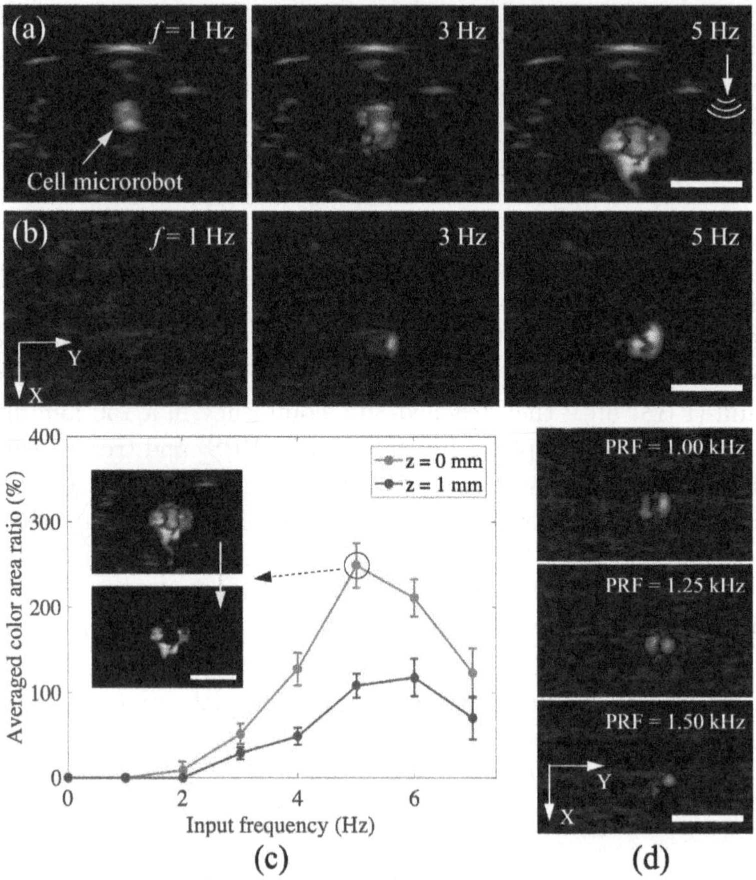

Figure 8.10 Ultrasound Doppler imaging of a rotating cell microrobot in blood. (a) Ultrasound images of the rotating microrobot at different input frequencies with a field strength of 12 mT (z = 0). (b) The imaging plane was positioned 1 mm above the pattern plane (z = 1 mm). The PRF for (a) and (b) was set to 0.70 kHz. (c) The average area of Doppler color in 3 s at input frequencies of 0–7 Hz and a PRF of 0.70 kHz. The inset images demonstrate the image processing used to extract the color area. The error bars indicate the standard deviation from three experiments. (d) Ultrasound images at PRFs of 1.00–1.50 kHz (z = 1 mm). The input frequency was 5 Hz. All scale bars are 2 mm.

of ultrasound pulses emitted per unit time. If two pulses are emitted to a moving reflector within a time interval of 1/PRF, there will be a phase difference between the two backscattered echoes. By emitting multiple pulses, the motion of the reflector can be detected. Increasing PRF from 1.00 kHz to 1.50 kHz results in a reduced sensitivity of the ultrasound system to low flow velocity, as shown in Figure 8.10d. Consequently, only the region near the rotating microrobot with relatively high flow velocity is detected, resulting in a decreased Doppler color area. The adjustment of PRF depends on the application requirements. In an environment with negligible flow or disturbances, a lower PRF could be used for acquiring better Doppler signals.

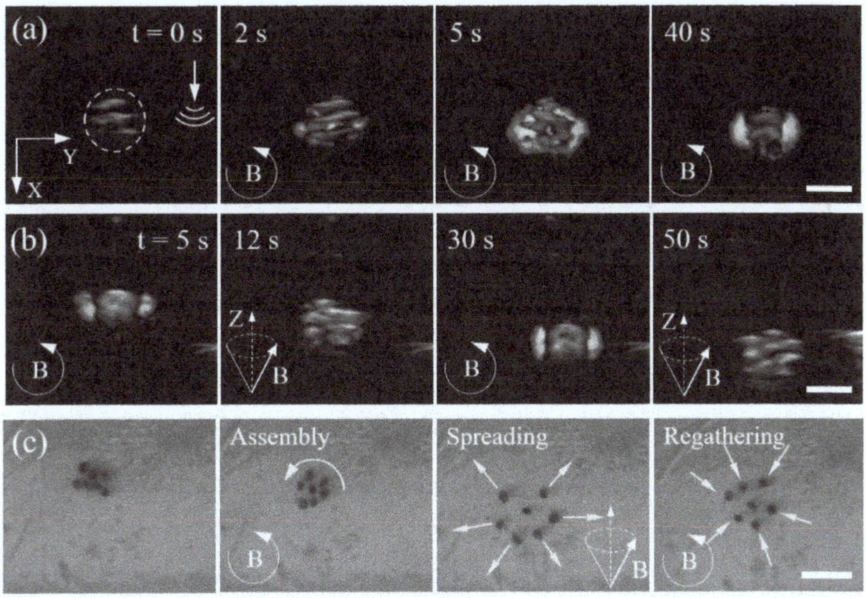

Figure 8.11 Collective pattern formation of cell microrobots in blood. (a) Formation of a pattern of seven microrobots under a rotating magnetic field. (b) Reversible pattern spreading and regathering under a precessing field and a rotating field, respectively. (c) Reversible formation under a light microscope in glycerol-water solution (viscosity: 4 mPa · s). The two fields have a frequency of 5 Hz, and the precessing field has a precession angle of 30°. All scale bars are 3 mm.

A high PRF should be considered when manipulating microrobots in a dynamic environment to avoid noise signals from background flow.

8.5.2 Pattern Formation and Navigation of Collective Microrobots in Stagnant Blood

The gathering of the microrobots was achieved through the use of a rotating magnetic field. As described in Eqs. (8.9)–(8.13), the pattern formation of the collective microrobots was governed by the balance between the magnetic and hydrodynamic interactions among the microrobots. The attractive magnetic force between the microrobots decreased the separation distance, while the hydrodynamic repulsive force prevented them from clustering together. The initial separation distance between the cell microrobots should be limited to allow for sufficient robot-robot interactions (Eqs. (8.9) and (8.10)). Through experimental trials, the initial mean separation distance among cell robots was limited below 3 mm (*i.e.*, five body lengths) before conducting pattern formation. Within 60 s, an ordered pattern of seven-cell robots could be obtained. At $t = 5$ s, a Doppler signal was observed in the space between microrobots (Figure 8.11a). After decreasing the separation distance ($t = 40$ s), the induced rotating flow between two microrobots canceled each other out (Figure 8.5), resulting in negligible Doppler signals inside the pattern. The collective pattern was reversibly

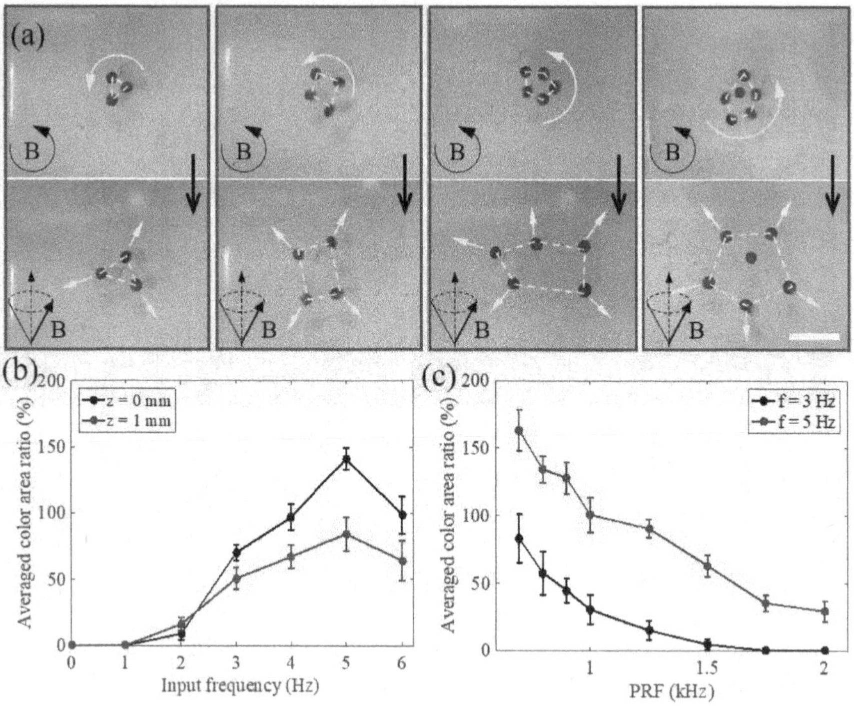

Figure 8.12 (a) Patterns formed and spread with different numbers of cell microrobots in the glycerolwater solution (viscosity: 4 mPa · s). The two field have a frequency of 5 Hz and the precessing field has a precession angle of 30°. The scale bar is 3 mm. (b) Average area of Doppler color in 3 s at input frequencies of 0–6 Hz and a PRF of 0.70 kHz. (c) Average area of Doppler color in 3 s at PRF of 0.70–2.00 kHz. Each error bar denotes the standard deviation from three experiments.

spread and regathered by adjusting the magnetic interaction (Figure 8.11b). A precessing field with a precession angle $\theta = 30°$ was applied to enlarge the separation distance between microrobots, resulting in the pattern spreading at $t = 12$ s. By setting θ to 90°, *i.e.*, changing the precessing field to a rotating field, the pattern regathered, and continuous Doppler signals were observed at $t = 30$ s. This reversible gathering-spreading manipulation can be on-demand controlled, demonstrating the controllability of the collective pattern. Figure 8.11c depicts the reversible process in a glycerol-water solution with a blood-like viscosity under a light microscope. By using different numbers of cell microrobots, gathered patterns were obtained and adjusted under external fields (Figure 8.12a). The relationship between the Doppler color area and the input frequency was investigated. The ratio was defined as the average color area in 3 s divided by the area of the collective pattern (Figure 8.12a). The results showed that the Doppler signals increased with the rotating frequency at imaging planes of z = 0 mm and 1 mm. However, the area ratio decreased with a larger PRF due to the reduced sensitivity to regions of low blood flow velocity (Figure 8.12b).

The collective microrobots were navigated by adding a tilt angle (pitch angle γ) to the rotating magnetic field. The locomotion was enabled by the friction asymmetry

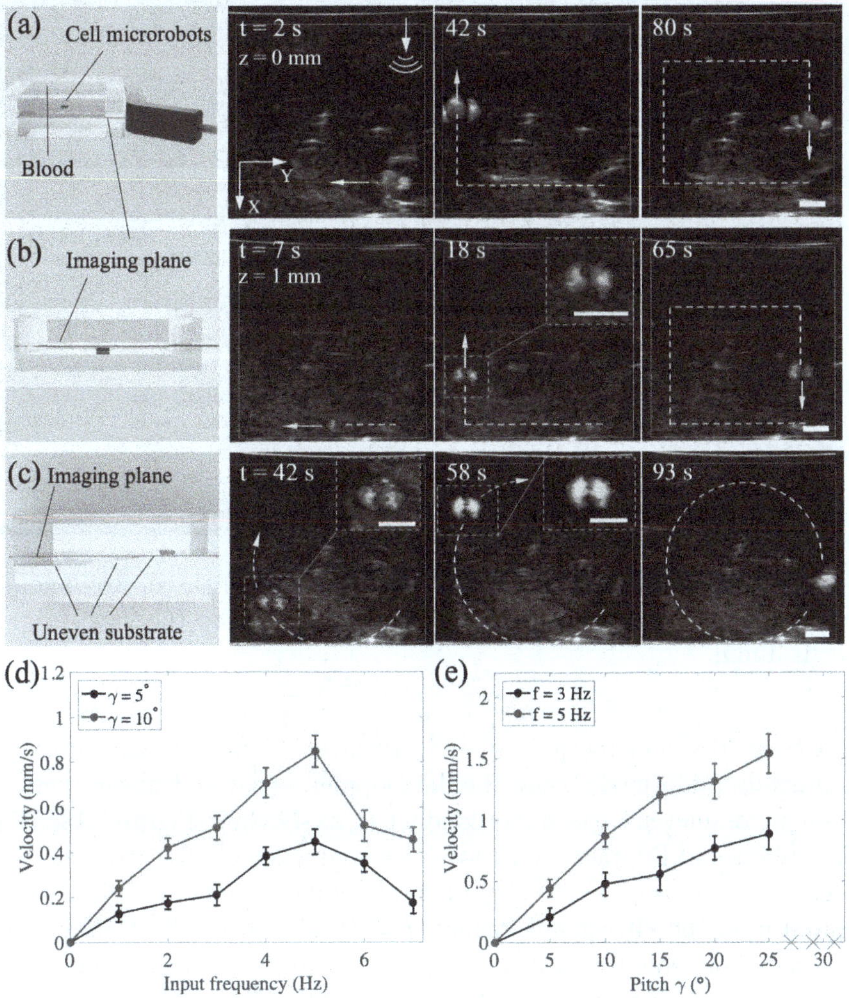

Figure 8.13 Navigation of collective microrobots on flat and uneven surfaces. (a) and (b) show the collective navigation along a rectangular trajectory with the imaging plane located at z = 0 mm and z = 1 mm, respectively. (c) Navigation of the collective microrobots on an uneven surface. The schematic drawing in (a)–(c) illustrates the position of the imaging plane, cell microrobots, and the substrate. All scale bars are 3 mm. (d) The relationship between locomotion velocity and the input frequency at pitch angle (γ) of 5° and 10°. (e) The relationship between locomotion velocity and γ at input frequencies of 3 Hz and 5 Hz. Each error bar denotes the standard deviation from three experiments.

near the substrate. Figure 8.13a shows the navigation process with the imaging plane at z = 0 mm. The navigation direction of the collective microrobots was open-loop controlled by adjusting the yaw angle β of the input field. Localization was performed based on the induced Doppler signals, and the microrobots were navigated along a rectangular trajectory. When the imaging plane was moved 1 mm above the microrobots, only Doppler signals were detected (Figure 8.13b). The position of the

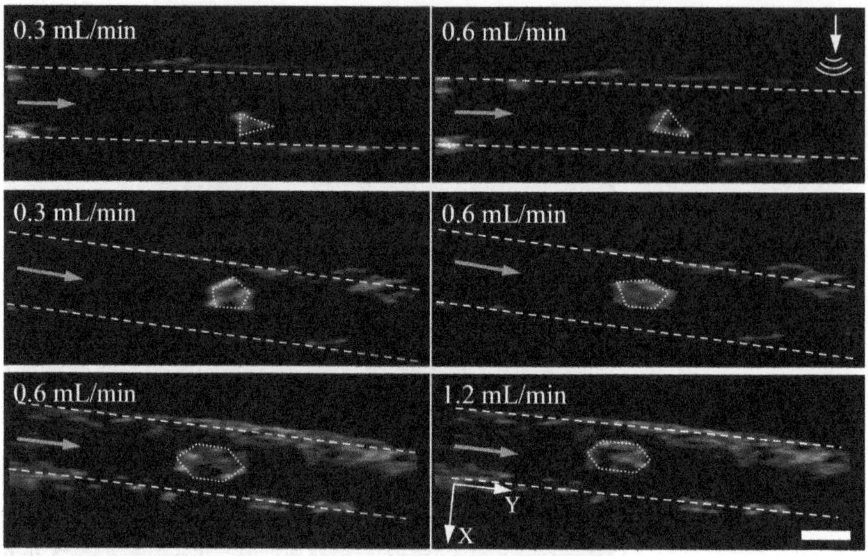

Figure 8.14 B-mode ultrasound images of the assembly of three, five, and seven cell microrobots in flowing conditions. The blue arrows denote the flow direction. The scale bar is 3 mm.

microrobots could still be recognized, and navigation along the rectangular trajectory was successfully performed. Using the 3D Doppler signal and navigation capability, navigation on an uneven surface was conducted, as shown in Figure 8.13c. The collective microrobots and Doppler signal were observed when the microrobots were within the imaging plane ($t = 42$ s). As the microrobots navigated downhill, they gradually disappeared from the ultrasound images ($t = 58$ s), and localization was conducted indirectly based on Doppler signals. The relationship between the navigation velocity and input frequency was investigated (Figure 8.13d). The velocity increased with the input frequency and γ before reaching the step-out frequency, which is in agreement with Eq. (8.5). Moreover, the navigation velocity also increased with pitch angle (Figure 8.13e). However, the pattern cannot remain stable when $\gamma > 25°$ due to the decreased magnetic attraction between microrobots (Eq. (8.9)).

8.5.3 Pattern Formation and Navigation of Collective Microrobots in Flowing Blood

Assembly of cell microrobots was conducted in flowing blood to investigate the requirements for pattern formation in dynamic environments. The experiments were conducted in a 4 mm-diameter tube with various flow rates. The tube was loaded with different numbers of cell microrobots (similar to the assembly in Figure 8.12), and then the rotating field and blood flow were turned on simultaneously (Figure 8.14). We applied two criteria to estimate the successful formation of pattern. First, the formation of an assembled pattern where the separation distance between microrobots did not change significantly. This criterion aimed to validate the interactions between microrobots in a dynamic environment. Second, the pattern was able to move as an entity without losing any microrobots, which is critical for maintaining access rate.

TABLE 8.1 Pattern assembly, formation, and collective navigation in flowing blood

Number of microrobots	Flow rate (mL/min)	γ (°)	Assembled pattern	γ' (°)	Collective motion
3	0.3	2	✓	4	✓
3	0.6	5	✓	7	✓
3	0.9	8	✓	10	✓
3	1.2	10	✓	13	✓
3	1.5	—	×	—	×
5	0.3	3	✓	5	✓
5	0.6	7	✓	10	✓
5	0.9	10	✓	—	×
5	1.2	—	×	—	×
7	0.3	3	✓	5	✓
7	0.6	5	✓	8	✓
7	0.9	8	✓	10	✓
7	1.2	10	✓	13	✓
7	1.5	13	✓	13	✓
7	1.7	15	✓	—	×
7	2.0	—	×	—	×

— not applicable; ✓ success; × failure

Due to the boundaries of the tube, the five- and seven-microrobot patterns displayed elongation during the assembly process. Table 8.1 shows the assembly results, where patterns of three, five, and seven were formed and actuated. In order to overcome blood flow, we added the pitch angle γ and γ' during the pattern formation and the following collective motion, respectively. In comparison with the patterns of three and five microrobots, the seven-robots pattern shows better stability when the input flow rate was higher than 1.2 mL/min. It was due to the existence of the central microrobot that provided magnetic attraction to surrounding microrobots, as analyzed in Figure 8.3a.

The ability to actuate microrobots in flowing conditions is crucial for applications in the vascular system. In order to study their collective navigation in blood flow, a tube with a 4 mm inner diameter was utilized, with flow rates ranging from 0 to 6 mL/min, corresponding to a mean velocity range of 0 to 7.956 mm/s. Navigation of a pattern of seven microrobots was investigated. Prior to turning on the blood flow, the microrobots were arranged into a pattern using a rotating magnetic field. After adding a pitch angle to the external field, the rotation of microrobot is to be separated into in-plane rotation (relative to the imaging plane) and out-of-plane rotation. The ability to navigate against blood flow was enabled by the out-of-plane rotation, while the in-plane rotation component provided Doppler signals. As illustrated in Figure 8.9b, the ultrasound wave propagated perpendicularly to the blood flow, denoted by an insonation angle of $\alpha = 90°$. Therefore, the Doppler

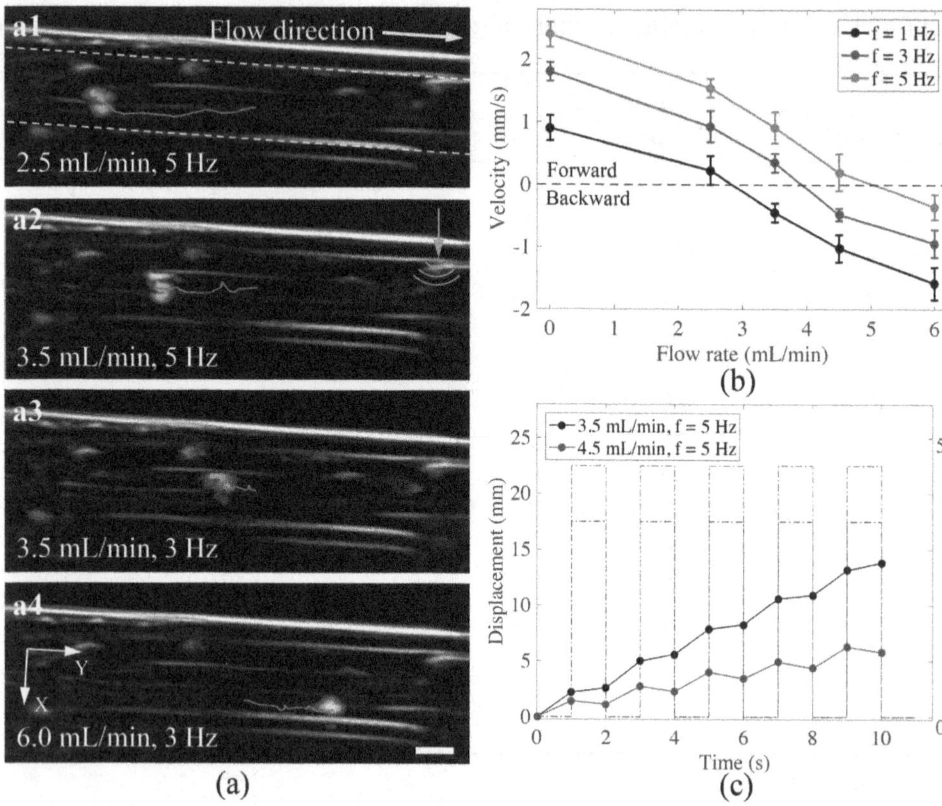

Figure 8.15 Magnetic actuation of collective cell microrobots in flowing blood. (a) Upstream navigation against flowing blood with the input flow rates of 0–6 mL/min. The tracking duration is 5 s in all cases. PRF is set at 1.00 kHz. The scale bar is 2 mm. (b) Actuation velocity against flowing blood with different flow rates. Each error bar represents the standard deviation of three experiments. (c) Upstream navigation against pulsating blood flow. Dashed lines denote the pulsating flow rate.

signal generated by the input blood flow was negligible, and only the Doppler signals resulting from the collective pattern were observed, as depicted in Figure 8.15a. The collective navigation was tested at various flow rates. Upon increasing the flow rate from 2.5 mL/min to 3.5 mL/min, the actuation velocity decreased to around 0.92 mm/s. Further decreasing the input frequency to 3 Hz resulted in a velocity of 0.32 mm/s (Figures 8.15a1 – a3). If the flow rate exceeded a certain threshold, the microrobots were unable to navigate upstream due to insufficient actuation force and were instead dragged by the blood flow (Figure 8.15a4). If the flow rate decreased again, the microrobots resumed forward navigation. We investigated the relationship between navigation velocity under different flow rates was investigated (Figure 8.15b). The forward velocity decreased with the frequency, whereas the backward velocity increased after reaching the threshold flow velocity. To investigate the navigation capability in pulsating flow conditions, the blood flow was programmed to change periodically. Figure 8.15c shows the forward displacement of the collective

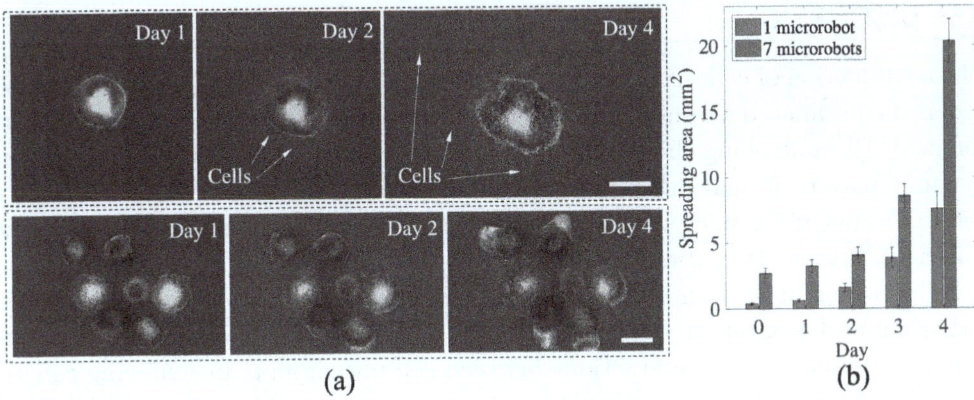

Figure 8.16 Cell proliferation and spreading. (a) Fluorescence images of the spreading cells around a single and seven collective microrobots. The scale bars are 500 μm. (b) The relationship between cell spreading area and culture time. Each error bar represents the standard deviation from five trials.

microrobots navigating against pulsatile blood flow. The microrobots exhibited forward displacement at a flow rate of 3.5 mL/min in both high-flow and no-flow regions. During five cycles of perfusions, the microrobots moved forward a distance of 13.83 ± 2.86 mm (three trials). After increasing the flow rate to 4.5 mL/min, the microrobots were unable to maintain forward motion in high-flow regions. Nonetheless, they were able to move forward between two perfusions, reaching a net displacement of 5.79 ± 1.37 mm in total (three trials). During the experiments, the ultrasound wave propagation direction was perpendicular to the flow direction, with an insonation angle of $\alpha = 90°$. Therefore, no significant Doppler signal created by the flow was observed. After the navigation process, the assembly status was checked by adjusting the imaging plane to $z = 0$ mm using B-mode ultrasound. The results showed that no pattern disruption occurred in either flowing or pulsatile flow conditions, indicating the vital role played by robot-robot interactions in maintaining pattern stability in dynamic environments.

The cell microrobots are live bio-hybrid agents with the capability for cell proliferation. Following the collective formation and navigation process, the cell microrobots were collected into a 6-well plate (with a hydrophilic surface) and cultured in DMEM with 10% FBS to investigate the proliferation of the loaded stem cells. After 2–4 days of culture, the cells exhibited significant proliferation, as observed using an inverted fluorescence microscope (Figure 8.16a). Compared to the cell spreading area around a single microrobot, a larger area was observed around the collective microrobots (Figure 8.16b). The delivery of collective microrobots could increase the access rate to the target region and improve the efficiency of stem cell-based therapy, such as cardiovascular disease therapy [36], blood development [37], and vascular tissue engineering [38].

8.6 DISCUSSION

The introduction of collective behavior to microrobots enables simpler agents to organize in a coordinated manner and increases their disturbance to the surrounding environment. By controlling the interactions between the building blocks, we can achieve dynamic pattern formation and navigation. To gain a fundamental understanding of collective control for microrobots, we used time-dependent magnetic fields to achieve collective pattern formation and navigation. The magnetic interaction can be adjusted between attraction and repulsion, which has been used for reversible pattern formation and separation. The comparison between Table 8.1 and Figure 8.15 highlights the importance of interactions between cell microrobots in achieving collective control in flowing environments. Once assembled into a stable pattern, the collective microrobots were navigated against a relatively higher flow rate and simultaneously avoided pattern disruption. Our strategy can be integrated with balloon catheter intervention to temporally control blood flow and release microrobots, reducing the impact of blood flow during pattern formation and navigation [39]. Then the collective cell robots can be magnetically navigated to the region that is hard to reach for medical catheters, benefiting cell delivery to hard-to-reach, tortuous sites.

Medical imaging is crucial for accurately localizing collective microrobots. In this study, we utilized power Doppler ultrasound imaging modality for localization. Power Doppler ultrasound is a noninvasive, magnetic field-compatible technique that is widely used in clinics for measuring blood flow. Compared to typical B-mode ultrasound imaging, power Doppler ultrasound is more sensitive to low flow velocity, which enables indirect localization based on the rotating microrobot-induced flow. Moreover, the experimental results demonstrate that the use of collective microrobots enlarged the color area of Doppler signals in the ultrasound system. The integration of magnetic control and ultrasound imaging systems can also be used in the delivery of small-scale agents, such as drug carriers and imaging contrast agents (*e.g.*, for ultrasound imaging and magnetic resonance imaging).

8.7 CONCLUSION

In summary, our study demonstrated the Doppler ultrasound imaging and magnetic navigation of collective cell microrobots in stagnant and flowing blood. We showed that the cell microrobots could be reversibly gathered and spread under external magnetic fields, enabling controlled navigation in a collective state. Under power Doppler ultrasound imaging, Doppler signals were observed around the pattern and affected by the input field frequency and PRF of the ultrasound waves. Moreover, Doppler signals were observed when the imaging plane was above the collective microrobots, which confirmed the simulation results. By utilizing the real-time 3D Doppler signals, the collective cell microrobots were able to be navigated and localized on flat and uneven surfaces in whole blood environments. Experiments also demonstrated that different collective patterns were formed in flowing blood, and the collective microrobots were able to exhibit upstream locomotion with a mean flow velocity up to 5.97 mm/s. The study presents an approach for real-time navigation and localization of collective bio-hybrid microagents in bio-fluid environments. The integration of medical imaging and magnetic actuation systems provides a solution for active delivery applications.

Bibliography

[1] Metin Sitti, Hakan Ceylan, Wenqi Hu, Joshua Giltinan, Mehmet Turan, Sehyuk Yim, and Eric D Diller. Biomedical applications of untethered mobile milli/microrobots. *Proceedings of the IEEE*, 103(2):205–224, 2015.

[2] Jinxing Li, Berta Esteban-Fernandez de Avila, Wei Gao, Liangfang Zhang, and Joseph Wang. Micro/nanorobots for biomedicine: Delivery, surgery, sensing, and detoxification. *Science Robotics*, 2(4), 2017, Art. no. eaam6431.

[3] Jiachen Zhang, Ziyu Ren, Wenqi Hu, Ren Hao Soon, Immihan Ceren Yasa, Zemin Liu, and Metin Sitti. Voxelated three-dimensional miniature magnetic soft machines via multimaterial heterogeneous assembly. *Science Robotics*, 6(53), 2021. Art. no. eabf0112.

[4] Mi Li, Ning Xi, Yuechao Wang, and Lianqing Liu. Progress in nanorobotics for advancing biomedicine. *IEEE Transactions on Biomedical Engineering*, 68(1):130–141, 2021.

[5] Tiantian Xu, Jia Liu, Chenyang Huang, Tianfu Sun, and Xinyu Wu. Discrete-time optimal control of miniature helical swimmers in horizontal plane. *IEEE Transactions on Automation Science and Engineering*, 2021. DOI: 10.1109/TASE.2021.3079958.

[6] Jiangfan Yu, Dongdong Jin, Kai-Fung Chan, Qianqian Wang, Ke Yuan, and Li Zhang. Active generation and magnetic actuation of microrobotic swarms in bio-fluids. *Nature Communications*, 10, 2019, Art. no. 5631.

[7] Yunus Alapan, Ugur Bozuyuk, Pelin Erkoc, Alp Can Karacakol, and Metin Sitti. Multifunctional surface microrollers for targeted cargo delivery in physiological blood flow. *Science Robotics*, 5(42), 2020, Art. no. eaba5726.

[8] Ania Servant, Famin Qiu, Mariarosa Mazza, Kostas Kostarelos, and Bradley J Nelson. Controlled in vivo swimming of a swarm of bacteria-like microrobotic flagella. *Advanced Materials*, 27(19):2981–2988, 2015.

[9] Zhiqiang Zheng, Huaping Wang, Lixin Dong, Qing Shi, Jianing Li, Tao Sun, Qiang Huang, and Toshio Fukuda. Ionic shape-morphing microrobotic end-effectors for environmentally adaptive targeting, releasing, and sampling. *Nature Communications*, 12, 2021. Art. no. 411.

[10] Daniel Ahmed, Alexander Sukhov, David Hauri, Dubon Rodrigue, Gian Maranta, Jens Harting, and Bradley J Nelson. Bioinspired acousto-magnetic microswarm robots with upstream motility. *Nature Machine Intelligence*, 3:116–124, 2021.

[11] Dongdong Jin, Ke Yuan, Xingzhou Du, Qianqian Wang, Shijie Wang, and Li Zhang. Domino reaction encoded heterogeneous colloidal microswarm with on-demand morphological adaptability. *Advanced Materials*, 2021. DOI: 10.1002/adma.202100070.

[12] Qianqian Wang, Dongdong Jin, Ben Wang, Neng Xia, Ho Ko, Bonaventure Yiu Ming Ip, Thomas Wai Hong Leung, Simon Chun Ho Yu, and Li Zhang. Reconfigurable magnetic microswarm for accelerating tPA-mediated thrombolysis under ultrasound imaging. *IEEE/ASME Transactions on Mechatronics*, 2021. DOI: 10.1109/TMECH.2021.3103994.

[13] Hui Xie, Mengmeng Sun, Xinjian Fan, Zhihua Lin, Weinan Chen, Lei Wang, Lixin Dong, and Qiang He. Reconfigurable magnetic microrobot swarm: Multimode transformation, locomotion, and manipulation. *Science Robotics*, 4(28), 2019, Art. no. eaav8006.

[14] Ana C Hortelao et al. Swarming behavior and in vivo monitoring of enzymatic nanomotors within the bladder. *Science Robotics*, 6(52), 2021. Art. no. eabd2823.

[15] Qianqian Wang, Lidong Yang, Jiangfan Yu, Philip Chiu, Y.-P Zheng, and Li Zhang. Real-time magnetic navigation of a rotating colloidal microswarm under ultrasound guidance. *IEEE Transactions on Biomedical Engineering*, 67(12):3403–3412, 2020.

[16] Haifeng Xu, Mariana Medina-Sánchez, Manfred F Maitz, Carsten Werner, and Oliver G Schmidt. Sperm micromotors for cargo delivery through flowing blood. *ACS Nano*, 14(3):2982–2993, 2020.

[17] Azaam Aziz, Stefano Pane, Veronica Iacovacci, Nektarios Koukourakis, Jürgen Czarske, Arianna Menciassi, Mariana Medina-Sánchez, and Oliver G Schmidt. Medical imaging of microrobots: Toward in vivo applications. *ACS Nano*, 14(9):10865–10893, 2020.

[18] Qianqian Wang and Li Zhang. External power-driven microrobotic swarm: From fundamental understanding to imaging-guided delivery. *ACS Nano*, 15(1):149–174, 2021.

[19] Qiyang Chen, Fang-Wei Liu, Zunding Xiao, Nitin Sharma, Sung Kwon Cho, and Kang Kim. Ultrasound tracking of the acoustically actuated microswimmer. *IEEE Transactions on Biomedical Engineering*, 66(11):3231–3237, 2019.

[20] Veronika Magdanz et al. Ironsperm: Sperm-templated soft magnetic microrobots. *Science Advances*, 6(28), 2020, Art. no. eaba5855.

[21] Qianqian Wang and Li Zhang. Ultrasound imaging and tracking of micro/nanorobots: From individual to collectives. *IEEE Open Journal of Nanotechnology*, 1:6–17, 2020.

[22] Islam SM Khalil, Anke Klingner, Youssef Hamed, Yehia S Hassan, and Sarthak Misra. Controlled noncontact manipulation of nonmagnetic untethered microbeads orbiting two-tailed soft microrobot. *IEEE Transactions on Robotics*, 36(4):1320–1332, 2020.

[23] Qianqian Wang et al. Ultrasound doppler-guided real-time navigation of a magnetic microswarm for active endovascular delivery. *Science Advances*, 7, 2021. Art. no. eabe5914.

[24] Ben Wang, Kai Fung Chan, Ke Yuan, Qianqian Wang, Xianfeng Xia, Lidong Yang, Ho Ko, J. Yi-Xiang Wang, Joseph Jao Yiu Sung, Philip Wai Yan Chiu, and Li Zhang. Endoscopy-assisted magnetic navigation of biohybrid soft microrobots with rapid endoluminal delivery and imaging. *Science Robotics*, 6, 2021. Art. no. eabd2813.

[25] Andras Z Szeri. *Fluid Film Lubrication.* Cambridge University Press, 2010.

[26] TO Tasci, PS Herson, KB Neeves, and DWM Marr. Surface-enabled propulsion and control of colloidal microwheels. *Nature Communications*, 7, 2016, Art. no. 10225.

[27] John P Tanzosh and Howard A Stone. Transverse motion of a disk through a rotating viscous fluid. *Journal of Fluid Mechanics*, 301:295–324, 1995.

[28] Sonia Melle, Oscar G Calderón, Miguel A Rubio, and Gerald G Fuller. Microstructure evolution in magnetorheological suspensions governed by mason number. *Physical Review E*, 68(4), 2003, Art. no. 041503.

[29] Stefano Giovanazzi, Axel Görlitz, and Tilman Pfau. Tuning the dipolar interaction in quantum gases. *Physical Review Letters*, 89(13), 2002, Art. no. 130401.

[30] Jeffrey A Schonberg and EJ Hinch. Inertial migration of a sphere in poiseuille flow. *Journal of Fluid Mechanics*, 203:517–524, 1989.

[31] Qianqian Wang, Lidong Yang, and Li Zhang. Micromanipulation using reconfigurable self-assembled magnetic droplets with needle guidance. *IEEE Transactions on Automation Science and Engineering*, 2021. DOI: 10.1109/TASE.2021.3062779.

[32] Bartosz A Grzybowski, Xingyu Jiang, Howard A Stone, and George M Whitesides. Dynamic, self-assembled aggregates of magnetized, millimeter-sized objects rotating at the liquid-air interface: Macroscopic, two-dimensional classical artificial atoms and molecules. *Physical Review E*, 64(1):011603, 2001.

[33] Eric Climent, Kyongmin Yeo, Martin R Maxey, and George E Karniadakis. Dynamic self-assembly of spinning particles. *Journal of Fluids Engineering*, 129(4):379–387, 2007.

[34] K Namdee, M Carrasco-Teja, MB Fish, P Charoenphol, and O Eniola-Adefeso. Effect of variation in hemorheology between human and animal blood on the binding efficacy of vascular-targeted carriers. *Scientific Reports*, 5(1):1–14, 2015.

[35] Kwitae Chong, Scott D Kelly, Stuart Smith, and Jeff D Eldredge. Inertial particle trapping in viscous streaming. *Physics of Fluids*, 25(3), 2013, Art. no. 033602.

[36] Luiza Bagno, Konstantinos E Hatzistergos, Wayne Balkan, and Joshua M Hare. Mesenchymal stem cell-based therapy for cardiovascular disease: progress and challenges. *Molecular Therapy*, 26(7):1610–1623, 2018.

[37] Elaine Dzierzak and Anna Bigas. Blood development: hematopoietic stem cell dependence and independence. *Cell Stem Cell*, 22(5):639–651, 2018.

[38] H-H Greco Song, Rowza T Rumma, C Keith Ozaki, Elazer R Edelman, and Christopher S Chen. Vascular tissue engineering: progress, challenges, and clinical promise. *Cell Stem Cell*, 22(3):340–354, 2018.

[39] Mengdi Han, Lin Chen, Kedar Aras, Cunman Liang, Xuexian Chen, Hangbo Zhao, Kan Li, Ndeye Rokhaya Faye, Bohan Sun, Jae-Hwan Kim, et al. Catheter-integrated soft multilayer electronic arrays for multiplexed sensing and actuation during cardiac surgery. *Nature Biomedical Engineering*, 4:997–1009, 2020.

IV

Application

CHAPTER 9

Reconfigurable Collective Nanorobots for Accelerating Thrombolysis

9.1 INTRODUCTION

Blood clots caused by blood clotting disrupt normal circulation within the living vascular system. It can even lead to life-threatening problems such as coronary artery infarction, ischaemic stroke, pulmonary embolism and so on [1]. Blood clots can form in both veins and arteries, even deep vein thrombosis and pulmonary embolism. The formation of a blood clot usually begins with the aggregation of platelets as clotting factors are activated and fibrin aggregates around the platelets, thus the fibrin network gradually traps more red blood cells (RBCs) and platelets. Infusion of thrombolytic drugs and mechanical removal using imaging-guided catheters are the traditional methods of thrombosis treatment. Revascularisation and prevention of early and late thrombosis can be achieved with thrombolytic and anticoagulant drugs [2, 3]. However, the current treatment methods have some defects and safety problems. For example, the use of a large number of thrombolytic drugs may cause problems such as bleeding and unstable blood pressure [4, 5], and drug injection therapy has the problem of low target hit rate [6]. The use of catheters is difficult to perform clinically because friction at vessel boundaries increases the probability of injury, especially during insertion and retraction of small vessels [7, 8]. Some researchers have recently put forward the idea of combining thrombolytic drugs with mini-robot or microrobots [9, 10, 11, 12]. Mechanical grinding can increase the lysis rate. However, since thrombus formation usually occurs in confined environments, the use of millimeter-scale robots may narrow the scope of application because mechanical friction would increase the probability of disintegration of smaller thrombus fragments, which would lead to the risk of secondary vascular occlusion. In addition, because of its small size, it is difficult to track a single small robot for further *in vivo* applications.

DOI: 10.1201/9781032665788-9

Swarming microrobots offer a possibility to tackle the above issues. The cluster of microrobots provides a way to solve the above problems. Recently, different collective behavior and microswarm control techniques have been presented [13, 14, 15]. Compared with using a single miniature robot [16, 17, 18, 19, 20], swarming micro/nanorobots can deliver larger doses of drugs or energy delivery in batches, and have been applied in medical imaging-guided delivery and targeted therapy [21, 22]. Swarming microrobots have two advantages in favor of thrombolysis. First of all, the reconfigurable swarm formation and pattern transformation of agent-agent interaction control are very beneficial to local delivery and adaptability. The building blocks can be injected into the desired position as needed, and the formation of the microswarm can be remotely controlled by the external magnetic field. The reversible deformation or transformation of a swarm pattern makes it more adaptable to the environment, especially in limited and narrow lumens such as blood vessels and bile ducts. The reconfigurable and regathering capability of the microswarm avoids the mechanical injury of blood vessels and enhances the accessibility of small vessels. Secondly, the water flow induced by microswarms can have an impact on the surrounding environment. We can make a reasonable hypothesis that a driven microswarm disturbs the surrounding fluid, which might accelerate mass transfer near the clot-blood interface. In addition, when the microswarm performs the actual delivery task, the medical imaging system must participate in the *in vivo* tracking of micro/nanorobots. Aggregated building blocks will increase the concentration or areal density of micro/nanorobots, which will improve the contrast of medical imaging [23]. So far, various imaging techniques have been used to locate microswarms, including magnetic resonance imaging (MRI) [24], positron emission tomography/computed tomography (PET/CT) [25], and infrared fluorescence imaging [26]. Among many imaging techniques, ultrasound imaging is favored because of its low cost, no radiation, deep imaging depth, and high time resolution (that is, fast imaging speed), and has become one of the most promising tools for locating micro/nanorobots. Through the feedback of ultrasound images, the motion control of robot microswarm can be carried out in blood vessels or opaque tissues. So a thrombolysis method which integrates swarm control and ultrasound imaging is worth studying.

In this chapter, we propose a scheme to accelerate tissue plasminogen activator (tPA)-mediated thrombolysis by using magnetite nanoparticles (Fe_3O_4) microswarms in ultrasound imaging. TPA is an FDA-approved thrombolytic drug for the treatment of ischemic stroke. We have achieved the following objectives:

(1) Pig whole blood formed nanoparticle microswarms in an oscillating magnetic field. Because the working environment is in a viscous blood environment, the aggregation ability of microswarms is crucial, which is different from colloidal swarms formed in low-viscosity media.

(2) We can reversibly affect the aspect ratio of the microswarm by adjusting the input field. Controlling the elongation or shortening of microclusters can make them adapt to different restricted environments and clot areas.

(3) In the blood environment, microswarms are localized by ultrasound imaging and can be performed in two switchable modes of motion.

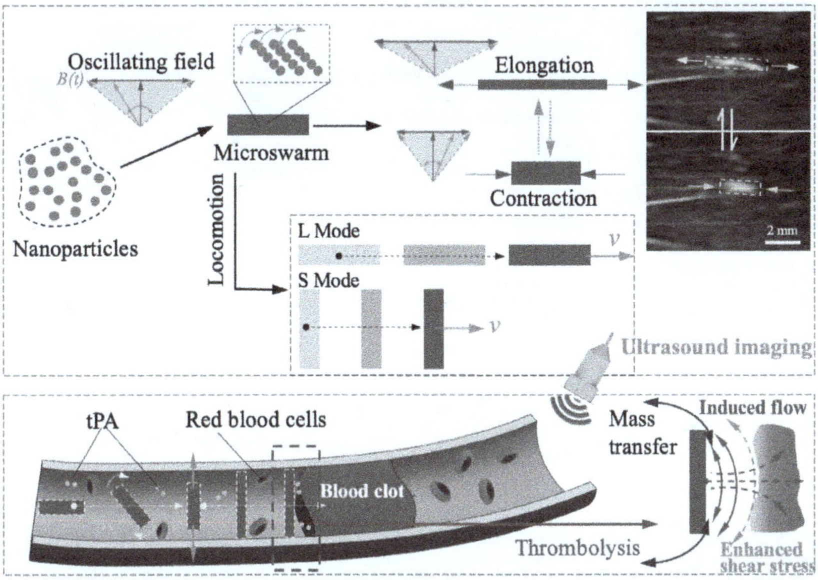

Figure 9.1 Schematic illustration of the tissue plasminogen activator (tPA)-mediated thrombolysis using magnetic microswarms. Microswarms form and navigate in blood with two modes of motion under an oscillating magnetic field, and can autonomously adjust their aspect ratios to adapt to confined environments and clot areas. Swarm formation, reversible deformation, and navigation during thrombolysis can be accomplished under ultrasound imaging.

(4) We also conducted simulations to study the effect of swarm-induced blood flow on the clot-blood interface, including shear stress analysis.

(5) We also studied and compared pure tPA lysis and microswarm-assisted lysis. The cleavage rates were quantitatively compared, analyzed and discussed.

The thrombolysis strategy is shown in Figure 9.1. tPA and nanoparticles are implanted, and microswarms are formed in an oscillating magnetic field. Then the microswarm navigates in two motion modes and stretches to adapt to the clot area. At last, under the influence of fluid convection caused by microswarm and enhanced shear stress at the clot-blood interface, the clot gradually dissolves.

9.2 MATHEMATICAL MODELING AND SIMULATION

According to the induced dipole interaction between magnetic nanoparticles, nanoparticle chains can be formed under an oscillating magnetic field, and the formation of clusters is determined by the interaction between the chains. Here, we propose a mathematical model to estimate the state of the chain. We study the influence of the flow caused by the microswarm on the blood clot by establishing simulation, but the chain state data, like driving frequency and length, are defined according to the modeling results.

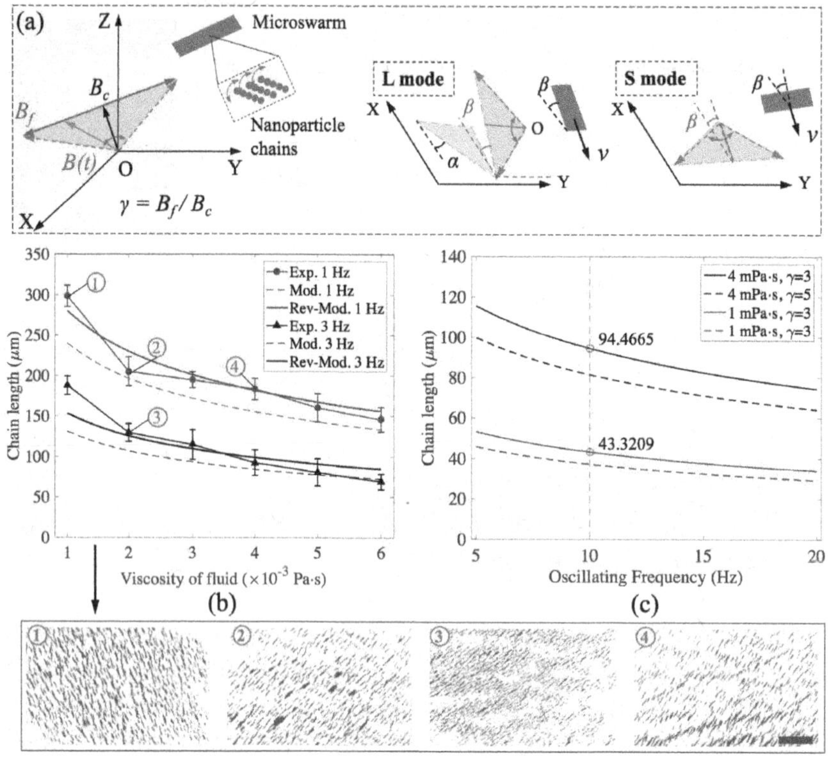

Figure 9.2 Using an oscillating magnetic field to drive nanoparticle microswarms. (a) The schematic diagram of the oscillation field $B(t)$ is shown in the figure. Blue and black arrows represent alternating field $B_f(t)$ and static field B_c, respectively. The two figures on the right show two modes of translation along the long axis and the short axis. α and β are the yaw angle relative to the X axis and the pitch angle relative to the XY plane, respectively. (b) The figure shows experimental and simulated results for chain lengths in aqueous glycerol solutions of different viscosities. Exp., Mod., and Rev-Mod. represent the results of experiments, mathematical models, and revised models, respectively. Each error bar represents the standard deviation of the results of three experiments. Images ①-④ show the chain of nanoparticles in the driving process accordingly. The scale bar is 300 μm. (c) The graph shows the relationship between chain length and input frequency under different γ and viscosity.

9.2.1 Mathematical Modeling of Nanoparticle Chains

A three-axis Helmholtz coil system generates an oscillating magnetic field, which is used to pool nanoparticles and form magnetic microclusters. Superposition of uniform field B_c and alternating field B_f to form and control oscillating magnetic field, as

$$\mathbf{B} = \mathbf{B}_f + \mathbf{B}_c = B_f \sin(2\pi f t)\hat{\mathbf{i}} + B_c\hat{\mathbf{j}} \tag{9.1}$$

where f is the frequency of the alternating field, and $\hat{\mathbf{i}}$, $\hat{\mathbf{j}}$ denote the unit vectors (Figure 9.2a). The angle between the alternating field B_f and the uniform field B_c is 90°. The magnetic interaction between the nanoparticles and the nanoparticle chain is the main reason for the formation of the microswarm. By applying a magnetic field, the nanoparticle chain will be formed on the XY plane because of the magnetic force between the nanoparticles. The interaction among the oscillating chains further aggregates the nanoparticles into a smaller area and then forms a banded microcluster with a long axis parallel to B_f. The field ratio $\gamma = B_f/B_c$ is defined as the ratio of the two field strengths, and it is the key parameter to adjust the aspect ratio of the microswarm. When the γ is increased, the microswarm shows elongation, and can shrink again by decreasing the γ. We have explained the details and mechanisms in previous work [27]. The microswarm can realize the translational motion by adding a small tilt angle (pitch angle) β to the oscillation field, and the direction of motion can be controlled by adjusting the yaw angle α (Figure 9.2a). In addition, microswarms have two modes of translational movement: movement along the long axis (L mode) and movement along the short axis (S mode). Switch between the two modes by adding an inclination angle to B_f (L mode) or B_c (S mode).

The magnetic chain-chain interaction is the main reason for the formation of microswarms, so we take the nanoparticle chain as the basic unit for analysis. In the process of driving, the oscillation angle $\varphi(t)$ between the field and the Y-axis is $\varphi(t) = \arctan[\gamma \sin(2\pi f t)]$ (L mode). If the jump-out frequency of the nanoparticle chain is higher than the driving frequency, then the angular velocity of the chain can be obtained by deriving time, as

$$\omega(t) = \frac{d}{dt}\varphi(t) = \frac{2\pi\gamma f \cos(2\pi f t)}{1 + \gamma^2 \sin^2(2\pi f t)}. \tag{9.2}$$

During the drive at an angular velocity $\omega(t)$, the magnetic moment Γ_m and the hydrodynamic resistance moment Γ_d applied on a chain cancel each other out at low Reynolds number, that is, the Re is estimated to be in the range of 10^{-2}. The magnetic moment at the center of the chain is calculated by adding all the torques from the other nanoparticles, which means that it can be simplified by only considering the magnetic moment of the nearest nanoparticle. For a nanoparticle chain with N particles, the driving magnetic moment is expressed as [28]

$$\Gamma_m = \frac{3\mu_0 m^2(t)(N-1)}{4\pi(2R)^3}\sin(2\theta) \tag{9.3}$$

where μ_0 is the permeability of free space, and R is the particle radius. θ represents the phase lag between the applied field $B(t)$ and the long axis of the particle chain. $m(t) = V_p\chi_p B(t)/\mu_o$ is the induced dipole moment of a particle, where $V_p = \frac{4}{3}\pi R^3$ is the volume of the nanoparticle and χ_p is the magnetic susceptibility of nanoparticles. So the magnetic torque can be expressed as $\Gamma_m = \pi R^3 \chi_p^2 B^2(t)(N-1)/6\mu_0$. Considering the shape factor, the resistance moment of the nanoparticle chain is expressed as [29]

$$\Gamma_d = \frac{8\pi R^3}{3}\frac{N^3}{\ln\frac{N}{2} + \frac{2.4}{N}}\eta\omega(t) \tag{9.4}$$

where η is the viscosity of the surrounding fluid. In order to evaluate the stability of the nanoparticle chain, the Mason number is used as the ratio between viscous resistance and driving magnetic torque [30]. By definition, the modified Mason number in this example can be expressed as

$$R_T = \frac{\Gamma_d}{\Gamma_m} = 16\frac{\mu_0 \eta \omega(t)}{\chi_p^2 B^2(t)} \frac{N^3}{(N-1)(\ln\frac{N}{2} + \frac{2.4}{N})}. \tag{9.5}$$

To express the relationship between the field strength over time and the oscillation angle $\varphi(t)$, the applied electric field can be expressed as $B(t) = B_c/\cos\varphi(t) = B_f/\gamma\cos\varphi(t)$. If B_f remains the same (10 mT during experiments), the Mason number becomes

$$R_T \propto \eta\omega(t)\gamma^2\cos\varphi(t)^2 \frac{N^2}{\ln\frac{N}{2} + \frac{2.4}{N}} \tag{9.6}$$

where take $N \approx N-1$ for simplification because the chain length is in tens of microns. From the above analysis, we can see that two time-dependent parameters are the main reasons that affect the stability of the chain: the field strength $B(t)$ and angular velocity $\omega(t)$. If $R_T > 1$, the resistance moment is greater than the magnetic moment, causing the chain to break. Otherwise, the chain will remain stable during the drive process. When $R_T = 1$, a critical situation occurs at which the resistance torque is equal to the maximum driven magnetic torque. So the number of nanoparticles in the chain (N) can be given by $R_T = 1$, and the chain length can be calculated by

$$L = 2NR. \tag{9.7}$$

The calculated chain lengths in fluids with different viscosity are shown by the two dotted lines in Figure 9.2b, where the average angular velocity $\overline{\omega} = \int_0^{1/f} |\omega(t)| dt/(1/f)$ is used to study the change of chain length under the field strength varying with time. In order to verify the validity of the mathematical model, we carried out experiments on the formation of chains in glycerol-water solution at different viscosities. In order to simulate the ionic environment of whole blood, phosphate buffered saline (PBS) was added to the solution. The ionic strength of all liquids is 0.18 mol/L (180 mM), which is very close to that of human blood (0.15–0.18 mol/L) [31]. The average length of the nanoparticle chain is calculated by MATLAB software [32]. Compared with the simulation results, we analyze from the experimental results that under the same input parameters, the nanoparticle chains have a larger length (Figure 9.2b). The above phenomenon is mainly caused by the interaction between the electrostatic torque on the chain and the flux chain. The nanoparticles we synthesized are dispersed in an ionic environment, and they can avoid repulsion caused by electrostatic charge and get together [33]. After the addition of ionic fluids, the partially neutralized charges lead to a decrease in the repulsion between nanoparticles. This change in electrostatic force can be regarded as an equivalent electrostatic attraction, which mainly depends on the distance between nanoparticles and ion concentration (C_{ion}). So during the driving process, a constant electrostatic torque (Γ_e) is added to the chain. The interaction between magnetic chains is caused by the

TABLE 9.1 Key Parameters in Mathematical Modeling

Parameters [unit]	Definition	Value
μ_0 [V · s/(A · m)]	Magnetic permeability (vacuum)	1.257×10^{-6}
χ_p	Magnetic susceptibility of nanoparticle	0.8
B [T]	Applied field strength	1×10^{-2}
R [m]	Radius of nanoparticle	2×10^{-7}
V_p [m^3]	Volume of nanoparticle	3.35×10^{-20}
C_{ion} [mol/L]	Ion strength of fluids	0.18

magnetization of chains, as [34]

$$\mathbf{m}(t) = \frac{V_c \chi_\alpha}{\mu_0(1+\chi)} \mathbf{B}(t) \tag{9.8}$$

where $\mu_0(1+\chi)$ is the penetration rate of the particle chain and χ_α is the apparent susceptibility tensor related to shape [35]. If we regard the nanoparticle chain as an ellipsoid, the magnetic dipole moment of the chain in the in-plane oscillating field can be expressed as $[m_x \ m_y]^T = \frac{V_c\chi}{\mu_0(1+\chi)}[\frac{B_x}{1+n_a\chi} \ \frac{B_y}{1+n_b\chi}]^T$, where n_a and n_b is the demagnetization factor along the major axis and the minor axis. The induced magnetic field at point P of the ith particle chain (located at O_{ci} with dipole moment m_{ci}) is given by $B_{ci}(P) = \frac{\mu_0}{4\pi}(3m_{ci} \cdot \hat{n_{ci}} - m_{ci})$ with $\hat{n_{ci}}$ the unit vector of the separation distance between $\hat{n_{ci}}$ and P [36]. So the magnetic force exerted by the ith chain on the jth chain is expressed as

$$\mathbf{F}_{ij} = -\frac{\mu_0}{4\pi}\nabla(\nabla\frac{\mathbf{m}_i \cdot \mathbf{d}_{ij}}{d_{ij}^3} \cdot \mathbf{m}_j) \tag{9.9}$$

where $\mathbf{d}_{ij} = d_{ij}\hat{\mathbf{n}_{ci}}$ is the separation distance between the two chains. From the above analysis, we can see that the flux-chain interaction is mainly affected by the external field strength. Driven by the oscillation field, this interaction can be simplified to part of the magnetic torque, as $\Gamma_{inter} = \kappa\Gamma_m$ with κ the coefficient. So the modified Mason number is redefined as

$$\begin{aligned} R_T &= \frac{\Gamma_d(\eta,\omega)}{(1+\kappa)\Gamma_m(B) + \Gamma_e(C_{ion})} \\ &= \frac{16\pi R^3 N^3 \eta\omega(t)}{(\ln\frac{N}{2} + \frac{2.4}{N})[(\frac{1+\kappa}{\mu_0})\pi R^3 N \chi_p^2 B^2(t) + 6\Gamma_e]}. \end{aligned} \tag{9.10}$$

According to the parameters in Table 9.1, Γ_e is estimated in the range of 10^{-14}–10^{-16} N · m, and $(1+\kappa/\mu_0)\pi R^3 N \chi_p^2 B^2(t)$ is calculated in the range of 10^{-12}–10^{-13} N · s. So in this case, the electrostatic torque is relatively negligible and we adopt $\Gamma_e = 1 \times 10^{-15}$ N · m in the calculation. In order to gain the optimization model with the least error from the experimental results, κ needs to be reevaluated. We take κ = [0.1, 1], the interval is 0.01 to carry on the calculation, finally take $\kappa = 0.33$ as the optimized value. Based on Eq. (9.10), the modified chain length distribution is plotted in Figure 9.2b (Rev-mod). According to the modified model, the relationship between chain length and input frequency is shown in Figure 9.2c. During the thrombolysis experiment, we used an input frequency of 10 Hz and γ of 3–5. So in PBS with the viscosity of 1 mPa · s and blood with 4 mPa · s at a shear rate of 10 s^{-1}, the chain lengths driven by 10 Hz field are calculated to be 94.4665 μm and 43.3209 μm, respectively. These values are then used in the simulation to study the flow caused by microswarms near the clot area. Blood is a non-Newtonian fluid, and its viscosity is different in time and space in a dynamic environment [37]. The experiments were performed in a stagnant blood environment with static channel boundaries, and only blood near excited microswarms exhibited flow, so we assumed constant blood viscosity.

9.2.2 Simulations of Induced Fluid Flow

We set up two finite element model-based simulations to study the induced flow around the microswarm and the clot-blood interface. According to the modeling results, the length of the nanoparticle chain driven by 10 Hz field in the blood is set to 45 μm (Figure 9.3a). The chain distance along the X and Y axes is set to 90 μm, which is twice the length of the chain. The viscosity of the fluid is 4 mPa · s, and its density is 1.05 $\times 10^3$ kg/m^3. It can be used to simulate the blood environment. In the first model (case I, Figures 9.3a and 9.3b), the swarm pattern is initiated near the anti-skid wall on the left to simulate the interaction between the microswarm and the blood clot. The distance between the wall and the mode is set to 45 μm. In the second model (case II, Figures 9.3c–e), The swarm pattern is limited by three no-slip walls, which simulates the situation that the microswarm transformation has the same width as the clot area. Simulation results on the top view in show that 3D fluid flow is induced around the pattern, and the in-plane convection between the microswarm and the clot is actively formed (yellow arrows). The simulation results of the first view in Figures 9.3b and 9.3c display that the 3D fluid flow is induced around the pattern and an in-plane convection is actively formed between the microcluster and the clot, as indicated by the yellow arrow. At a distance from the microswarm mode 200 μm, the induced velocity is above 100 μm/s. The side view of Figures 9.3d and 9.3e shows the existence of out-of-plane convection in the vertical direction, where the flow interacts with the top and bottom of the clot area. We can see from these results that if the thickness of the clot is greater than that of the microswarm mode, then the mass transfer may affect the whole clot-blood interface. In addition, boundary conditions affect flow distribution near the clot-blood interface. The average velocity distribution near the interface with a driving period of 0.1 s is shown in Figure 9.3f, where the step interval is set to 0.002 s. The comparison of the above two cases shows that microswarm deformation can be adapted to the clot area, which can further enhance the induced convection, and in the second case the whole clot-blood interface area can be affected by the mode-induced convection.

9.2.3 Simulations of Motion of RBCs and Shear Stress

We have established a simulation of red blood cell movement to study the mass transfer around the swarm pattern and the clot-blood interface. In Figure 9.4a, the

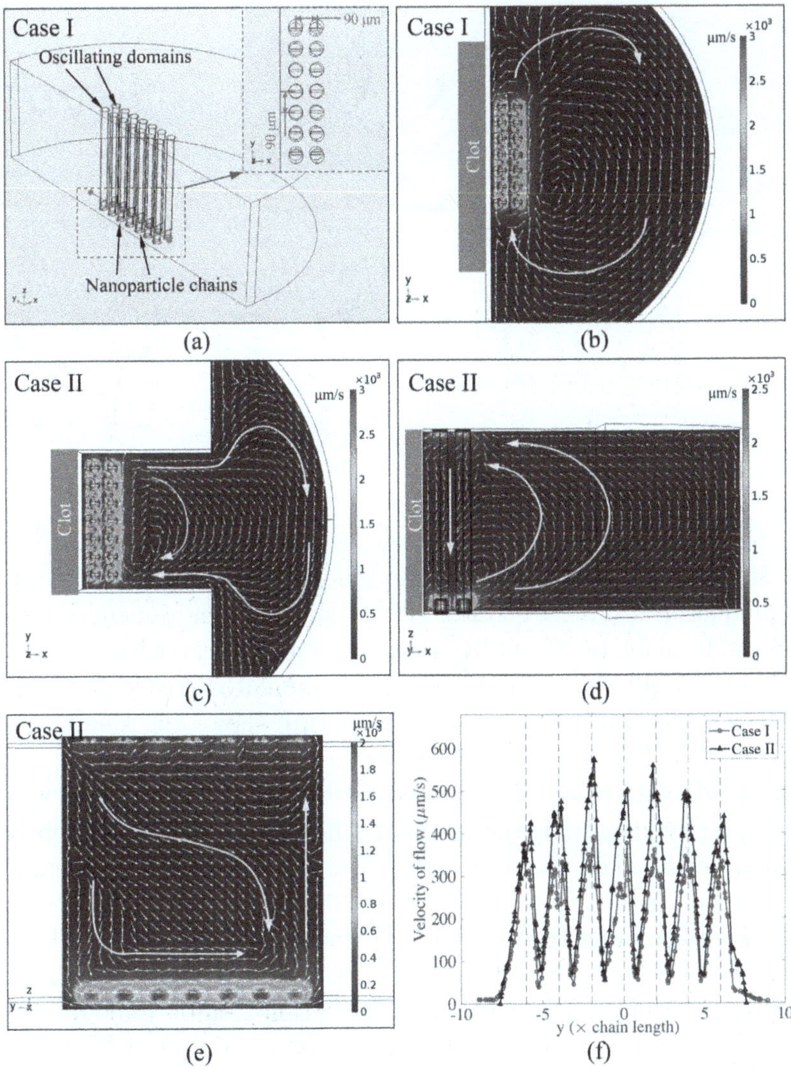

Figure 9.3 Simulation of swarm pattern-induced flow near the clot area. (a) Design of the model in case I. The chain-chain separation distance is set to twice the chain length as shown. (b, c) Fluid flow induced around the pattern on the cross section of the XY plane of the z = 30 μm. The color profile represents the velocity, as shown in the color legend on the right. The white arrow indicates the direction of flow. (d), (e) represent the traffic distribution on the XY- and YZ-planes, respectively. The yellow arrows in (b)–(e) indicate convection caused by the pattern and boundaries. (f) This section shows the average velocity distribution along the red cut line in (a) during a drive period of 0.1 seconds. Each dotted line indicates the position of the center of the chain in (f).

simulated red blood cell particles with a diameter of 6 μm and a density of 1.09 $\times 10^3$ kg/m^3 were released from five release points in the blood, each with 50 release points. The distance between each point and the flow pattern is 45 μm. The motion

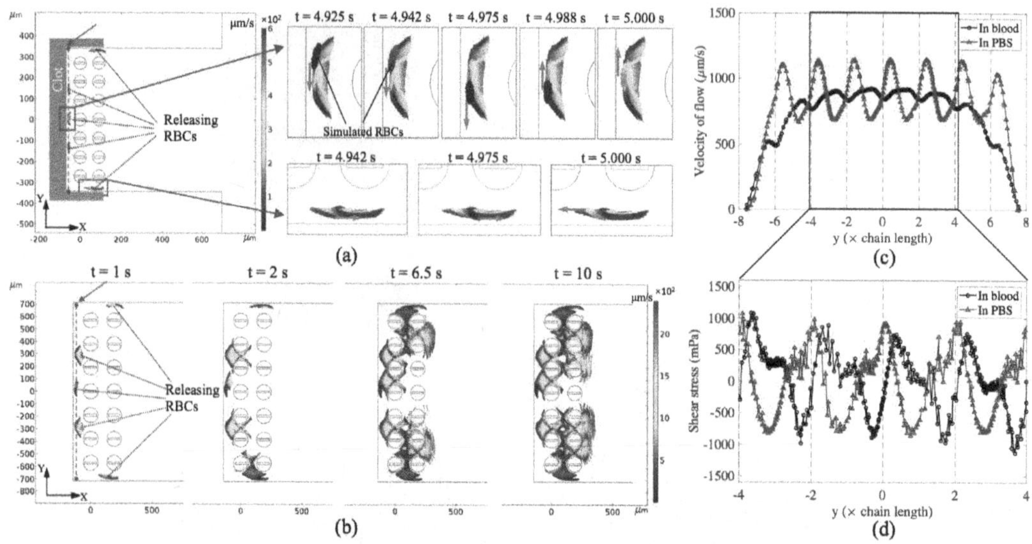

Figure 9.4 Simulation of red blood cell movement and shear stress. (a) This section shows the simulation results of 250 free simulation of the movement of red blood cells (particles 6 μm in diameter) from five release points (50 particles each) in the blood. The figure on the right shows the trajectory of simulated RBCs between the swarm pattern and clot-blood interfaces. (b) This picture shows the simulation results of 250 RBCs in PBS. In (a, b), the particles are released at $t = 0.2$ s. The input frequency is 10 Hz with $\gamma = 3$. Fluid viscosity in (a), (b) are 4 mPa · s and 1 mPa · s, respectively. (c) This part is the mode and flow velocity distribution between the clot-fluid interface for the two cases at $t = 5$ s. The cutting line is parallel to the Y axis, with coordinates of X axis = 45 μm and 95 μm in blood and PBS environment, respectively, corresponding to the purple dotted line in (a, b). (d) This illustration is the shear stress distribution along two cutting lines. The curve in this figure is reproduced using MATLAB based on the simulation results. Each dotted line in (c, d) indicates the position of the center of the chain.

of SRBCs is determined by the resistance of induced flow. The SRBC moves back and forth at the same motion frequency as the chain oscillation frequency. They move along -Y and Y directions at $t = 4.9235$–4.975 s and $t = 4.975$–5 s, respectively, and their velocities reach the maximum at $t = 4.95$ s and 5 s. In order to further study the mass transfer between the pattern and the clot-fluid interface, a simulation was established in PBS (Figure 9.4b). At this point, the SRBCs came from the dissolved clot and were released at a distance of 95 μm from the pattern. From the results, we can see that the SRBCs gradually move out of the area between the clot and the pattern, and the new liquid will flow to this area. We can see from the simulation results in Figures 9.4a and 9.4b that the mass transfer at the clot-fluid interface is enhanced and the dissolved clots or fragments will be removed from the area between the clot and the pattern. At the same time, new tPA molecules are transferred to the thrombus-fluid interface, which allows for sustained thrombus dissolution. Therefore, this approach can improve the expected lysis efficiency. Figure 9.4c shows the induced speed between the clot and the pattern. At the same input frequency, the longer chain in the PBS in Figure 9.4b provides a higher flow velocity, where the flow disturbance is caused by the distributed oscillation chain. In addition to enhancing mass transfer, the effect of the rapidly changing flow profile near the clot-fluid interface on the rate of thrombolysis needs to be studied. As Chong *et al.* proposed, we know that the first order of the velocity gradient is the shear rate, but the local shear stress near the interface can be calculated as the product of the shear rate and fluid viscosity [38]. Figure 9.4d displays the shear stress near the interface between simulated blood and PBS. Although the velocity gradient in the case of PBS is higher than that in the case of blood, we all know that the blood viscosity is relatively high and the shear stress can be maintained at the same order of magnitude. The average absolute values of shear stress in blood and PBS are 401.580 mPa and 458.982 mPa, respectively. It can be known that microswarms in the blood environment can also produce relatively high shear stress for blood clots. In the process of clot lysis, plasminogen is activated by tPA molecules into plasmin, which dissolves the fibrin network into degraded fibrin. The shear stress accelerated the removal rate of the reaction products and exposed the new fibrin network to tPA molecules. So the enhanced shear stress is helpful to the cracking efficiency. In addition, compared with the normal physiological level of shear stress, that is, intra-arterial 1–7 Pa, it is considered biologically that the shear stress caused by microswarms is safe [39]. From the simulation results, it is concluded that the convection and shear stress near the clot-fluid interface caused by microswarms can increase the cracking rate. Higher driving frequency can enhance the effect of microswarms on the clot area. The relatively low field frequency will reduce the effect of microswarms on the clot-fluid interface and results in a lower cracking rate. In the course of the experiment, the driving frequency is set to 10 Hz so as to obtain the microswarm with a fast oscillation chain.

9.3 EXPERIMENTAL SETUP AND METHODS

The three-axis Helmholtz coil system is controlled by a control PC through a LabVIEW program, and coil pairs are driven by three servo amplifiers (ADS 50/5 4-Q-DC, Maxon Inc.) through an I/O card (Model 826, Sensoray Inc.). An ultrasound system (Terason t3200, Teratech Corporation, USA) with a linear array probe (16HL7, Teratech Corporation, USA) was integrated into a magnetic drive system for microswarm imaging (Figure 9.5a). We placed the Eco-Flex PDMS channel in the center of the coil and filled it with pig whole blood. Blood was maintained at 37°C using a heating plate. The temperature of the heating plate is based on the calibration of the thermal imager (FLIR One Pro). 1 mL blood was mixed with 20 μL calcium chloride solution (0.5 mol/L), and then injected into the clot area of the blood filling channel (5 mm long, 1.5 mm high with 1.5 mm, 2 mm, and 2.5 mm wide). After 20 minutes, the clot of 11.3–18.8 mm^3 forms and fills the channel (Figure 9.5b). In the thrombolysis experiments, only one clot area was filled with blood clots. The Fe_3O_4 magnetic nanoparticles are prepared by the solvothermal method [40], Then a silicon dioxide layer is synthesized on the surface. After that, the surface of the nanoparticles

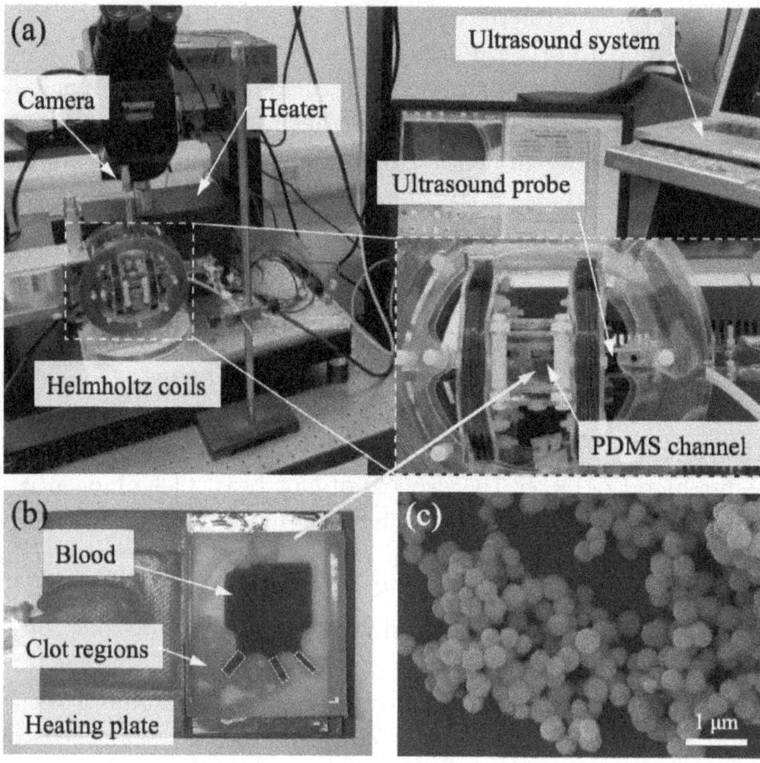

Figure 9.5 Experimental equipment and materials. (a) The ultrasound probe is placed in the central area of the three-axis Helmholtz coil. The coil is controlled by the control box and the laboratory computer. A miniature camera is installed at the top of the coil to check the assembly of the container and probe. (b) Place the PDMS channel filled with blood and thrombus on a heating plate to maintain at 37°C. (c) Scanning electron microscope images of hydrophobic Fe_3O_4@SiO_2 nanoparticles.

is hydrophobic by silanization. The diameter of the nanoparticles was measured from scanning electron microscope (SEM) images (Figure 9.5c).

9.4 EXPERIMENTAL RESULTS AND DISCUSSION

9.4.1 Formation and Reversible Elongation of a Microswarm

First, a drop of about 3 μL nanoparticle water suspension with a concentration of 5 mg/mL was added to the PDMS tank containing pig whole blood. Driven by the oscillation field, nanoparticle chains are formed, and then the magnetic and hydrodynamic interactions between the chains produce patterns (Figure 9.6a). The ultrasound contrast of the microswarm is stronger than that of the diffused nanoparticles, which is beneficial to the swarm localization. This is mainly due to the high area density of nanoparticles (5.9–8.2 $\mu g/mm^2$) [41]. The aspect ratio of the microswarm can be adjusted reversibly by adjusting the field ratio γ. The microswarm shows elongation by gradually increasing γ from 3 to 7 and shrinking by lowering γ back to 3. The

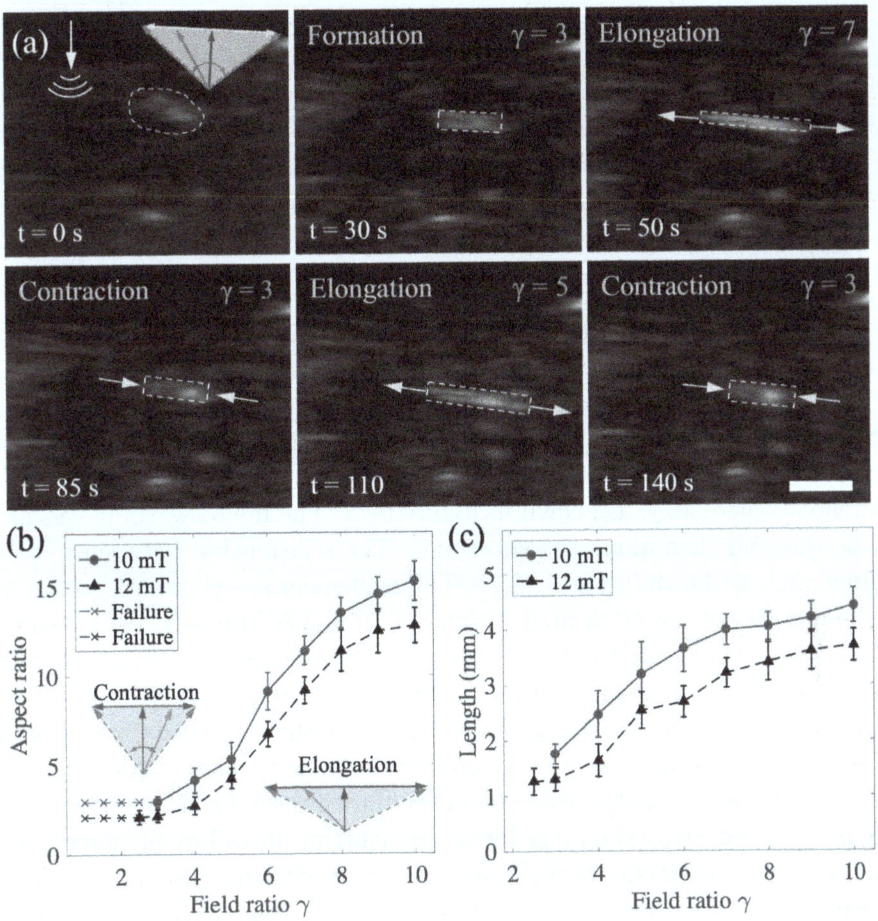

Figure 9.6 Reversible elongation of a microswarm in blood. (a) Ultrasound images show the elongation and contraction of microswarm. Arrows indicate the direction of stretching and contraction, and the figure shows the propagation direction of ultrasound waves. The scale bar is 2 mm. (b) The relationship between the aspect ratio of a microswarm and the input field ratio γ when the input field strengths of 10 mT and 12 mT. (c) The relationship between the length (major axis) of microswarms and γ. Each error bar in (c) and (d) represents the standard deviation from three trials.

recombination process in the blood is about three times faster than in water due to the relatively high viscous environment [27]. The fluid resistance of blood slows down the aggregation efficiency of nanoparticles. At the same time, blood cells could affect the hydrodynamic interaction between chains. Because of the strong ability of aggregation, the pattern was successfully formed and deformed in the blood. Figure 9.6b displays the relationship between the aspect ratio and the input field ratio, where the aspect ratio can reach the upper limit of 15.26 ± 1.10 and the input field strength is 10 mT. In addition, when the input strength increases from 10 mT to 12 mT, the larger magnetic attraction between the nanoparticle chains shrinks the swarm pattern, the aspect ratio decreases, and the upper limit decreases to 12.75 ±

1.28. In the process of reversible elongation, the length of the microswarm changes from 1.26 ± 0.24 mm to 4.43 ± 0.31 mm (Figure 9.6c). In the process of swarm formation and deformation, the influence of ultrasound on swarm stability can be ignored. The controllable reconfiguration ability provides the microswarm with the ability to adapt to a variety of constrained environments. This is very important for performing thrombolysis in blood vessels of different diameters.

9.4.2 Magnetic Navigation of a Microswarm

The motion of the microswarm is induced by adding a tilt angle (pitch angle β) to the oscillation field, in which the difference of friction between the top and bottom side (near the substrate) leads to translation motion. As analyzed in Section II, L-mode and S-mode motions can be achieved by adding pitch angles to the alternating and electrostatic field components, respectively (Figure 9.2a). The two motion modes can be switched controllably, as shown in Figure 9.7a. The microswarm moves first along the long axis and then along the short axis. The relationship between motion speed and pitch angle is shown in Figure 9.7b. The movement speed of both modes increases with the increase of the pitch angle, up to 35.80 ± 3.86 μm/s (L mode) and 23.97 ± 3.07 μm/s (S mode). But the larger dragging forces caused by relatively high speed may disturb the internal interaction between structural elements and even lead to pattern damage. When γ >10°, the speed driven by the L mode decreases because the increased fluid resistance affects the interaction between nanoparticle chains. When γ >7°, such speed loss is also observed in the S mode-driving state. When γ >10° the swarm pattern is destroyed by resistance, resulting in the failure of swarm navigation. Based on the resistance equation $F_D = 0.5C_D\rho u^2 A$ with dimensionless coefficient C_D, fluid density ρ, relative speed u, and reference area A, compared with the mircoswarm driven by L mode, the microswarm driven by S mode increases more resistance and has the same velocity. So the L mode provides the better motor ability and mode stability.

The two motion modes have their own advantages. The microswarm driven by L mode can navigate to the clot area more efficiently. In the process of thrombolysis, it is necessary to drive the microswarm in S mode to make the long edge face the blood clot for the following two reasons. Firstly, as shown in the simulation results in Figure 9.3 and Figure 9.4, there is a rapidly changing fluid flow near the long axis of the microswarm, which causes enhanced convection of tPA molecules and enhanced shear stress in the clot area. Next, along the long axis of the microswarm controls the reversible elongation. In order to adapt to the clot area, the length of the microswarm should be adjusted to the width of the clot area. So the S mode meets the requirements of thrombolysis in a restricted environment. Figure 9.7c shows the swarm navigation to the 1.5 mm wide clot area, in which the L mode is first used to drive the microswarm when t = 0–80 s. After reaching the selected clot area, the direction of the microswarm is changed by controlling the yaw angle α (t = 120 s). The driver is then changed to S mode, and then the swarm shrinks to accommodate the blood clot. No significant ultrasound interference was observed in the process of pattern formation, reversible elongation and navigation.

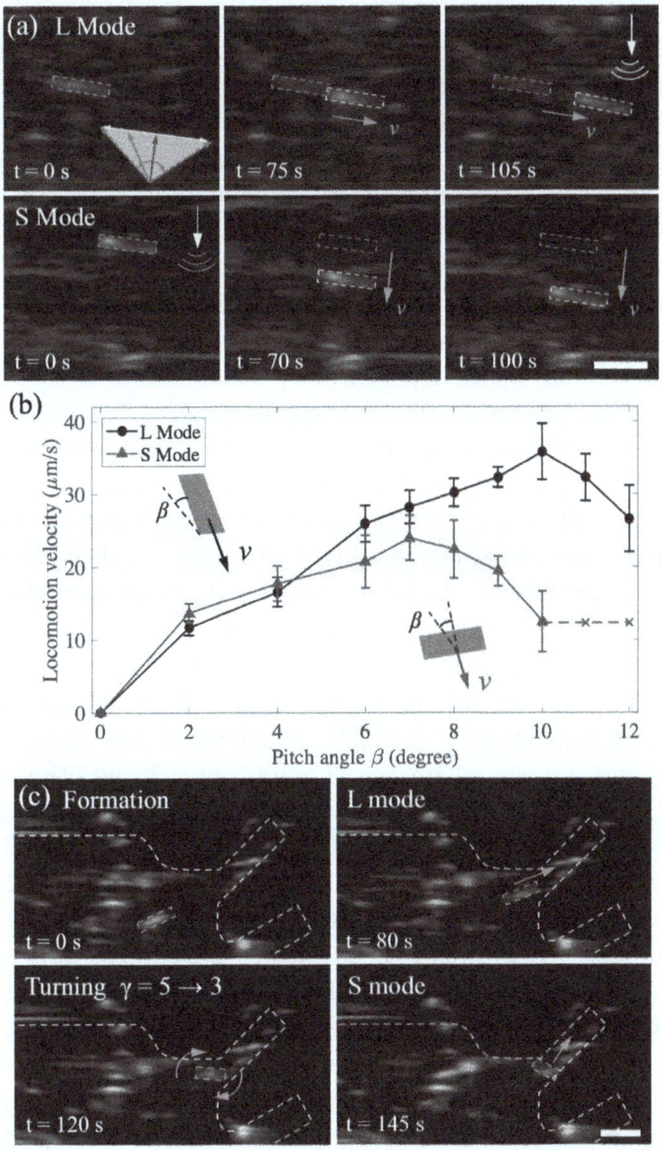

Figure 9.7 Magnetic navigation of microbiota in the blood. (a) There are two forms of microswarm movement: L-type and S-type, and the translation speed is along the long axis and the short axis, respectively, as shown by the blue arrow in the figure. The scale bar is 2 mm. (b) The figure shows the relationship between the input pitch angle β and the motion speed. The blue cross denotes the failure of the movement. Each error bar represents the standard deviation from three trials. (c) Magnetic navigation to the clot area. The drive, direction, and aspect ratio of the microswarm were adjusted to reach and fit the clot area. The scale bar is 3 mm.

9.4.3 Thrombolysis Using a Microswarm under Ultrasound Imaging

Here, we used commercial tPA injection (Actilyse 50 mg, Boehringer Ingelheim Pharma Gmbh & Co. KG, Germany) to perform microswarm assisted thrombolysis in PBS and blood environment. Figure 9.8a displays that thrombus was dissolved in tPA-PBS solution (drug concentration: 3 mg/ml). The transparent environment enables simultaneous observation with cameras and ultrasound imaging. The microswarm is guided and deformed to adapt the clot area and then activated in S mode with $\beta = 1°$. At first, the movement of the microswarm is blocked by the clot when $t = 10$ min. Due to the influence of the flow induced by the microswarm and the interaction with the repulsive fluid at the clot-PBS boundary, the microswarm does not mechanically rub the clot. The model remained stable during thrombolysis. The residual volume of thrombus is measured according to the images of camera and ultrasound imaging system (Figure 9.8b). Because of the hypoechoic nature of blood clots, the ultrasound contrast of blood clots is too low to be visualized. So the residual volume in the ultrasound image is calculated on the assumption that the clot is uniformly dissolved in the thickness direction (z-direction), as $V_{res} = (|P_s(t) - P_e|)/(|P_e - P_0|) \times 100\%$, where $P_s(t)$ is the real-time tracking location of the microswarm, P_0 and P_e are the positions of both ends of the thrombus. At $t = 40$–60 minutes, the blood clot gradually dissolves, resulting in the translational movement of the microswarm. As Figure 9.8a shows, because of the existence of microclusters, the clot area at the bottom dissolves faster. Affected by 3D induced flow (Figure 9.3), the top clot area is also affected and dissolves at a higher cracking rate than pure tPA. The average difference between camera-based and ultrasound image-based residual clot measurement is 5.32%, which shows the effectiveness of indirect measurement using ultrasound images (Figure 9.8b). In addition, the two control groups carried out experiments in pure PBS and tPA-PBS solutions with different drug concentrations (Figure 9.8c). The average dissolution rate increases with the drug dose, and a higher rate is observed in the wide clot area of 2.5 mm, which is because of the larger area of the clot-fluid interface.

Microswarm-assisted thrombolysis in blood environment is performed in ultrasound imaging. Blood clots with widths of 1.5 mm, 2.0 mm, and 2.5 mm was targeted (Figure 9.9). In each trial, only one clot area was full of blood clots. For the clot regions with 1.5 mm-, 2.0 mm-, and 2.5 mm-widths, the initial clot volumes are 11.25 mm^3, 15 mm^3, and 18.75 mm^3, respectively. The microswarm in S mode is blocked at $t = 0$ min of tachycardia and moves to the end of the clot area when part of the clot dissolves. In the 1.5 mm-, 2.0 mm-, and 2.5 mm-wide area of the blood clot, the average velocity during the dissolution of the blood clot was 58.20 ± 14.39 μm/s, 63.18 ± 7.56 μm/s, and 76.67 ± 9.93 μm/s, respectively. When the microswarm reaches the end of the clot area ($P_s(t) = P_e$), the blood is drawn and filtered through a 100-mesh filter with a pore diameter of 150 μm). Finally, we observed neither small blood clots nor residual blood lots adhering to the channel, showing that this non-contact interaction between microswarms and blood clots reduces the chances of disintegration of smaller blood clot fragments. From these results, we can see that the proposed method can reduce the risk of secondary vascular occlusion caused by small flowing blood clots or clot fragments.

The cleavage rate as a function of time is shown in Figure 9.10. The cleavage rate of tPA increased in all three cases before $t = 40$ min, and tPA reached its peak at 30–50 min after administration. After about 86 minutes, 80 minutes, and 69 minutes,

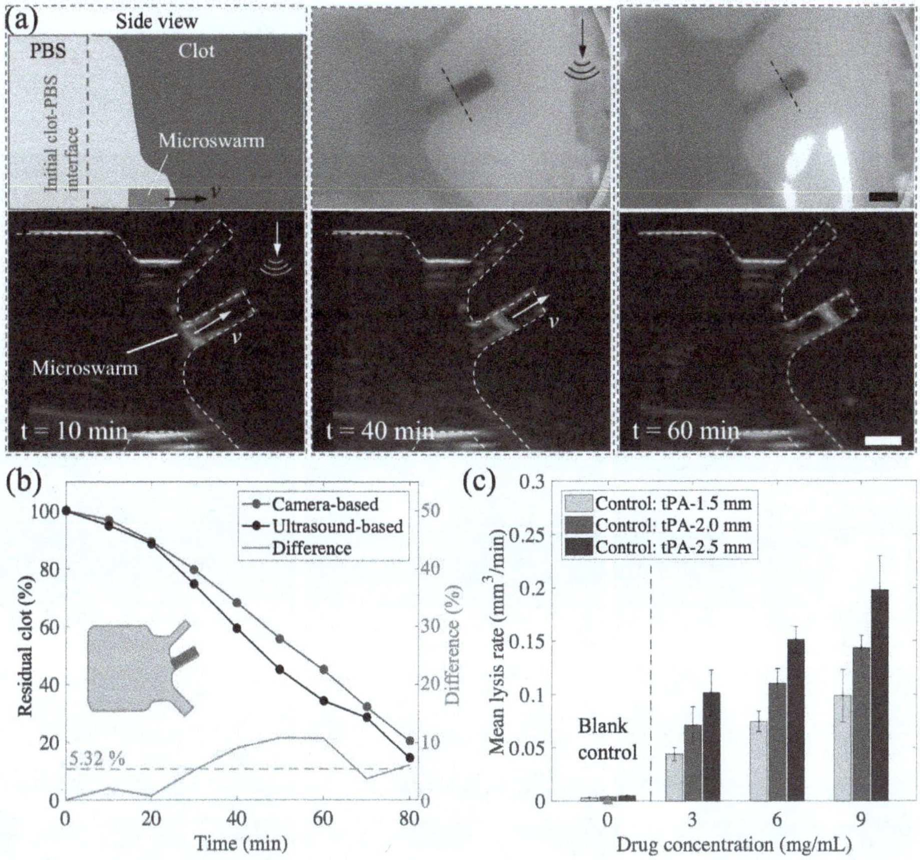

Figure 9.8 Microswarm assisted thrombolysis in PBS. (a) The process of thrombolysis was monitored by video camera and ultrasound imaging, which were displayed accordingly. Yellow dashed lines in ultrasound images indicate channel boundaries. The scale bar is 3 mm. (b) Comparison of residual blood clot estimation based on camera and ultrasound image in the process of microswarm assisted thrombolysis. (c) The average cleavage rate of the control groups using different doses of tPA without microswarm. Each error bar represents the standard deviation from three trials. The blank control group shows the volume change of clot in pure PBS.

the blood clot area was dredged, and the thrombolytic rates of the 1.5 mm-, 2.0 mm-, and 2.5 mm-width areas were 0.1310 ± 0.0324 mm^3/min, 0.1895 ± 0.0227 mm^3/min, and 0.2669 ± 0.0372 mm^3/min, respectively. Compared to the tPA alone (that is, 1.5 mm: 0.0418 ± 0.0041 mm^3/min, 2.0 mm: 0.0710 ± 0.0175 mm^3/min, 2.5 mm: 0.1013 ± 0.0214 mm^3/min), the microswarm-assisted lysis rates increased by 3.13 times (1.5 mm), 2.67 times (2.0 mm), and 2.63 times (2.5 mm), respectively. This enhancement is analyzed from three aspects. First of all, the blood flow caused by microswarms enhances the convection of tPA molecules. Mass transfer in-plane and out-of-plane near the clot-blood interface is accelerated. Fresh molecules continue to spread to the clot-blood interface, and tPA activates plasminogen into plasmin, leading to the fibrin network dissolving into degraded fibrin. Secondly, the shear stress on the

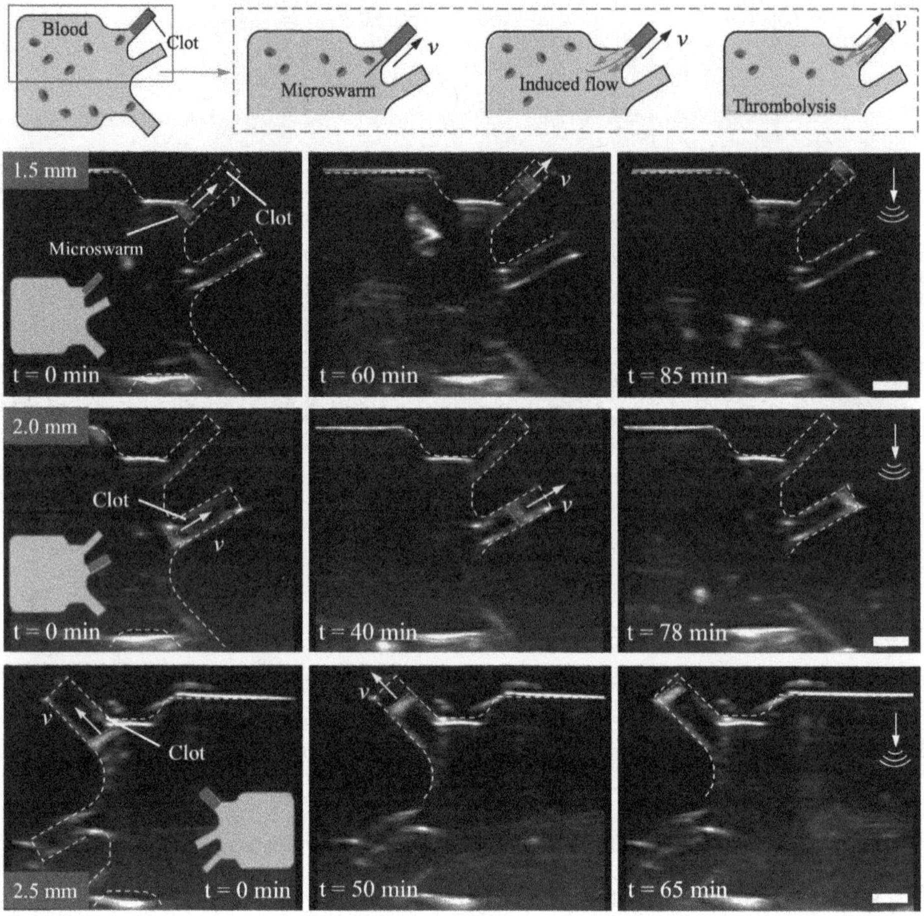

Figure 9.9 The results of microswarm assisted blood thrombolysis experiment, in which the concentration of the drug is 3 mg/mL. The dissolution process takes place in three thrombus areas with widths of 1.5 mm, 2.0 mm, and 2.5 mm, respectively. The position of the microswarm is marked with a red rectangle. All scale bars are 3 mm.

thrombus-blood interface increases. As shown in Figures 9.4b and 9.4c, there is a similar increase in shear stress in both PBS and the blood environment. The mass transfer efficiency in blood is lower than that in PBS (Figures 9.4a–c), the comparison of the *PBS+swarm-* and *Blood+swarm-*cases in Figure 9.10b shows that the shear force has a significant effect on the cleavage rate. When the plasmin molecule is located on the surface of the thrombus and activated by fibrin, the increased shear force accelerates the removal of the reaction product, exposing new fibrin that reacts continuously with plasmin at the lysine site. Third, the clot-blood interface area increases. As analyzed in Figure 9.8a, the cracking of the clot exposes more areas to tPA molecules, resulting in an increase in the reaction area and cracking rate.

tPA is a thrombolytic drug approved by FDA. However, if tPA spreads throughout the body, high doses of tPA may cause symptomatic intracranial hemorrhage.

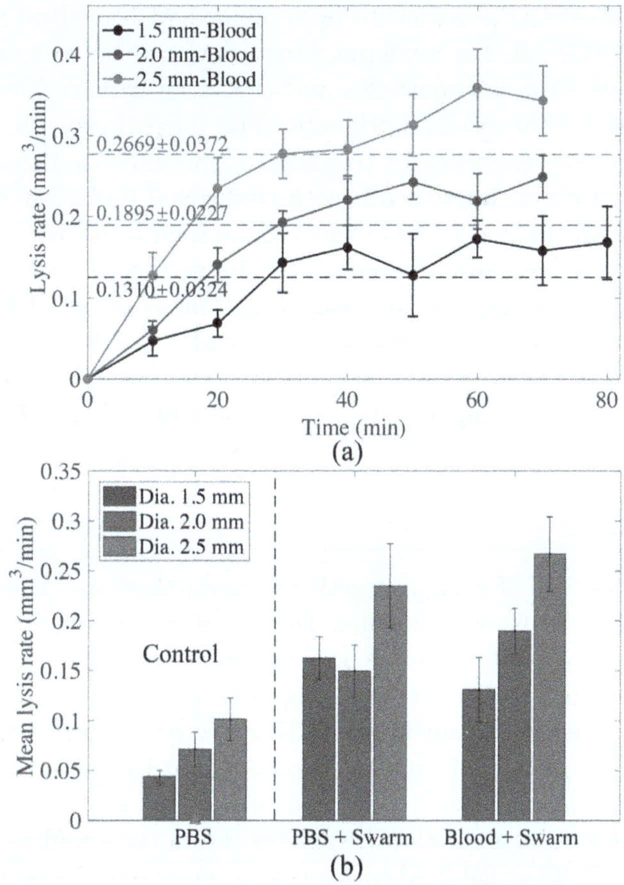

Figure 9.10 Dissolution rate of microswarm assisted thrombolysis under ultrasound imaging. (a) Changes of dissolution rate during thrombolysis in blood when the drug concentration is 3 mg/mL. Three clot areas with different widths were studied experimentally. The average rate is marked by a dotted line. (b) Average dissolution rates of three clot regions in PBS and blood environment. The drug concentration of the three groups was 3 mg/mL. Each error bar represents the standard deviation of three experiments.

The results in Figure 9.8c and Figure 9.10b display that the microswarm assisted cleavage rate is higher than that of pure tPA with three times drug concentration (9 mg/mL). The efficiency of thrombolysis is improved, the dose of tPA drug is reduced, and the risk of side effects and bleeding is reduced. In order to further improve the proposed *in vivo* verification strategy, several factors need to be considered. Firstly, the effects of blood flow should be reduced. Magnetic gradients can be used for swarm navigation in the bloodstream. The out-of-plane (swarm plane) magnetic field gradient keeps the microswarm near the boundary of the container. In this process, the resistance to the microswarm is reduced because of the parabolic distribution of fluid velocity [42]. Furthermore, the in-plane magnetic field gradient favors the aggregation of nanoparticles, increasing the access of nanoparticles to the clot area. The proposed scheme also represents the potential to be combined with medical procedures, such as catheterization [43, 44]. For example, blood flow can be stopped by inflating a balloon catheter, and the nanoparticles and tPA drug can be released together to the thrombus area for thrombolytic therapy. The microswarm integration strategy is also beneficial to the efficiency of treatment, especially for thrombosis in zigzag blood vessels that are difficult to reach with traditional tools. After completing the thrombolysis task, the magnetic guide wire can be used to recover the nanoparticles through the catheter. Secondly, the interaction between nanoparticles and endothelial cells of blood vessels needs to be evaluated. This is essential for the formation of microflora and navigation in blood vessels. Finally, the toxicity of nanoparticles needs to be tested before they are injected into the body. Particles with functional layers are required for biocompatibility, such as polydopamine (PDA) coated Fe_3O_4 nanoparticles and particles [45].

9.5 CONCLUSION

We have shown a method of using magnetic microswarms to accelerate tPA-mediated thrombolysis under ultrasound imaging. Driven by the oscillation magnetic field, microswarm formation, switchable navigation and reversible elongation are realized in the blood. The microswarm moves along the long axis and short axis and the moving speed can reach 35.82 μm/s and 23.97 μm/s, respectively. It shows reversible elongation by adjusting the external electric field, and the aspect ratio is about 16. We also established an analytical model to estimate the state of nanoparticle chains in blood and used it as a simulation parameter. From the simulation results, it can be seen that three-dimensional fluid convection is generated around the microcluster, and the shear stress near the clot-fluid interface is further enhanced. The experiments in this paper show that microswarms can be formed, navigated and deformed under ultrasound imaging, and then can adapt to different clot areas. When combined with microswarm, the cracking rate can be increased to 3.13 times, which is higher than that when the concentration of pure tPA is 3 times higher. This study offers an idea of using ultrasound-located micromachines as a tool to accelerate thrombolysis, indicating that microswarm adjuvant therapy has a great prospect in biomedical applications guided by medical imaging.

Bibliography

[1] John A Heit. Epidemiology of venous thromboembolism. *Nature Reviews Cardiology*, 12(8):464–474, 2015.

[2] Alina Zenych, Louise Fournier, and Cédric Chauvierre. Nanomedicine progress in thrombolytic therapy. *Biomaterials*, 258, 2020. Art. no. 120297.

[3] Mimi Wan et al. Platelet-derived porous nanomotor for thrombus therapy. *Science Advances*, 6(22), 2020, Art. no. eaaz9014.

[4] Göt Thomalla et al. Outcome and symptomatic bleeding complications of intravenous thrombolysis within 6 hours in MRI-selected stroke patients: comparison

of a german multicenter study with the pooled data of atlantis, ecass, and ninds tPA trials. *Stroke*, 37(3):852–858, 2006.

[5] Maya Juenet, Rachida Aid-Launais, Bo Li, Alice Berger, Joël Aerts, Véronique Ollivier, Antonino Nicoletti, Didier Letourneur, and Cédric Chauvierre. Thrombolytic therapy based on fucoidan-functionalized polymer nanoparticles targeting p-selectin. *Biomaterials*, 156:204–216, 2018.

[6] Zhoujiang Chen, Tian Xia, Zhanlin Zhang, Songzhi Xie, Tao Wang, and Xiaohong Li. Enzyme-powered janus nanomotors launched from intratumoral depots to address drug delivery barriers. *Chemical Engineering Journal*, 375, 2019. Art. no. 122109.

[7] Lawrence R Wechsler. Intravenous thrombolytic therapy for acute ischemic stroke. *New England Journal of Medicine*, 364(22):2138–2146, 2011.

[8] Netanel Korin, Mathumai Kanapathipillai, Benjamin D Matthews, Marilena Crescente, Alexander Brill, Tadanori Mammoto, Kaustabh Ghosh, Samuel Jurek, Sidi A Bencherif, Deen Bhatta, Ahmet U Coskun, Charles L Feldman, Denisa D Wagner, and Donald E Ingber. Shear-activated nanotherapeutics for drug targeting to obstructed blood vessels. *Science*, 337(6095):738–742, 2012.

[9] Islam SM Khalil, Dalia Mahdy, Ahmed El Sharkawy, Ramez R Moustafa, Ahmet Fatih Tabak, Mohamed E Mitwally, Sarah Hesham, Nabila Hamdi, Anke Klingner, Abdelrahman Mohamed, and Metin Sitti. Mechanical rubbing of blood clots using helical robots under ultrasound guidance. *IEEE Robotics and Automation Letters*, 3(2):1112–1119, 2018.

[10] Tonguc O Tasci, Dante Disharoon, Rogier M Schoeman, Kuldeepsinh Rana, Paco S Herson, David WM Marr, and Keith B Neeves. Enhanced fibrinolysis with magnetically powered colloidal microwheels. *Small*, 13(36), 2017, Art. no. 1700954.

[11] Julien Leclerc, Haoran Zhao, Daniel Bao, and Aaron T Becker. In vitro design investigation of a rotating helical magnetic swimmer for combined 3-d navigation and blood clot removal. *IEEE Transactions on Robotics*, 36(3):975–982, 2020.

[12] Ben Wang, K Kostarelos, Bradley J Nelson, and Li Zhang. Trends in micro-/nano-robotics: Materials development, actuation, localization, and system integration for biomedical applications. *Advanced Materials*, 33(4), 2021. Art. no. 2002047.

[13] Daniel Ahmed, Thierry Baasch, Nicolas Blondel, Nino Läubli, Jürg Dual, and Bradley J Nelson. Neutrophil-inspired propulsion in a combined acoustic and magnetic field. *Nature Communications*, 8, 2017. Art. no. 770.

[14] Hui Xie, Xinjian Fan, Mengmeng Sun, Zhihua Lin, Qiang He, and Lining Sun. Programmable generation and motion control of a snakelike magnetic microrobot swarm. *IEEE/ASME Transactions on Mechatronics*, 24(3):902–912, 2019.

[15] Jiangfan Yu, Dongdong Jin, Kai-Fung Chan, Qianqian Wang, Ke Yuan, and Li Zhang. Active generation and magnetic actuation of microrobotic swarms in bio-fluids. *Nature Communications*, 10:Art. no. 5631, 2019.

[16] Sajad Salmanipour, Omid Youssefi, and Eric D Diller. Design of multi-degrees-of-freedom microrobots driven by homogeneous quasi-static magnetic fields. *IEEE Transactions on Robotics*, 37(1):246–256, 2021.

[17] Lidong Yang, Qianqian Wang, and Li Zhang. Model-free trajectory tracking control of two-particle magnetic microrobot. *IEEE Transactions on Nanotechnology*, 17(4):697–700, 2018.

[18] Tiantian Xu, Jiangfan Yu, Chi-Ian Vong, Ben Wang, Xinyu Wu, and Li Zhang. Dynamic morphology and swimming properties of rotating miniature swimmers with soft tails. *IEEE/ASME Transactions on Mechatronics*, 24(3):924–934, 2019.

[19] Xinyu Wu, Jia Liu, Chenyang Huang, Meng Su, and Tiantian Xu. 3-d path following of helical microswimmers with an adaptive orientation compensation model. *IEEE Transactions on Automation Science and Engineering*, 17(2):823–832, 2020.

[20] Jia Yang, Chuang Zhang, XiaoDong Wang, WenXue Wang, Ning Xi, and Lian-Qing Liu. Development of micro- and nanorobotics: A review. *Science China Technological Sciences*, 62(1):1–20, 2019.

[21] Qianqian Wang and Li Zhang. External power-driven microrobotic swarm: From fundamental understanding to imaging-guided delivery. *ACS Nano*, 15(1):149–174, 2021.

[22] Mi Li, Ning Xi, Yuechao Wang, and Lianqing Liu. Progress in nanorobotics for advancing biomedicine. *IEEE Transactions on Biomedical Engineering*, 68(1):130–141, 2021.

[23] Jiangfan Yu, Qianqian Wang, Mengzhi Li, Chao Liu, Lidai Wang, Tiantian Xu, and Li Zhang. Characterizing nanoparticle swarms with tuneable concentrations for enhanced imaging contrast. *IEEE Robotics and Automation Letters*, 4(3):2942–2949, 2019.

[24] Xiaohui Yan, Qi Zhou, Melissa Vincent, Yan Deng, Jiangfan Yu, Jianbin Xu, Tiantian Xu, Tao Tang, Liming Bian, Yi-Xiang Wang, Kostas Kostarelos, and Li Zhang. Multifunctional biohybrid magnetite microrobots for imaging-guided therapy. *Science Robotics*, 2(12), 2017, Art. no. eaaq1155.

[25] Diana Vilela, Unai Cossío, Jemish Parmar, Angel M Martínez-Villacorta, Vanessa Gómez-Vallejo, Jordi Llop, and Samuel Sánchez. Medical imaging for the tracking of micromotors. *ACS Nano*, 12(2):1220–1227, 2018.

[26] Ania Servant, Famin Qiu, Mariarosa Mazza, Kostas Kostarelos, and Bradley J Nelson. Controlled in vivo swimming of a swarm of bacteria-like microrobotic flagella. *Advanced Materials*, 27(19):2981–2988, 2015.

[27] Jiangfan Yu, Ben Wang, Xingzhou Du, Qianqian Wang, and Li Zhang. Ultra-extensible ribbon-like magnetic microswarm. *Nature Communications*, 9, 2018, Art. no. 3260.

[28] Ioannis Petousis, Erik Homburg, Roy Derks, and Andreas Dietzel. Transient behaviour of magnetic micro-bead chains rotating in a fluid by external fields. *Lab on a Chip*, 7(12):1746–1751, 2007.

[29] C Wilhelm, J Browaeys, A Ponton, and J-C Bacri. Rotational magnetic particles microrheology: the maxwellian case. *Physical Review E*, 67(1), 2003, Art. no. 011504.

[30] Y Gao, MA Hulsen, TG Kang, and JMJ Den Toonder. Numerical and experimental study of a rotating magnetic particle chain in a viscous fluid. *Physical Review E*, 86(4), 2012, Art. no. 041503.

[31] Sung Il Han, Yong Kyoung Yoo, Junwoo Lee, Cheonjung Kim, Kyungjae Lee, Tae Hoon Lee, Hyungsuk Kim, Dae Sung Yoon, Kyo Seon Hwang, Rhokyun Kwak, and Jeong Hoon Lee. High-ionic-strength pre-concentration via ion concentration polarization for blood-based biofluids. *Sensors and Actuators B: Chemical*, 268:485–493, 2018.

[32] Qianqian Wang, Jiangfan Yu, Ke Yuan, Lidong Yang, Dongdong Jin, and Li Zhang. Disassembly and spreading of magnetic nanoparticle clusters on uneven surfaces. *Applied Materials Today*, 18, 2020, Art. no. 100489.

[33] Jiangfan Yu and Li Zhang. Reversible swelling and shrinking of paramagnetic nanoparticle swarms in biofluids with high ionic strength. *IEEE/ASME Transactions on Mechatronics*, 24(1):154–163, 2018.

[34] Jake J Abbott, Eric Diller, and Andrew J Petruska. Magnetic methods in robotics. *Annual Review of Control, Robotics, and Autonomous Systems*, 3:57–90, 2020.

[35] Harpreet Singh, Paul E Laibinis, and T Alan Hatton. Rigid, superparamagnetic chains of permanently linked beads coated with magnetic nanoparticles. synthesis and rotational dynamics under applied magnetic fields. *Langmuir*, 21(24):11500–11509, 2005.

[36] Robert A Schill. General relation for the vector magnetic field of a circular current loop: a closer look. *IEEE Transactions on Magnetics*, 39(2):961–967, 2003.

[37] A. Dutta and J. M. Tarbell. Influence of Non-Newtonian Behavior of Blood on Flow in an Elastic Artery Model. *Journal of Biomechanical Engineering*, 118(1):111–119, 02 1996.

[38] Kwitae Chong, Scott D Kelly, Stuart Smith, and Jeff D Eldredge. Inertial particle trapping in viscous streaming. *Physics of Fluids*, 25(3), 2013, Art. no. 033602.

[39] Jacek J Paszkowiak and Alan Dardik. Arterial wall shear stress: observations from the bench to the bedside. *Vascular and Endovascular Surgery*, 37(1):47–57, 2003.

[40] Dongdong Jin, Ke Yuan, Xingzhou Du, Qianqian Wang, Shijie Wang, and Li Zhang. Domino reaction encoded heterogeneous colloidal microswarm with on-demand morphological adaptability. *Advanced Materials*, 2021. DOI: 10.1002/adma.202100070.

[41] Qianqian Wang, Lidong Yang, Jiangfan Yu, Philip WY Chiu, Yong-Ping Zheng, and Li Zhang. Real-time magnetic navigation of a rotating colloidal microswarm under ultrasound guidance. *IEEE Transactions on Biomedical Engineering*, 67(12):3403–3412, 2020.

[42] Qianqian Wang, Kai Fung Chan, Kathrin Schweizer, Xingzhou Du, Dongdong Jin, Simon Chun Ho Yu, J. Bradley Nelson, and Li Zhang. Ultrasound Doppler-guided real-time navigation of a magnetic microswarm for active endovascular delivery. *Science Advances*, 7, 2021. Art. no. eabe5914.

[43] Kim Tien Nguyen, Seok-Jae Kim, Hyun-Ki Min, Manh Cuong Hoang, Gwangjun Go, Byungjeon Kang, Jayoung Kim, Eunpyo Choi, Ayoung Hong, Jongoh Park, and Chang-Sei Kim. Guide-wired helical microrobot for percutaneous revascularization in chronic total occlusion in-vivo validation. *IEEE Transactions on Biomedical Engineering*, 68(8):2490–2498, 2021.

[44] Sungwoong Jeon, Ali Kafash Hoshiar, Kangho Kim, Seungmin Lee, Eunhee Kim, Sunkey Lee, Jin-young Kim, Bradley J Nelson, Hyo-Jeong Cha, Byung-Ju Yi, et al. A magnetically controlled soft microrobot steering a guidewire in a three-dimensional phantom vascular network. *Soft Robotics*, 6(1):54–68, 2019.

[45] Ben Wang, Kai Fung Chan, Ke Yuan, Qianqian Wang, Xianfeng Xia, Lidong Yang, Ho Ko, J. Yi-Xiang Wang, Joseph Jao Yiu Sung, Philip Wai Yan Chiu, and Li Zhang. Endoscopy-assisted magnetic navigation of biohybrid soft microrobots with rapid endoluminal delivery and imaging. *Science Robotics*, 6, 2021. Art. no. eabd2813.

CHAPTER 10

Microrobotic Collective Nanoparticles for Selective Embolization

10.1 INTRODUCTION

Collective behaviors are prevalent in nature and offer significant advantages over individual entities. Swarms, in particular, exhibit remarkable capabilities in performing complex tasks. For example, fish schools exhibit collective behavior to evade predators [1], while insect swarms collaborate to construct nests [2]. Drawing inspiration from the collective intelligence observed in natural swarms, researchers have developed various robotic swarm systems. These include Kilobots [3], swarm-bots [4], and loosely coupled robots [5]. These swarm systems have been designed to accomplish tasks such as targeted locomotion [3, 4, 5], obstacle avoidance [4, 5], and object transport [4, 5, 6]. By emulating the principles of natural swarms, these robotic systems aim to achieve similar levels of efficiency and adaptability in various applications.

At micro-nanoscale, agents rely on physical and chemical interactions to form microrobotic swarms. Various external stimuli, such as magnetic fields [7, 8, 9], electric fields [10, 11, 12], acoustic fields [13, 14, 15], optical fields [16, 17, 18], and chemical signals [19, 20, 21], are applied to facilitate swarm formation. Due to their uncomplicated structure and effective manipulation, magnetic colloids have been employed to create groups of particles, by implementing various control methods [22, 23, 24]. Additionally, they have been utilized in biomedical applications including precise administration of medications [25, 26, 27], improved imaging techniques [28], and hyperthermia treatment [29]. Magnetic particle swarms, propelled by rotating magnetic fields and magnetic field gradients, have demonstrated the ability to navigate within bovine eyes [25] and blood vessels [26] for targeted drug delivery. Additionally, magnetic swarms induced by oscillating magnetic fields have been utilized for hyperthermia in cancer treatment [29, 30]. In contrast to these extensively studied tasks, embolization is a clinical technique used to block blood vessels for treating various diseases, such as tumors, fistulas, and arteriovenous malformations [31]. In current

DOI: 10.1201/9781032665788-10

clinical practices, embolic agents are deployed through catheters. Large vessels are occluded using millimeter-sized platinum or tungsten coils [31, 32], while polymeric particles and gelling solutions are released upstream to block downstream vessels [33]. However, these passive agents lack selectivity, leading to unintended blockage of non-targeted blood vessels and resulting in severe complications like stroke and blindness [31, 32, 34]. Magnetic particles, on the other hand, hold promise as embolic agents since they can form swarms on demand by applying magnetic fields. To achieve selective embolization, it is crucial to maintain swarm integrity within the targeted region while breaking the swarm integrity outside of it. This necessitates maintaining sufficiently high magnetic field strength within the targeted region while abruptly reducing it outside. Existing magnetic micromanipulation strategies are inadequate for achieving this goal as they either use uniform magnetic fields lacking selectivity within the workspace [9, 22, 23, 24, 25] or magnetic field gradients where the field strength monotonically decreases from the external magnetic source to the workspace center [26, 27, 35]. To achieve the desired spatial distribution of magnetic field strength for selective embolization, dynamic planning of magnetic field gradients is required.

In this chapter, we introduce an actuation strategy aimed at preserving the cohesiveness of magnetic particle swarms to accurately obstruct blood flow within specific regions, enabling selective embolization. To establish a foundation, we propose an analytical model that elucidates the relationship between magnetic field strength and swarm integrity. Building upon this model, we devise a dynamic magnetic field that facilitates the formation of particle swarms and sustains their integrity at targeted junctions within microchannels, even under fluidic flow conditions. By utilizing thrombin-coated magnetic particles in conjunction with the proposed strategy, we successfully achieve selective embolization in *ex vivo* porcine omentums and *in vivo* porcine kidneys. This research not only enhances our fundamental comprehension of microrobotic swarm behaviors within physiological settings but also serves as a proof of concept for the practical application of selective embolization.

10.2 MAINTENANCE OF SWARM INTEGRITY IN FLOW

To achieve targeted embolization, swarms of microrobots can be generated on demand to block specific blood vessels within a desired area, as depicted in Figure 10.1a. By releasing microrobotic agents near the intended region through a catheter, the required dosage can be minimized. To ensure distribution within blood capillaries, we utilized superparamagnetic particles measuring 1 μm in diameter, which is smaller than red and white blood cells. These particles were coated with thrombin, an enzyme that converts soluble fibrinogen in the blood into fibrin meshes, effectively trapping red blood cells (RBCs) with the particles. Through experimental fine-tuning of the thrombin concentration on the particles, we were able to activate the particles, causing them to assemble into clotting swarms at targeted junctions. However, in the presence of blood flow, weak interactions between particles could lead to swarm fragmentation at the junctions. Therefore, we investigated the maintenance of swarm integrity under physiologically relevant conditions, such as microfluidic channels with

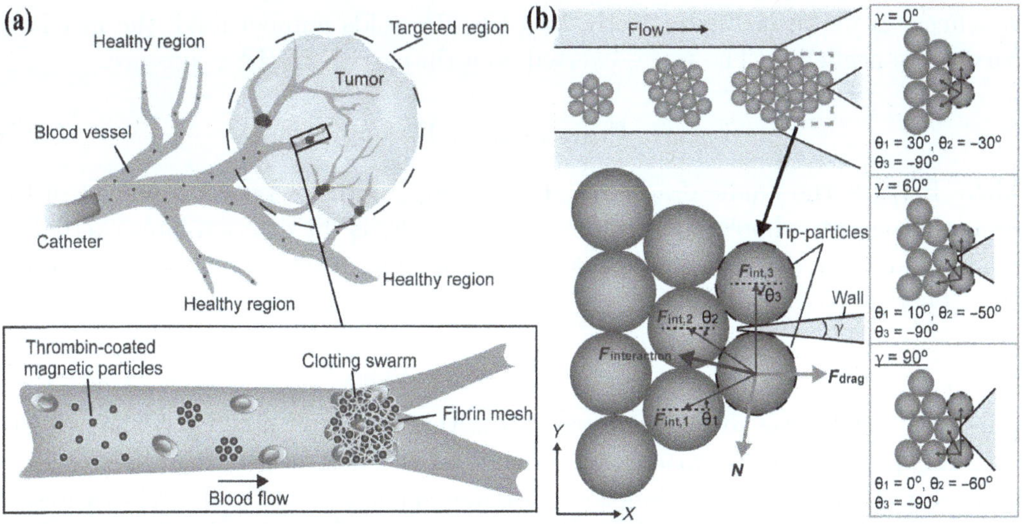

Figure 10.1 Maintenance of swarm integrity at targeted junctions. (a) Schematics illustrating the use of magnetic particle swarms to block the junctions inside a targeted region. (b) Schematic analysis of the forces exerted on tip-particles. The brown circles indicate magnetic particles. The black dashed circles denote the tip-particles. The magnetic interaction forces and their resultant interaction force are indicated by thin blue arrows and a thick blue arrow, respectively. The fluidic drag force and the reaction force are indicated by thick red arrows. γ is the branching angle of the junction. θ is the angle between the magnetic interaction force and the x axis. The configurations of particles at junctions with different branching angles are demonstrated in the green boxes. Purple regions represent the walls of junctions.

branching blood vessels and blood flow. We injected a suspension of magnetic particles into a y-shaped microfluidic channel featuring branching angles of 120°, while maintaining flow rates of up to 120 μm/s. By applying a rotating magnetic field with a frequency of 20 Hz, we induced swarm formation. Upon reaching a junction, the swarm's integrity was sustained if the interactions between magnetic agents were sufficiently strong. Otherwise, the swarms split and were carried away by the flow. As the split swarms moved outside the region influenced by the magnetic field, the flow further disassembled them.

To investigate the relationships between the branching angle, flow rate, magnetic field strength, and swarm integrity, the swarm at a junction is modeled. The particles on the front are taken as representative ones (named tip-particles, as shown in Figure 10.1b. Tip-particles are exerted with the strongest constraining magnetic interactions in the swarm. Thus, the maintenance of the tip-particle configuration indicates that the swarm integrity can also be achieved. In contrast, if the tip-particles are disassembled by the flow, some of the remaining particles of the swarm would serve as the new tip-particles with weaker constraining magnetic interactions, which would still be disassembled until the entire swarm is split. In our analysis, the coordinate system is defined as shown in Figure 10.1b. In a low–Reynolds number fluid, the inertia of particles is negligible. The forces exerted on a tip-particle in the x axis are:

$$\mathbf{F_{drag}} + \mathbf{F_{interaction,x}} + \mathbf{F_r} \sin \frac{\gamma}{2} = 0 \tag{10.1}$$

where $\mathbf{F_{drag}}$ is the fluidic drag force, $\mathbf{F_{interaction,x}}$ is the x-axial component of the resultant magnetic dipole-dipole interaction force, $\mathbf{F_r}$ is the reaction force exerted by the wall, and γ is the branching angle of the junction. The fluidic drag force exerted on a spherical particle is

$$\mathbf{F_{drag}} = -C_d(\mathbf{v_p} - \mathbf{v_f}) \tag{10.2}$$

where C_d is the drag force coefficient, $\mathbf{v_f}$ is the flow rate, and $\mathbf{v_p}$ is the velocity of the tip-particle. For compacted inner particles within a swarm, their average drag coefficient is less than that of uniformly distributed particles [36] and can be expressed as $C_d = 3\pi\eta dk$, where η is the dynamic viscosity of the fluid, d is the diameter of the particle, and k is a drag coefficient correction factor. The magnetic interaction force exerted between particles can be expressed as [37]

$$\mathbf{F_{int,ij}} = \frac{3V^2\chi_p^2}{4\pi\mu_0 r_{ij}^4}\left[\left(1 - 5\left(\hat{\mathbf{B}} \cdot \hat{\mathbf{r}}_{\mathbf{ij}}\right)^2\right)\hat{\mathbf{r}}_{\mathbf{ij}} + 2\left(\hat{\mathbf{B}} \cdot \hat{\mathbf{r}}_{\mathbf{ij}}\right)\hat{\mathbf{B}}\right] B^2 = \mathbf{c_{int,ij}} B^2 \tag{10.3}$$

where $\mathbf{F_{int,ij}}$ is the interaction force exerted on tip-particle j by particle i, V is the volume of the particle, r_{ij} and $\hat{\mathbf{r}}_{\mathbf{ij}}$ are the distance and unit vector between the center of particle i and that of tip-particle j, respectively, χ_p is the effective magnetic susceptibility of the particle, μ_0 is the permeability of free space, B is the magnetic field strength, $\hat{\mathbf{B}}$ is the unit vector of the magnetic field, and the coefficient can be expressed as $\mathbf{c_{int,ij}} = \frac{3V^2\chi_p^2}{4\pi\mu_0 r_{ij}^4}[(1 - 5(\hat{\mathbf{B}} \cdot \hat{\mathbf{r}}_{\mathbf{ij}})^2)\hat{\mathbf{r}}_{\mathbf{ij}} + 2(\hat{\mathbf{B}} \cdot \hat{\mathbf{r}}_{\mathbf{ij}})\hat{\mathbf{B}}]$.

With Eq. (10.3), the x-axial component of the resultant magnetic interaction force exerted on a tip-particle can be calculated as

$$\begin{aligned} \mathbf{F_{interaction,x}} &= \begin{bmatrix} \mathbf{F_{int,1}} & \mathbf{F_{int,2}} & \mathbf{F_{int,3}} \end{bmatrix} \begin{bmatrix} \cos\theta_1 \\ \cos\theta_2 \\ \cos\theta_3 \end{bmatrix} \\ &= B^2 \begin{bmatrix} \mathbf{c_{int,1}} & \mathbf{c_{int,2}} & \mathbf{c_{int,3}} \end{bmatrix} \begin{bmatrix} \cos\theta_1 \\ \cos\theta_2 \\ \cos\theta_3 \end{bmatrix}. \end{aligned} \tag{10.4}$$

where indexes 1, 2, and 3 indicate the neighboring particles that are exerting on the tip-particle, and θ is the angle between $\mathbf{F_{int,ij}}$ and the x axis. By analyzing the configurations of particles at junctions with different branching angles, θ_1, θ_2, and θ_3 are estimated, as shown in Figure 10.1b. Balancing the forces in the y axis, the reaction force is

$$\mathbf{F_r} = -\frac{1}{\cos\frac{\gamma}{2}} \begin{bmatrix} \mathbf{F_{int,1}} & \mathbf{F_{int,2}} & \mathbf{F_{int,3}} \end{bmatrix} \begin{bmatrix} \sin\theta_1 \\ \sin\theta_2 \\ \sin\theta_3 \end{bmatrix}$$
$$= -\frac{B^2}{\cos\frac{\gamma}{2}} \begin{bmatrix} \mathbf{c_{int,1}} & \mathbf{c_{int,2}} & \mathbf{c_{int,3}} \end{bmatrix} \begin{bmatrix} \sin\theta_1 \\ \sin\theta_2 \\ \sin\theta_3 \end{bmatrix} \tag{10.5}$$

where $0 \leq \gamma < \pi$. By substituting Eqs. (10.2), (10.4), and (10.5) into Eq. (10.1), the critical magnetic field strength $B_{critical}$ maintaining the configuration of tip-particles in the swarm can be derived as

$$B_{critical} = \left(3\pi\eta dk(\mathbf{v_p} - \mathbf{v_f}) \left(\begin{bmatrix} \mathbf{c_{int,1}} & \mathbf{c_{int,2}} & \mathbf{c_{int,3}} \end{bmatrix} \begin{bmatrix} \cos\theta_1 \\ \cos\theta_2 \\ \cos\theta_3 \end{bmatrix} - \tan\frac{\gamma}{2} \begin{bmatrix} \mathbf{c_{int,1}} & \mathbf{c_{int,2}} & \mathbf{c_{int,3}} \end{bmatrix} \begin{bmatrix} \sin\theta_1 \\ \sin\theta_2 \\ \sin\theta_3 \end{bmatrix} \right)^{-1} \right)^{\frac{1}{2}}. \tag{10.6}$$

From Eq. (10.6), it can be predicted that $B_{critical}$ becomes higher when the viscosity of fluid η and flow rate $\mathbf{v_f}$ are higher, and $B_{critical}$ has a negative relationship with the branching angle γ. When a dynamic magnetic field is applied, the component $\hat{\mathbf{B}}$ in the coefficient $\mathbf{c_{int,ij}}$ varies with time, resulting in different Bcritical over time. Therefore, an average value of Bcritical is calculated via numerical simulation.

We then experimentally investigated the influence of flow rate, branching angle, and fluid viscosity on Bcritical. In experiments, y-shaped microfluidic channels with branching angles of 30°, 60°, 90°, and 120° were used, which cover the range of physiological branching angles of vascular networks [38]. Magnetic particles suspended in porcine whole blood were injected into the channels at flow rates of up to 120 μm/s. The flow rates were quantified by measuring the speed of tracing particles in the fluid. As discussed above, $B_{critical}$ is the minimum field strength that can maintain swarm integrity at a junction. Figure 10.2a shows the experimental results (black dots), from which one can see that a higher $B_{critical}$ was required when the flow rate was higher, and with the same flow rate, $B_{critical}$ was lower when the branching angle was larger. To quantify the influence of fluid viscosity on $B_{critical}$, magnetic particles suspended in phosphate-buffered saline (PBS) solution were used (PBS's viscosity: $\approx$ 1 cP versus porcine blood plasma's viscosity: 1.4 cP [39]), and the results are shown in Figure 10.2b. Compared to the data in Figure 10.2a, with the same flow rate and branching angle, Bcritical was lower when the viscosity of the fluid was lower. The calculated $B_{critical}$ values in porcine blood plasma and PBS solution were plotted as the red lines in Figures 10.2a and 10.2b, respectively. Relative errors were calculated by dividing the result differences between the model and experiments by the model. In porcine whole blood and PBS solution, the average relative errors were

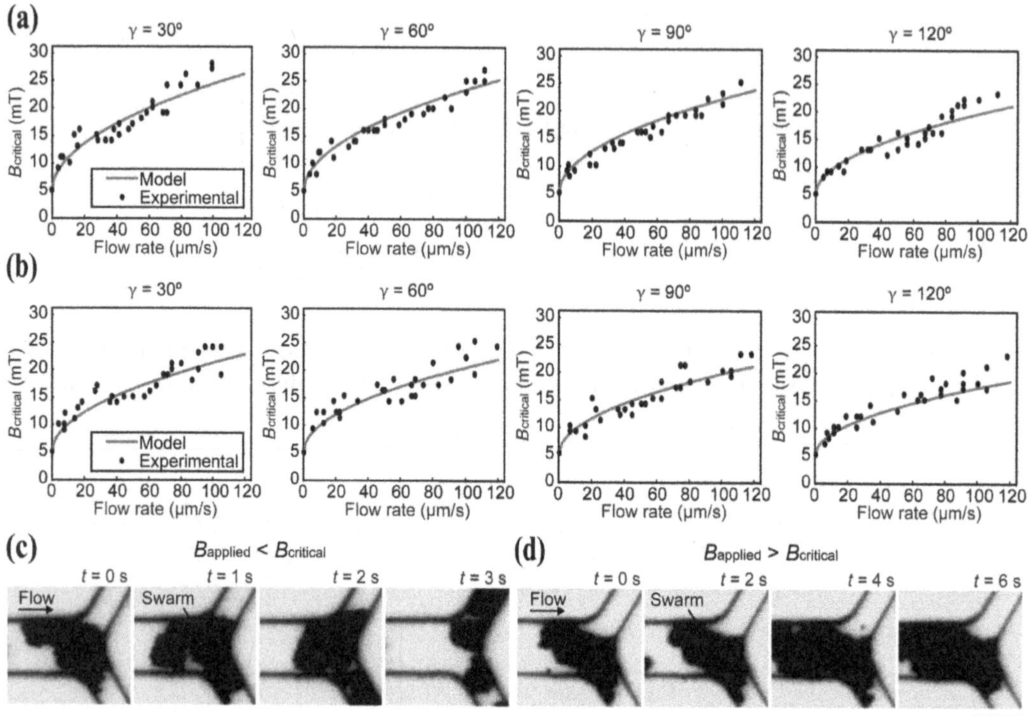

Figure 10.2 Experimental validations for the model. (a and b) The relationship between critical magnetic field strength $B_{critical}$ and flow rate at junctions with different branching angles γ in porcine whole blood and PBS, respectively. (c and d) The integrity of swarms when the magnetic field strength applied was lower and higher than $B_{critical}$, respectively. Scale bar, 20 μm.

8.0% and 9.1%, respectively. These errors can be attributed to the proposed model that was built based on the two-dimensional (2D) model of swarms; however, swarms have multiple layers of particles along the z axis, resulting in the change of magnetic interaction forces and thus causing the approximately 9% errors.

10.3 ACTUATION STRATEGY FOR SELECTIVE MAINTENANCE OF SWARM INTEGRITY

When a rotating magnetic field with a strength exceeding a critical value ($B_{critical}$) is applied, swarms become immobilized at all the junctions within the magnetic field's coverage. However, in the context of selective embolization, it is preferable to have a low magnetic field strength outside the targeted region to disrupt swarm integrity and prevent unintended blockages. To achieve high selectivity, we have developed an actuation strategy that ensures swarm integrity is maintained solely within the targeted region. This strategy involves creating a dynamic magnetic field by multiplexing the magnetic fields generated by individual coils over time, as illustrated in Figure 10.3a. During the first quarter of an actuation cycle (0 to 1/4 T, where T represents the full cycle), two adjacent coils, acting as dominant coils (depicted as brown coils in

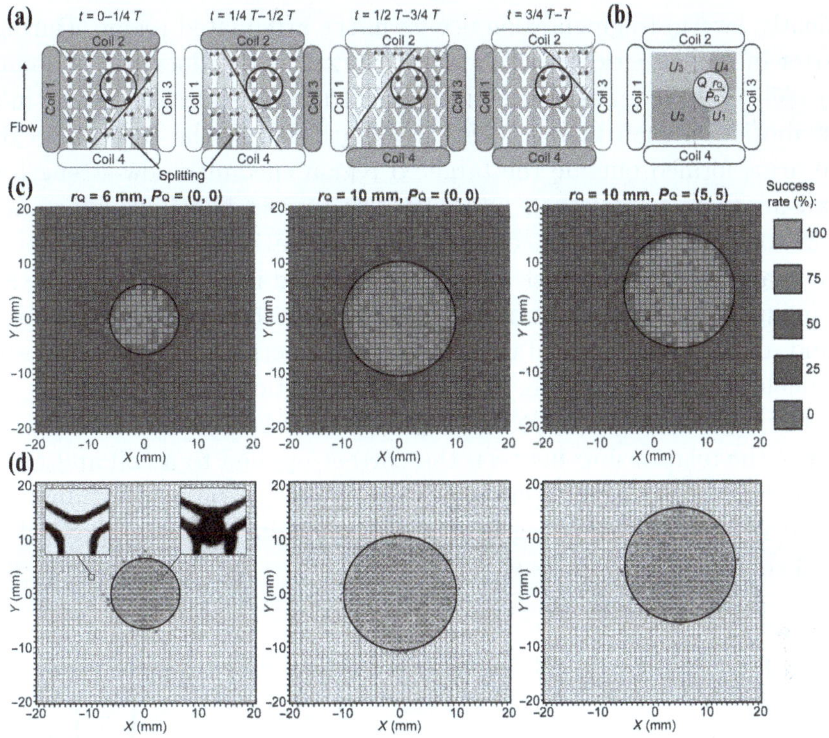

Figure 10.3 Actuation strategy for selective maintenance of swarm integrity and experimental validation. (a) Schematic illustration of the proposed actuation strategy. The black circles indicate the targeted region. The brown and white coils are the dominant and auxiliary coils, respectively. The black lines separate the workspace into regions with the magnetic field strengths higher and lower than $B_{critical}$. The black arrowhead denotes the flow direction. (b) Schematic illustration of the targeted and nontargeted regions described in the brute-force search. The black circle indicates the targeted region. The radius r_Q and the center position P_Q of the targeted region are labeled. The nontargeted subregions U_1, U_2, U_3, and U_4 are highlighted with different colors. (c) Experimental success rate of the proposed strategy in maintaining the swarm integrity in three cases. The experimental data in each small square were measured from independent microfluidic channels, and four experiments were repeated to determine the success rate. The black circles indicate the targeted regions. (d) Experimental spatial distribution of locations with a success rate of 75% and above in three cases. The left inset shows an empty junction indicating that swarms were split, and the right inset shows a swarm successfully maintained at a junction. The black circles indicate the targeted regions.

Figure 10.3a), receive higher currents to increase the magnetic field strength within the targeted region. Simultaneously, the other two coils, serving as auxiliary coils, are subjected to relatively lower currents. Importantly, the currents in the dominant and auxiliary coils flow in opposite directions, resulting in a reduction of the magnetic field strength outside the targeted region (indicated by black circles in Figure 10.3a).

Consequently, swarm fragmentation occurs in the attenuated region. During the second quarter of the actuation cycle (1/4 T to 1/2 T), the allocation of dominant and auxiliary coils is altered, as depicted in Figure 10.3a. Despite the change in magnetic field distribution, a high magnetic field strength within the targeted region is ensured. Swarms formed outside the targeted region encounter low-strength magnetic fields, causing them to lose their integrity. The current distribution among the four coils undergoes four changes to complete a full actuation cycle (T). Throughout the cycle, the magnetic field strength within the targeted region always exceeds $B_{critical}$, thereby maintaining swarm integrity at junctions within the intended area. On the other hand, outside the targeted region, swarms experience periodic exposure to low magnetic field strength, resulting in their fragmentation at junctions.

To determine the magnetic field strength produced by an electromagnetic system, we explored the relationship between the current applied to a coil and the resulting magnetic field. In the case of a circular loop, the magnetic field exhibits axial symmetry. The magnetic field strength at a specific point can be expressed using the cylindrical coordinate system as equation [40]

$$\begin{bmatrix} B_{\rho,m} \\ B_{\theta,m} \\ B_{z,m} \end{bmatrix} = \begin{bmatrix} \frac{\mu z_m}{2\pi\rho_m\sqrt{(a+\rho_m)^2+{z_m}^2}}\left(\frac{a^2+{z_m}^2+{\rho_m}^2}{{z_m}^2+(\rho_m-a)^2}E(k_m)-K(k_m)\right)I_m \\ 0 \\ \frac{\mu}{2\pi\sqrt{(a+\rho_m)^2+{z_m}^2}}\left(\frac{a^2-{z_m}^2-{\rho_m}^2}{{z_m}^2+(\rho_m-a)^2}E(k_m)+K(k_m)\right)I_m \end{bmatrix} = \begin{bmatrix} R_m I_m \\ 0 \\ Q_m I_m \end{bmatrix} \tag{10.7}$$

where m is the index indicating the coils in a system, $B_{\rho,m}$, $B_{\theta,m}$, and $B_{z,m}$ are the components of magnetic field strength generated along the unit vectors $\hat{e}_\rho$, $\hat{e}_\theta$, and $\hat{e}_z$, respectively, ρ_m, θ_m, and z_m are the cylindrical coordinates of the analyzed point relative to the coordinate frame of the coil m, a is the radius of the coil, μ is the permeability of the coil, $K(k)$ and $E(k)$ are the elliptic integrals of first and second kind, respectively, and the argument of the elliptic integrals is ${k_m}^2 = \frac{4\rho_m a}{(a+\rho_m)^2+{z_m}^2}$, and I_m is the current applied in the coil m. These magnetic field strength components are then transformed to the Cartesian coordinate system of the coil m as

$$\begin{bmatrix} B_{x,m} \\ B_{y,m} \\ B_{z,m} \end{bmatrix} = \begin{bmatrix} B_{\rho,m}\cos\theta_m \\ B_{\rho,m}\sin\theta_m \\ B_{z,m} \end{bmatrix} = \begin{bmatrix} R_m I_m \cos\theta_m \\ R_m I_m \sin\theta_m \\ Q_m I_m \end{bmatrix} \tag{10.8}$$

where $B_{x,m}$, $B_{y,m}$, and $B_{z,m}$ are the components of magnetic field strength along the x axis, the y axis, and the z axis of the coil m, respectively. Our electromagnetic system consists of four coils. By transforming the magnetic field strength generated by each coil to the Cartesian coordinate system of our workspace, the resulting magnetic field strength of a point can be calculated as

$$B_{(X,Y,Z)} = \begin{bmatrix} B_X \\ B_Y \\ B_Z \end{bmatrix} = \begin{bmatrix} Q_1 & R_2\cos\theta_2 & -Q_3 & -R_4\cos\theta_4 \\ R_1\cos\theta_1 & -Q_2 & -R_3\cos\theta_3 & Q_4 \\ R_1\sin\theta_1 & R_2\sin\theta_2 & R_3\sin\theta_3 & R_4\sin\theta_4 \end{bmatrix} \begin{bmatrix} I_1 \\ I_2 \\ I_3 \\ I_4 \end{bmatrix}. \tag{10.9}$$

Our workspace is in the xz plane of coils ($i.e.$, θ_1, θ_2, θ_3, and θ_4 are 0°). The model in Eq. (10.8) was validated by experiments. Experimentally measured magnetic field strength was compared to the model-calculated magnetic field strength distribution. The percentage difference of magnetic field strength between the experiment and the model was smaller than 10% within the workspace. To obtain the quantitative current sequences that generate the required dynamic magnetic fields for realizing the actuation strategy, a brute-force search algorithm [41] was implemented, which generates and tests all the possible current sequences. The targeted region Q was set to be a circular region with its center position P_Q and radius r_Q, as shown in Figure 10.3b. The nontargeted region U consisted of four subregions that were sequentially exposed to magnetic fields with strengths lower than $B_{critical}$ in an actuation cycle T. For example, the nontargeted subregions U_1 and U_2 were exposed to low-strength magnetic fields during 0 to 1/4 T and 1/4 T to 1/2 T, respectively. The current sequences must fulfill the following constraints to generate the required dynamic magnetic fields.

(1) Currents applied in both dominant coils are sinusoidal, and they have a phase difference of 90° between each other to generate a nonuniform rotating magnetic field

$$\begin{cases} I_{i,D1}(t) = I\sin(\omega t) \\ I_{i,D2}(t) = I\sin\left(\omega t + \frac{\pi}{2}\right) \end{cases}, t \in T_i \quad (10.10)$$

where I_{i,D_1} and $_{i,D_2}$ are the currents applied in the dominant coils, i indexes each quarter of the actuation cycle, I is the amplitude of the testing current and $I \in [0\text{ A}, 5\text{ A}]$ in our experimental setup, ω is the angular frequency, t is the time, and T_i indicates the quarter of the cycle. Under this condition, no additional requirement is needed for the currents applied in the auxiliary coils I_{i,A_1} and I_{i,A_2}.

(2) The magnetic field strength B inside the targeted region Q is higher than or equal to the calculated $B_{critical}$ in every quarter of the cycle.

$$B(t, p, I_{i,D1}, I_{i,D2}, I_{i,A1}, I_{i,A2}) \geq B_{critical}, \forall p \in Q, t \in T_i \quad (10.11)$$

where p indicates the point inside the workspace.

(3) The magnetic field strength B inside the nontargeted subregions U_i is lower than the calculated $B_{critical}$ during the corresponding quarter of the cycle

$$B(t, p, I_{i,D1}, I_{i,D2}, I_{i,A1}, I_{i,A2}) < B_{critical}, \forall p \in U_i, t \in T_i. \quad (10.12)$$

The brute-force search outputs a series of current sequences that fulfill the constraints. Using the actuation strategy, no blockage should be formed outside the targeted region. Therefore, we apply the following function to determine the current sequence that generates the weakest magnetic field strength inside the nontargeted region U to ensure the swarms are split

$$\begin{bmatrix} I_1 & I_2 & I_3 & I_4 \end{bmatrix} = \underset{I_1, I_2, I_3, I_4}{\arg\min} \sum_{t=0}^{T} \sum_{p=1}^{U} B(t, p, I_1, I_2, I_3, I_4), \forall p \in U, t \in T \quad (10.13)$$

where I_1, I_2, I_3, and I_4 are the current sequences applied in coils 1, 2, 3, and 4, respectively.

The proposed actuation strategy was validated by experiments. Microfluidic channels with 120° branching angles were placed 1 mm apart from each other inside the workspace. Magnetic particles suspended in PBS solution were injected into the channels individually at a flow rate of 80 μm/s. From the model in Eq. (10.5), $B_{critical}$ was calculated to be 16 mT. Three targeted regions were set sequentially, (i) $P_{Q1} =$ (0 mm, 0 mm), $r_{Q1} = 6$ mm; (ii) $P_{Q2} =$ (0 mm, 0 mm), $r_{Q2} = 10$ mm; and (iii) $P_{Q3} =$ (5 mm, 5 mm), $r_{Q3} = 10$ mm. Three corresponding current sequences were obtained from the brute-force search, and then three different dynamic magnetic fields were generated. Figure 10.3c shows the success rate of maintaining swarm integrity at different locations (each square represents a location) inside the workspace, under the actuation of dynamic magnetic fields. At each location, experiments were repeated four times to determine the success rate (*e.g.*, a 50% success rate means successfully maintaining swarm integrity two times out of four trials). Experimental results showed that the average success rates were 91 and 6% inside and outside the targeted region, respectively, as summarized in Figure 10.3c. Figure 10.3d shows the experimental spatial distribution of locations with the success rate of 75% and above. We further used the Jaccard index [42] I_{JAC} to evaluate the selectivity of the proposed strategy

$$I_{JAC} = \frac{T_s}{T_s + T_{NS} + N_s} \tag{10.14}$$

where T_s is the number of targeted junctions with swarms, T_{NS} is the number of targeted junctions without swarms, and N_s is the number of nontargeted junctions with swarms. On the basis of the results in Figure 10.3d, the average index was determined to be 0.9, indicating a high selectivity of the proposed strategy.

10.4 EMBOLIZATION IN MICROFLUIDIC CHANNELS

In order to evaluate the effectiveness of using magnetic particle swarms to block blood flow, the blood flow rate was measured under different conditions and compared in Figure 10.4a. To ensure visibility under optical microscopy, porcine whole blood was diluted and injected into microfluidic channels with branching angles of 120°. The flow rate was quantified by measuring the velocity of red blood cells (RBCs), and 10 measurements were taken to determine the average flow rate. The injected flow rate was maintained at an average of 84 μm/s (represented by the red data points in Figure 10.4a). Based on the model described by Eq. (10.6), $B_{critical}$, the critical magnetic field strength, was calculated to be 16.6 mT.

Polystyrene particle suspension (represented by orange data points in Figure 10.4a) and magnetic particle suspension (represented by gray data points in Figure 10.4a) were introduced into the microfluidic channels. To maintain swarm integrity, a uniform rotating magnetic field with a strength of 20 mT was applied. Surprisingly, the average flow rate of 84 μm/s remained constant for both the polystyrene particle suspension and the magnetic particle suspension. The polystyrene particles, which

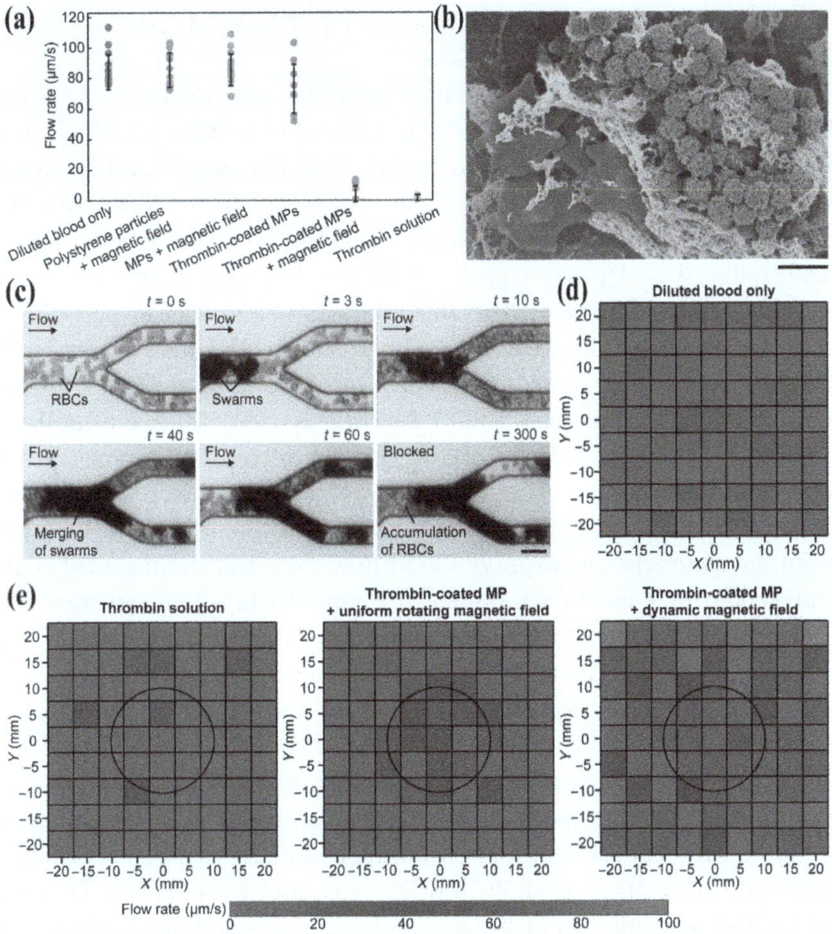

Figure 10.4 Embolization in microfluidic channels. (a) Different conditions for reducing blood flow rate. The flow rates were measured when the conditions were kept activated for 10 min. The error bars represent the SD of 10 trials. MPs denote magnetic particles. (b) Scanning electron microscopy image of a clotting swarm. For visualization, porcine RBCs, fibrin meshes, and magnetic particles were artificially colored in red, green, and blue, respectively. Scale bar, 2 μm. (c) Experimental results of embolization in microchannels using thrombin-coated magnetic particles. Scale bar, 20 μm. (d) The input flow rate of diluted porcine blood in the microfluidic channels (average flow rate: 83 μm/s). (e) Experimentally measured flow rate in the microfluidic channels under different embolization conditions. The flow rates were measured when the conditions were kept activated for 10 min. For (d) and (e), the data in each small square were measured from independent microfluidic channels, and three experiments were conducted to obtain an average flow rate. The black circles indicate the targeted region.

are non-responsive to magnetic fields, smoothly flowed along with the current without causing any blockages. On the other hand, the magnetic particles formed swarms at the junctions, but there was still enough space between the particles within the swarm. This allowed deformable red blood cells (RBCs) to pass through without significantly reducing the blood flow rate.

When magnetic particles coated with thrombin were utilized, the absence of a magnetic field resulted in a slight reduction in the average flow rate to 72 μm/s (represented by blue data points in Figure 10.4a). This decrease could be attributed to the formation of small clusters that had an impact on blood flow. However, when a uniform rotating magnetic field of 20 mT was applied, the average flow rate was significantly reduced to 4 μm/s (represented by green data points in Figure 10.4a). This reduction occurred because the thrombin-coated magnetic particles captured red blood cells (RBCs), filling the gaps and forming clotting swarms that blocked the flow. The scanning electron microscopy image in Figure 10.4b illustrates the entrapment of magnetic particles (blue) and RBCs (red) by fibrin meshes (green), forming a clotting swarm. Furthermore, experimental results demonstrating the occlusion of a branched channel using thrombin-coated magnetic particles are depicted in Figure 10.4c. In contrast, when a thrombin solution was directly injected into the microfluidic channels, the average blood flow rate was significantly reduced to 1 μm/s (represented by yellow data points in Figure 10.4a). This substantial decrease occurred because fibrinogen in the blood formed clots as anticipated. Compared to the passive embolization induced by a thrombin solution, the utilization of thrombin-coated magnetic particles allowed for active and on-demand blockage of channels. This activation was achieved by applying a rotating magnetic field with a strength higher than $B_{critical}$.

To confirm the effectiveness of our proposed strategy for selective embolization, we conducted validation experiments. Microfluidic channels with 120° branching angles were positioned 5 mm apart from each other within the workspace. Diluted porcine blood was individually injected into the microfluidic channels, maintaining an average flow rate of 83 μm/s, as depicted in Figure 10.4d. The blood flow rates under different embolization conditions are summarized in Figure 10.4e. The targeted region, indicated by black circles in Figure 10.4e, had a radius of 10 mm and was centered at (0 mm, 0 mm). At each location, the experiments were repeated three times to determine the average flow rate. When thrombin solution was injected, both inside and outside the targeted region, the average flow rate was significantly reduced to 2 μm/s. This result confirmed that thrombin solution caused nonselective embolization. Similarly, when thrombin-coated magnetic particles were actuated using a 20-mT uniform rotating magnetic field, the average flow rate was reduced to 4 μm/s throughout the entire workspace. This reduction occurred because clotting swarms formed at all junctions covered by the uniform rotating magnetic field. Through a brute-force search, we obtained the current sequence that satisfied Eqs. (10.10)– (10.13) and generated the corresponding dynamic magnetic field. Inside the targeted region, the average flow rate was reduced to 6 μm/s, representing a remarkable 93% reduction in flow rate. However, the flow rate outside the targeted region was minimally affected, remaining at approximately 79 μm/s. These results demonstrated that our actuation strategy, in combination with thrombin-coated magnetic particles, successfully achieved selective embolization with minimal unintended blockage outside the targeted region.

10.5 EMBOLIZATION IN PORCINE ORGANS

To validate the effectiveness of using magnetic particle swarms to block blood flow in tissues, we conducted experiments in an *ex vivo* porcine blood vessel. Figure 10.5a illustrates the blocking of a porcine blood vessel using microrobotic swarms. The

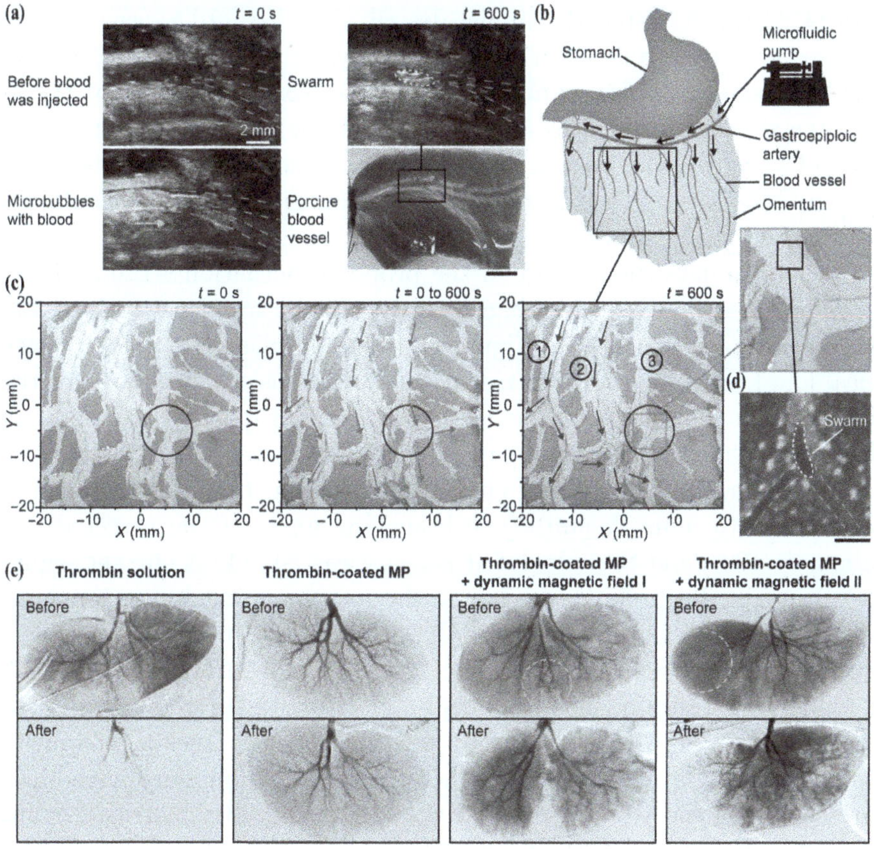

Figure 10.5 (a) Formation of a clotting swarm at the junction of an *ex vivo* porcine blood vessel. The red dashed lines outline the blood vessel and junction, and the yellow dashed line outlines the clotting swarm. The green arrow shows the flow direction of microbubbles. Scale bar, 10 mm. (b) Schematic illustrating the injection site of an *ex vivo* porcine omentum in experiments. Black arrows indicate the flow direction. (c) Selective embolization in the blood vessel network of an *ex vivo* porcine omentum with the targeted region centered at (5 mm, –5 mm). The black circles indicate the targeted region, the red arrows indicate the blood flow direction, and the blue arrows indicate the flow direction of blue dye. (d) Optical microscopy image showing a swarm formed at the targeted junction of an *ex vivo* porcine omentum. The red dashed lines outline the blood vessel and junction, and the yellow dashed lines outline the magnetic particle swarm. Scale bar, 200 μm. (e) Digital subtraction angiography results of *in vivo* porcine kidneys under different embolization conditions. The orange dotted circles indicate the targeted regions. Scale bar, 50 mm.

blood vessel, which had a branching angle of 30°, was visualized using an ultrasound imaging system (Vevo 3100, FUJIFILM VisualSonics). When microbubbles, which serve as ultrasound imaging contrasts, were injected with blood, they freely moved along with the blood, causing the blood vessel and junction to appear bright due to their high echogenicity. This indicated that the blood vessel was unobstructed. Next, thrombin-coated magnetic particles were injected into the blood vessel at a flow rate of 80 μm/s. Using the model described in Eq. (10.5), the corresponding $B_{critical}$ was calculated to be 23 mT. Subsequently, a uniform rotating magnetic field of 25 mT was maintained for 10 minutes to induce swarm formation at the junction. The brightened spot (outlined by a yellow dashed line) at the junction indicated the formation of a swarm. The presence of the swarm enhanced the contrast, resulting in the microbubbles ceasing their movement. This confirmed the successful blockage of the blood vessel by the swarm.

To further evaluate the efficacy of the proposed actuation strategy for selective embolization, we conducted experiments in the blood vessel network of an *ex vivo* porcine omentum, as depicted in Figures 10.5b and 10.5c. The greater omentum, a peritoneal fold known for tumor formation and metastasis, was chosen for this study [43]. Thrombin-coated magnetic particles were injected together with porcine blood into the greater omentum through the gastroepiploic artery, as illustrated in Figure 10.5b, at a flow rate of 80 μm/s. The targeted region had a radius of 6 mm and was centered at (5 mm, –5 mm). The branching angle of the targeted vessel was approximately 100°, and the calculated $B_{critical}$ was 20 mT. A current sequence was obtained through a brute-force search, and the corresponding dynamic magnetic field was sustained for 10 minutes. To assess the selectivity of embolization, blue dye was subsequently injected from the same site (gastroepiploic artery). The blood vessels outside the targeted region (blood vessels 1 and 2) were colored by the dye, while the blood vessel associated with the targeted junctions (blood vessel 3) remained red and unaffected, as shown in Figure 10.5c. When the targeted junctions were blocked, the fluidic resistance of the associated blood vessel 3 significantly increased compared to blood vessels 1 and 2 outside the targeted region. As a result, the blue dye bypassed blood vessel 3, confirming its blockage. Figure 10.5d presents an optical microscopy image revealing the swarm observed at the targeted junction, effectively blocking the blood vessel. This observation confirms the successful embolization achieved by the swarm.

We then tested the proposed actuation strategy for selective embolization in *in vivo* porcine kidneys, as shown in Figure 10.5e. Before embolization, blood vessels and kidneys appeared darker than backgrounds when iohexol (*i.e.*, an imaging contrast for digital subtraction angiography (DSA)) was injected into renal arteries. The kidneys were then embolized under different conditions for 10 min, after which iohexol was injected again to investigate the changes in the blood vessels and kidneys. Thrombin solution was supplied to the first kidney, and after embolization, the kidney and most of the blood vessels did not appear under DSA imaging, indicating that thrombin solution caused blockage without selectivity. Thrombin-coated magnetic particle solution was supplied to the second kidney, with no magnetic fields applied, and after 10 min, no change was observed in the blood vessels and kidney, indicating that thrombin-coated magnetic particles alone did not block the vessels. The third and the fourth kidneys were injected with thrombin-coated magnetic particle solution and were exposed to dynamic magnetic fields that corresponded to the targeted regions with 40 and 50 mm diameter, respectively (outlined by orange dotted circles). After 10 min, the targeted regions of the third kidney (middle portion) and the fourth kidney (left portion) did not appear under DSA imaging, while the other regions appeared darker, demonstrating that the proposed strategy was able to realize *in vivo* selective embolization.

10.6 DISCUSSION AND CONCLUSION

A method was devised to maintain the integrity of a swarm within a specific area by obstructing blood flow at intersections, thereby enabling targeted embolization. Analytical modeling was employed to establish the correlations among variables such as branching angle, fluid viscosity, flow rate, magnetic field strength, and swarm integrity. Building upon this model, an actuation strategy was devised, and a brute-force search algorithm was utilized to determine the optimal sequences of currents that produce the required dynamic magnetic fields. Through the use of thrombin-coated magnetic particles, the proposed strategy was validated in microfluidic channels. Experimental findings demonstrated the successful achievement of selective embolization while minimizing unintended blockages outside the intended region. Furthermore, the proposed strategy was effectively employed to achieve *in vivo* selective embolization in porcine kidneys.

The developed actuation strategy allows magnetic particle swarms to effectively embolize blood vessels within a specific region while selectively preserving their integrity. Although previous studies have demonstrated navigated locomotion of microrobotic swarms [7, 8, 9, 23, 24, 25, 26, 44, 45, 46, 47, 48], controlling the independent movement of multiple homogeneous swarms poses a challenge due to their identical behaviors in the same actuation field. Consequently, when dealing with tasks involving multiple scattered blood vessels, the swarms must be navigated sequentially, resulting in prolonged surgical procedures. Furthermore, navigating swarms *in vivo* remains difficult due to the ongoing investigation into effective *in vivo* swarm imaging techniques [46, 47, 48, 49, 50]. In contrast, our method eliminates the need for swarm navigation by leveraging blood flows to distribute the swarms and utilizing blood vessel junctions to confine their motion. Additionally, we designed dynamic magnetic fields to sustain swarm integrity within the targeted region while disrupting swarm cohesion outside of it.

In addition to embolization, the developed actuation strategy possesses a high degree of selectivity that opens up new possibilities for biomedical applications, including targeted hyperthermia. By employing this strategy for targeted hyperthermia, magnetic agents within the intended region can be propelled by strong magnetic fields, while agents outside the region experience weaker magnetic fields. Consequently, agents inside the targeted region will generate more heat over time compared to those outside, enhancing the efficacy of local hyperthermia while minimizing damage to surrounding healthy tissues. Furthermore, the strategy offers potential solutions for the design of intricate dynamic magnetic field-driven micromanipulation systems. For instance, magnetic agents within the targeted region can acquire greater rotational energy, enabling them to perform selective micromanipulation tasks with enhanced precision.

This study demonstrates the successful actuation of magnetic particle swarms to accomplish selective embolization. By employing the developed actuation strategy, microrobotic swarms offer a promising solution for achieving selective embolization, thereby addressing complications such as stroke and blindness (as observed in previous studies [31, 32, 34] associated with current passive and non-selective embolization techniques.

Bibliography

[1] Carl Anderson, Guy Theraulaz, and J-L Deneubourg. Self-assemblages in insect societies. *Insectes sociaux*, 49:99–110, 2002.

[2] Brian L Partridge. The structure and function of fish schools. *Scientific American*, 246(6):114–123, 1982.

[3] Michael Rubenstein, Alejandro Cornejo, and Radhika Nagpal. Programmable self-assembly in a thousand-robot swarm. *Science*, 345(6198):795–799, 2014.

[4] Roderich Groß, Michael Bonani, Francesco Mondada, and Marco Dorigo. Autonomous self-assembly in swarm-bots. *IEEE Transactions on Robotics*, 22(6):1115–1130, 2006.

[5] Shuguang Li, Richa Batra, David Brown, Hyun-Dong Chang, Nikhil Ranganathan, Chuck Hoberman, Daniela Rus, and Hod Lipson. Particle robotics based on statistical mechanics of loosely coupled components. *Nature*, 567(7748):361–365, 2019.

[6] Jianing Chen, Melvin Gauci, Wei Li, Andreas Kolling, and Roderich Groß. Occlusion-based cooperative transport with a swarm of miniature mobile robots. *IEEE Transactions on Robotics*, 31(2):307–321, 2015.

[7] Daniel Ahmed, Alexander Sukhov, David Hauri, Dubon Rodrigue, Gian Maranta, Jens Harting, and Bradley J Nelson. Bioinspired acousto-magnetic microswarm robots with upstream motility. *Nature Machine Intelligence*, 3(2):116–124, 2021.

[8] Fernando Martinez-Pedrero, Eloy Navarro-Argemí, Antonio Ortiz-Ambriz, Ignacio Pagonabarraga, and Pietro Tierno. Emergent hydrodynamic bound states between magnetically powered micropropellers. *Science Advances*, 4(1):eaap9379, 2018.

[9] Hui Xie, Mengmeng Sun, Xinjian Fan, Zhihua Lin, Weinan Chen, Lei Wang, Lixin Dong, and Qiang He. Reconfigurable magnetic microrobot swarm: Multimode transformation, locomotion, and manipulation. *Science Robotics*, 4(28):eaav8006, 2019.

[10] Bo Zhang, Andrey Sokolov, and Alexey Snezhko. Reconfigurable emergent patterns in active chiral fluids. *Nature Communications*, 11(1):4401, 2020.

[11] Antoine Bricard, Jean-Baptiste Caussin, Nicolas Desreumaux, Olivier Dauchot, and Denis Bartolo. Emergence of macroscopic directed motion in populations of motile colloids. *Nature*, 503(7474):95–98, 2013.

[12] Zuochen Wang, Zhisheng Wang, Jiahui Li, Changhao Tian, and Yufeng Wang. Active colloidal molecules assembled via selective and directional bonds. *Nature Communications*, 11(1):2670, 2020.

[13] Kai Melde, Andrew G Mark, Tian Qiu, and Peer Fischer. Holograms for acoustics. *Nature*, 537(7621):518–522, 2016.

[14] Sho C Takatori, Raf De Dier, Jan Vermant, and John F Brady. Acoustic trapping of active matter. *Nature Communications*, 7(1):10694, 2016.

[15] Zhichao Ma, Kai Melde, Athanasios G Athanassiadis, Michael Schau, Harald Richter, Tian Qiu, and Peer Fischer. Spatial ultrasound modulation by digitally controlling microbubble arrays. *Nature Communications*, 11(1):4537, 2020.

[16] Jeremie Palacci, Stefano Sacanna, Asher Preska Steinberg, David J Pine, and Paul M Chaikin. Living crystals of light-activated colloidal surfers. *Science*, 339(6122):936–940, 2013.

[17] Baohu Dai, Jizhuang Wang, Ze Xiong, Xiaojun Zhan, Wei Dai, Chien-Cheng Li, Shien-Ping Feng, and Jinyao Tang. Programmable artificial phototactic microswimmer. *Nature Nanotechnology*, 11(12):1087–1092, 2016.

[18] Zhuoran Zhang, Xian Wang, Jun Liu, Changsheng Dai, and Yu Sun. Robotic micromanipulation: Fundamentals and applications. *Annual Review of Control, Robotics, and Autonomous Systems*, 2:181–203, 2019.

[19] Jakia Jannat Keya, Ryuhei Suzuki, Arif Md Rashedul Kabir, Daisuke Inoue, Hiroyuki Asanuma, Kazuki Sada, Henry Hess, Akinori Kuzuya, and Akira Kakugo. Dna-assisted swarm control in a biomolecular motor system. *Nature Communications*, 9(1):453, 2018.

[20] Wei Gao, Allen Pei, Renfeng Dong, and Joseph Wang. Catalytic iridium-based janus micromotors powered by ultralow levels of chemical fuels. *Journal of the American Chemical Society*, 136(6):2276–2279, 2014.

[21] Changjin Wu, Jia Dai, Xiaofeng Li, Liang Gao, Jizhuang Wang, Jun Liu, Jing Zheng, Xiaojun Zhan, Jiawei Chen, Xiang Cheng, et al. Ion-exchange enabled synthetic swarm. *Nature Nanotechnology*, 16(3):288–295, 2021.

[22] Andreas Kaiser, Alexey Snezhko, and Igor S Aranson. Flocking ferromagnetic colloids. *Science Advances*, 3(2):e1601469, 2017.

[23] Berk Yigit, Yunus Alapan, and Metin Sitti. Programmable collective behavior in dynamically self-assembled mobile microrobotic swarms. *Advanced Science*, 6(6):1801837, 2019.

[24] Jiangfan Yu, Ben Wang, Xingzhou Du, Qianqian Wang, and Li Zhang. Ultra-extensible ribbon-like magnetic microswarm. *Nature Communications*, 9(1):3260, 2018.

[25] Jiangfan Yu, Dongdong Jin, Kai-Fung Chan, Qianqian Wang, Ke Yuan, and Li Zhang. Active generation and magnetic actuation of microrobotic swarms in bio-fluids. *Nature Communications*, 10(1):5631, 2019.

[26] Qianqian Wang, Kai Fung Chan, Kathrin Schweizer, Xingzhou Du, Dongdong Jin, Simon Chun Ho Yu, Bradley J Nelson, and Li Zhang. Ultrasound doppler-guided real-time navigation of a magnetic microswarm for active endovascular delivery. *Science Advances*, 7(9):eabe5914, 2021.

[27] Gwangjun Go, Sin-Gu Jeong, Ami Yoo, Jiwon Han, Byungjeon Kang, Seokjae Kim, Kim Tien Nguyen, Zhen Jin, Chang-Sei Kim, Yu Ri Seo, et al. Human adipose–derived mesenchymal stem cell–based medical microrobot system for knee cartilage regeneration in vivo. *Science Robotics*, 5(38):eaay6626, 2020.

[28] Jiangfan Yu, Qianqian Wang, Mengzhi Li, Chao Liu, Lidai Wang, Tiantian Xu, and Li Zhang. Characterizing nanoparticle swarms with tuneable concentrations for enhanced imaging contrast. *IEEE Robotics and Automation Letters*, 4(3):2942–2949, 2019.

[29] Ben Wang, Kai Fung Chan, Jiangfan Yu, Qianqian Wang, Lidong Yang, Philip Wai Yan Chiu, and Li Zhang. Reconfigurable swarms of ferromagnetic colloids for enhanced local hyperthermia. *Advanced Functional Materials*, 28(25):1705701, 2018.

[30] Xian Wang, Junhui Law, Mengxi Luo, Zheyuan Gong, Jiangfan Yu, Wentian Tang, Zhuoran Zhang, Xueting Mei, Zongjie Huang, Lidan You, et al. Magnetic measurement and stimulation of cellular and intracellular structures. *ACS Nano*, 14(4):3805–3821, 2020.

[31] Jingjie Hu, Hassan Albadawi, Brian W Chong, Amy R Deipolyi, Rahul A Sheth, Ali Khademhosseini, and Rahmi Oklu. Advances in biomaterials and technologies for vascular embolization. *Advanced Materials*, 31(33):1901071, 2019.

[32] Sandeep Vaidya, Kathleen R Tozer, and Jarvis Chen. An overview of embolic agents. In *Seminars in Interventional Radiology*, volume 25, pages 204–215. © by Thieme Medical Publishers, 2008.

[33] Riad Salem and Robert J Lewandowski. Chemoembolization and radioembolization for hepatocellular carcinoma. *Clinical Gastroenterology and Hepatology*, 11(6):604–611, 2013.

[34] Jose I Bilbao, Antonio Martínez-Cuesta, Femín Urtasun, and Octavio Cosín. Complications of embolization. In *Seminars in Interventional Radiology*, volume 23, pages 126–142. Copyright© 2006 by Thieme Medical Publishers, Inc., 333 Seventh Avenue, New . . . , 2006.

[35] Xian Wang, Clement Ho, Y Tsatskis, Junhui Law, Zhuoran Zhang, M Zhu, Changsheng Dai, F Wang, Min Tan, Sevan Hopyan, et al. Intracellular manipulation and measurement with multipole magnetic tweezers. *Science Robotics*, 4(28):eaav6180, 2019.

[36] Xi Wang, Kai Liu, and Changfu You. Drag force model corrections based on nonuniform particle distributions in multi-particle systems. *Powder Technology*, 209(1-3):112–118, 2011.

[37] Kar W Yung, Peter B Landecker, and Daniel D Villani. An analytic solution for the force between two magnetic dipoles. *Magnetic and Electrical Separation*, 9, 1970.

[38] GROVER M Hutchins, MARTIN M Miner, and JOHN K Boitnott. Vessel caliber and branch-angle of human coronary artery branch-points. *Circulation Research*, 38(6):572–576, 1976.

[39] Ursula Windberger, A Bartholovitsch, R Plasenzotti, KJ Korak, and G Heinze. Whole blood viscosity, plasma viscosity and erythrocyte aggregation in nine mammalian species: reference values and comparison of data. *Experimental Physiology*, 88(3):431–440, 2003.

[40] James C Simpson, John E Lane, Christopher D Immer, and Robert C Youngquist. Simple analytic expressions for the magnetic field of a circular current loop. Technical report, 2001.

[41] Wisnu Anggoro. *C++ Data Structures and Algorithms: Learn How to Write Efficient Code to Build Scalable and Robust Applications in C++*. Packt Publishing Ltd, 2018.

[42] Abdel Aziz Taha and Allan Hanbury. Metrics for evaluating 3d medical image segmentation: analysis, selection, and tool. *BMC Medical Imaging*, 15(1):1–28, 2015.

[43] Jiuyang Liu, Xiafei Geng, and Yan Li. Milky spots: omental functional units and hotbeds for peritoneal cancer metastasis. *Tumor Biology*, 37:5715–5726, 2016.

[44] Helena Massana-Cid, Fanlong Meng, Daiki Matsunaga, Ramin Golestanian, and Pietro Tierno. Tunable self-healing of magnetically propelling colloidal carpets. *Nature Communications*, 10(1):2444, 2019.

[45] Hongyue Zhang, Zesheng Li, Changyong Gao, Xinjian Fan, Yuxin Pang, Tianlong Li, Zhiguang Wu, Hui Xie, and Qiang He. Dual-responsive biohybrid neutrobots for active target delivery. *Science Robotics*, 6(52):eaaz9519, 2021.

[46] Ania Servant, Famin Qiu, Mariarosa Mazza, Kostas Kostarelos, and Bradley J Nelson. Controlled in vivo swimming of a swarm of bacteria-like microrobotic flagella. *Advanced Materials*, 27(19):2981–2988, 2015.

[47] Zhiguang Wu, Jonas Troll, Hyeon-Ho Jeong, Qiang Wei, Marius Stang, Focke Ziemssen, Zegao Wang, Mingdong Dong, Sven Schnichels, Tian Qiu, et al. A swarm of slippery micropropellers penetrates the vitreous body of the eye. *Science Advances*, 4(11):eaat4388, 2018.

[48] Ben Wang, Kai Fung Chan, Ke Yuan, Qianqian Wang, Xianfeng Xia, Lidong Yang, Ho Ko, Yi-Xiang J Wang, Joseph Jao Yiu Sung, Philip Wai Yan Chiu, et al. Endoscopy-assisted magnetic navigation of biohybrid soft microrobots with rapid endoluminal delivery and imaging. *Science Robotics*, 6(52):eabd2813, 2021.

[49] Zhiguang Wu, Lei Li, Yiran Yang, Peng Hu, Yang Li, So-Yoon Yang, Lihong V Wang, and Wei Gao. A microrobotic system guided by photoacoustic computed tomography for targeted navigation in intestines in vivo. *Science Robotics*, 4(32):eaax0613, 2019.

[50] Mariana Medina-Sánchez and Oliver G Schmidt. Medical microbots need better imaging and control. *Nature*, 545(7655):406–408, 2017.

V

Summary and Outlook

CHAPTER 11

Summary and Outlook

In the past decade, great progress has been made in the microrobotic swarms and their applications in robot delivery. This book focuses on the latest developments in swarm formation, navigation, positioning and their applications in imaging-guided targeted delivery. Although considerable efforts have been made to achieve controllable delivery *in vivo*, there are still some problems and further progress is needed to effectively control the micromachine population in order to achieve the purpose of targeted delivery. Therefore, in this chapter, we will summarize the main research contents of microswarms, and briefly describe the future research opportunities and challenges.

11.1 FUNDAMENTAL

For swarm control, the control logic is different from single-robot control or multi-robot operation. Swarm control algorithms need to consider more access rates, interactions between swarms and the environment, and even feedback from a statistical perspective [1, 2].

(1) One of the problems to be solved in swarm control is the realization of 3D navigation. Most current collective micro/nanorobots operate in two-dimensional Spaces close to substrates or boundaries, making them incapable of performing complex three-dimensional delivery tasks. Achieving three-dimensional navigation requires addressing topics like compensating for gravity and buoyancy and developing robust control algorithms that can handle multidimensional feedback. And the boundaries of the environment must be considered, which facilitates the control process.Adopting a two-dimensional swarm formation is an optional solution, followed by three-dimensional navigation, which requires a reassessment of the constraints imposed by the boundary and the controllability of the swarm [3, 4, 5].

(2) Remote delivery. Although combining swarm control with technologies including catheter intervention is promising. However, remote navigation for swarms is time consuming, and the efficiency of acquiring building blocks suffers. The combination of micro/nano objects is capable of being loaded onto the tip of the catheter and subsequently released before reaching the challenging anatomical position. This method allows the swarm to pass through the narrow tube cavity and reach the intended destination. In addition, by integrating miniature cameras/sensors, the catheter can

DOI: 10.1201/9781032665788-11

be used as a valuable imaging device to monitor the environment in real time and provide haptic feedback [6]. The integration of aided tool navigation and robot crowd is an important approach for research and exploration.

(3) Environmental adaptability. Swarm models are flexible and adjustable, which enables them to be used in limited and ever-changing environments. Their good adaptability requires a rapid response to external driving energy, the ability to reconfigure shapes, and consistent control over pattern formation. To achieve this level of swarm intelligence requires seamless integration of the control system, synchronous positioning and real-time environment registration to ensure effective operation. In addition, microrobot swarms need to move efficiently in complex media and need to penetrate biological barriers during navigation [7, 8, 9]. It is important to study control strategies that address biological barrier penetration and maintain swarm function.

11.2 CONTROL

The integration of swarm control units with *in vivo* imaging technologies is a fundamental challenge for performing delivery tasks in living organisms. In spite of a variety of imaging techniques can be used to localize micropopulations within opaque tissues or organs, challenges remain in integrating imaging and control systems and selecting the appropriate imaging method based on factors such as navigation location, actuation method, building block material, and specific delivery task [10, 11]. For example, optical-based imaging is not suitable for deep tissue navigation. Ultrasound imaging can penetrate deep tissue, but it is difficult to achieve sufficient imaging contrast in gas-filled body parts such as the lungs. In the case of magnetically controlled microrobot swarms, the ability to form patterns and navigate in multiple degrees of freedom is affected by the strength and bandwidth of the field generators, which can be electromagnetic coils or magnets for permanent magnet-based systems [12]. Therefore, it is not feasible to integrate these controller units with MRI systems as it would interfere with the MRI process. The trade-offs between imaging and control systems, and the development of swarm control schemes that can be integrated with existing imaging systems, present significant challenges. Research attention should be focused on the integration of navigation and imaging in swarms using the same energy source. A recent proposal to drive a small robot using MRI gradient coils demonstrates the potential of an integrated control and imaging system [13]. Using machine learning techniques to analyze image feedback and simultaneously achieve adaptive swarm control can enable integrated imaging swarm control schemes [14]. The control scheme described above can establish a correlation between the collective behavior of a microrobot swarm and the characteristics of the biological environment, facilitating the mapping of physical boundaries and the identification of navigation strategies under complex conditions. One approach employs deep neural networks to analyze medical image feedback and track crowds, followed by crowd switching control to adapt to constrained environments.

11.3 APPLICATION: FROM *IN VITRO* TO *IN VIVO*

Recent research endeavors have primarily concentrated on integrating robotic swarms with established techniques, such as closed-loop control systems and medical imaging systems, to conduct preliminary trials at the preclinical level. However, several important considerations must be addressed before the application of microrobotic swarms in clinical settings, particularly in imaging-guided therapy.

Firstly, substantial efforts should be devoted to the integration of various systems, encompassing hardware, software, and autonomous control. Existing techniques, including catheters and endoscopes, can be incorporated to assist in delivery and therapy procedures [15, 16]. To achieve real-time control of microswarms in living organisms and monitor therapeutic processes, it is necessary to develop user interfaces that integrate microrobot control and feedback processing systems. Autonomous control has the advantages of high operating efficiency and liberates doctors from tedious and repetitive work. However, the degree of autonomy required must be carefully considered, as fully automated systems may require complex coding efforts and may raise safety concerns.

Second, addressing safety concerns is critical for using microrobot swarms for targeted therapy. These issues include determining the appropriate dose for effective delivery (pharmacokinetics), ensuring the reliability of the integrated system, and ensuring that the population can effectively penetrate biological barriers encountered during treatment [17, 18]. Before designing therapeutic procedures, it is crucial to evaluate the biocompatibility and potential toxicity of microrobotic swarms. Recent studies have highlighted the biocompatibility and biomedical applications of hydrogels, including hydrogel micro/nanoparticles and hydrogel-based micro/nanostructures [19, 20]. These hydrogel-based agents can serve as building blocks to reduce the toxicity of microrobotic swarms. Additionally, the use of biohybrid agents, such as particles enclosed within the plasma membrane of human platelets, cell membrane-coated micro/nanorobots, and bio-hybrid microrobots, can enhance the biocompatibility of the swarm [21, 22, 23]. The specific site of application of an actual microrobot swarm plays an important role in determining acceptable levels of toxicity. For example, when microrobot swarms are delivered within the gastrointestinal tract of live mice, histological assessment of microrobot swarm toxicity can be performed in different regions such as the stomach, duodenum, jejunum, distal colon, and ileum. This evaluation aims to investigate the biocompatibility and safety of the oral population [24, 25]. Comprehensive toxicity evaluation from various perspectives, including materials, dosage, and size of building blocks, may be necessary for swarms in endovascular delivery applications. To test the feasibility of the proposed scheme, it is imperative to conduct *ex vivo* trials and animal tests, necessitating collaboration between roboticists, material specialists, and medical practitioners.

Thirdly, identifying a compelling application that aids medical doctors and collaborators in evaluating the procedures involving microrobotic swarms is crucial. Accumulating experiences through such applications can generate greater interest among medical practitioners regarding the use of microrobotic swarms in targeted diagnosis and therapy. The ultimate goal of active-delivery microrobot swarm applications is imaging-guided therapy. Currently, however, proof-of-concept and *in vivo* studies of swarming microrobots in imaging-guided therapy are still limited. Medical imaging systems have not been widely involved in targeted therapy tasks, and swarm control approaches integrating imaging mainly focus on swarm localization and navigation. Research opportunities exist to bridge the gap between targeted therapy/delivery and imaging-guided population control for clinical application.

Over the past these years, scientists have been focused on deploying microswarms in biomedicine as promising therapeutic platforms. These microswarms have been designed using different materials and are capable of performing various tasks in confined environments. These swarms possess powerful capabilities, such as long-distance and fast locomotion in biofluids, cargo loading, and visual navigation for targeted transport. As a result, the applications of microswarms have been broadened, ranging from targeted drug delivery and precise local hyperthermia to real-time sensing and removal of thrombus. Moreover, these swarms have been tested in both artificial solutions and complex *in vivo* environments. But there are still limitations that prevent microswarms from advancing toward clinical applications.

The cytotoxicity of microswarms is still being investigated, as scientists are exploring materials that have good biocompatibility, biodegradability, and stability in biological environments [26, 27]. Clinical trials have shown the effectiveness of different microswarms in various applications [28, 29, 30, 31, 32, 33, 34, 35, 36, 37, 38, 39]. However, most microswarms currently rely on passive motion based on blood circulation, and there is a need to integrate active locomotion and pattern reconfiguration capabilities to improve targeting efficiency [40, 41]. Advancements in actuation strategies and deep tissue imaging will be crucial in transitioning microswarms from the laboratory to clinical applications at the same time.

To enhance the safety of *in vivo* treatments and diagnostics using microswarms, it is important to minimize material cytotoxicity [42]. This can be achieved by prioritizing materials with better biocompatibility and exploring the integration of swarm agents with natural biological materials [43, 44]. While swarm actuation and control strategies can improve the efficiency of targeted drug delivery [45, 46, 47], there is still a risk of agents being captured by organs or remaining in vessels during locomotion. Ensuring the preservation of human health is a challenge, and efforts should be made to improve the biodegradability of microswarms [48, 49].

In the field of actuation and control of microswarms, both external power sources and internal biological powers have been utilized effectively in small animal models [50, 51, 52, 53, 54, 55]. However, further development is needed in terms of devices, mechanisms, and control strategies to enable actuation in human-sized areas [56, 57]. This progress would facilitate precise operation, which is crucial for the movement of swarms. Currently, control methods rely mainly on open-loop techniques [41, 58], but due to the complex and unknown nature of *in vivo* environments, closed-loop automated control strategies should be developed to adapt to these conditions [59]. While many demonstrations of actuation and control approaches have been conducted in two-dimensional (2D) planes such as substrates, microchannels, and vessel boundaries, it is essential to explore three-dimensional (3D) operations of swarms [55]. Validating the formation and behavior of 2D swarms in 3D spaces is necessary to fully understand their capabilities. Additionally, selective control of microswarms offers the potential for high-efficiency task completion [60]. While some tasks can be accomplished by globally controlling all developed microswarms within a single field [47], adopting selective control methods among multiple swarms can enhance overall efficiency, especially for tasks requiring collective coordination, such as microassembly [61].

During the treatment of various diseases, it is necessary for microswarms to navigate toward targeted regions. Some swarms rely on passive methods, such as blood circulation, to reach target areas, which can result in high uncertainties and low targeting rates [62]. To improve the targeting rate, a combination of passive-specific binding (*e.g.*, antibody and antigen) and active remote actuation methods should be employed [63]. Some studies have shown promising drug delivery capabilities of swarms [27, 64], but the drug releasing rate and effectiveness still need to be systematically evaluated. Additionally, current microswarms primarily rely on external environmental changes, such as pH and temperature [65, 66, 67], to release drugs. However, these methods may have limitations when applied inside living bodies. Therefore, it is important to develop triggering factors that are applicable for *in vivo* applications. Visualization of microswarms is crucial for real-time imaging-guided locomotion [68, 69]. By obtaining clear vision feedback, an optimized path can be planned toward the target, such as a tumor. Currently, most experiments are conducted in small mice [70, 71], and efforts should be made to enhance imaging penetration depth in thicker human tissues [72, 73, 74]. The presence of blood cells can also blur the clinical imaging contrast for swarms in the bloodstream. Integrating machine learning algorithms with various imaging modalities can be a way to enhance imaging feedback [75, 76].

To facilitate clinical translation, it is crucial to address the regulatory and bioethical challenges associated with microswarms to ensure patient safety [77]. Measures should be taken to minimize harm and discomfort to patients by limiting the use of fabrication materials, actuation methods, and sensing mechanisms within a safe range. It is important for the swarms to degrade into harmless products or be cleared out of the body to prevent organ damage [40]. Additionally, organisms in living and hybrid swarms should undergo pretreatment before *in vivo* deployment to prevent proliferation and the production of harmful byproducts to normal tissues [26, 78].

In the next ten years, several promising developments can be expected in the field of microswarms. Firstly, there will be advancements in magnetic materials that exhibit improved biocompatibility and biodegradability, ensuring their safe use within the human body. Secondly, there will be a focus on developing actuation setups and automated swarm control strategies that are suitable for human-sized applications, enabling precise control over the swarms. Additionally, there will be advancements in imaging modalities that allow for real-time guidance and operation of the swarms in deeper tissues, overcoming current limitations. These developments will be made possible through intense efforts and close collaboration among different fields. Ultimately, with continued research and innovation, microswarms will be translated from the laboratory to practical clinical settings, serving as precise therapeutic and diagnostic platforms.

Bibliography

[1] Lidong Yang, Jiangfan Yu, and Li Zhang. Statistics-based automated control for a swarm of paramagnetic nanoparticles in 2-d space. *IEEE Transactions on Robotics*, 36(1):254–270, 2020.

[2] Qianqian Wang, Jiachen Zhang, Jiangfan Yu, Ji Lang, Zhiyang Lyu, Yunfei Chen, and Li Zhang. Untethered small-scale machines for microrobotic manipulation: From individual and multiple to collective machines. *ACS Nano*, page DOI: 10.1021/acsnano.3c05328, 2023.

[3] Shihao Yang, Qianqian Wang, Dongdong Jin, Xingzhou Du, and Li Zhang. Probing fast transformation of magnetic colloidal microswarms in complex fluids. *ACS Nano*, 16(11):19025–19037, 2022.

[4] Daniel Ahmed, Thierry Baasch, Nicolas Blondel, Nino Láubli, Júrg Dual, and Bradley J Nelson. Neutrophil-inspired propulsion in a combined acoustic and magnetic field. *Nature Communications*, 8:770, 2017.

[5] Fengtong Ji, Dongdong Jin, Ben Wang, and Li Zhang. Light-driven hovering of a magnetic microswarm in fluid. *ACS Nano*, 14(6):6990–6998, 2020.

[6] Yoonho Kim, German A Parada, Shengduo Liu, and Xuanhe Zhao. Ferromagnetic soft continuum robots. *Science Robotics*, 4(33):eaax7329, 2019.

[7] Zhiguang Wu, Ye Chen, Daniel Mukasa, On Shun Pak, and Wei Gao. Medical micro/nanorobots in complex media. *Chemical Society Reviews*, 49:8088–8112, 2020.

[8] Hakan Ceylan, Immihan C Yasa, Ugur Kilic, Wenqi Hu, and Metin Sitti. Translational prospects of untethered medical microrobots. *Progress in Biomedical Engineering*, 1(1):012002, 2019.

[9] Dongdong Jin and Li Zhang. Microrobotics-embodied intelligence weaves a better future. *Nature Machine Intelligence*, 2(11):663–664, 2020.

[10] Guido T van Moolenbroek, Tania Patiño, Jordi Llop, and Samuel Sánchez. Engineering intelligent nanosystems for enhanced medical imaging. *Advanced Intelligent Systems*, 2(10):2000087, 2020.

[11] Qianqian Wang, Nan Xiang, Ji Lang, Ben Wang, Dongdong Jin, and Li Zhang. Reconfigurable liquid-bodied miniature machines: Magnetic control and microrobotic applications. *Advanced Intelligent Systems*, page DOI: 10.1002/aisy.202300108, 2023.

[12] Lidong Yang and Li Zhang. Motion control in magnetic microrobotics: From individual and multiple to swarm. *Annual Review of Control, Robotics, and Autonomous Systems*, 4:1–26, 2021.

[13] Onder Erin, Hunter B Gilbert, Ahmet Fatih Tabak, and Metin Sitti. Elevation and azimuth rotational actuation of an untethered millirobot by mri gradient coils. *IEEE Transactions on Robotics*, 35(6):1323–1337, 2019.

[14] Frank Cichos, Kristian Gustavsson, Bernhard Mehlig, and Giovanni Volpe. Machine learning for active matter. *Nature Machine Intelligence*, 2(2):94–103, 2020.

[15] James W Martin, Bruno Scaglioni, Joseph C Norton, Venkataraman Subramanian, Alberto Arezzo, Keith L Obstein, and Pietro Valdastri. Enabling the future of colonoscopy with intelligent and autonomous magnetic manipulation. *Nature Machine Intelligence*, 2:595–606, 2020.

[16] Guillaume Lapouge, Philippe Poignet, and Jocelyne Troccaz. Towards 3d ultrasound guided needle steering tobust to uncertainties, noise and tissue heterogeneity. *IEEE Transactions on Biomedical Engineering*, page DOI: 10.1109/TBME.2020.3022619, 2020.

[17] Changyong Gao, Yong Wang, Zihan Ye, Zhihua Lin, Xing Ma, and Qiang He. Biomedical micro-/nanomotors: From overcoming biological barriers to *in Vivo* imaging. *Advanced Materials*, page DOI: 10.1002/adma.202000512, 2020.

[18] Ben Wang, K Kostarelos, Bradley J Nelson, and Li Zhang. Trends in micro-/nano-robotics: Materials development, actuation, localization, and system integration for biomedical applications. *Advanced Materials*, page DOI: 10.1002/adma.202002047, 2020.

[19] Kun Xue, Xiaoyuan Wang, Pei Wern Yong, David James Young, Yun-Long Wu, Zibiao Li, and Xian Jun Loh. Hydrogels as emerging materials for translational biomedicine. *Advanced Therapeutics*, 2(1):1800088, 2019.

[20] Mohammad Hosein Ayoubi-Joshaghani, Khaled Seidi, Mehdi Azizi, Mehdi Jaymand, Tahereh Javaheri, Rana Jahanban-Esfahlan, and Michael R Hamblin. Potential applications of advanced nano/hydrogels in biomedicine: Static, dynamic, multi-stage, and bioinspired. *Advanced Functional Materials*, 30(45):2004098, 2020.

[21] Jia Zhuang, Hua Gong, Jiarong Zhou, Qiangzhe Zhang, Weiwei Gao, Ronnie H Fang, and Liangfang Zhang. Targeted gene silencing *in Vivo* by platelet membrane-coated metal-organic framework nanoparticles. *Science Advances*, 6(13):eaaz6108, 2020.

[22] Berta Esteban-Fernández de Ávila, Weiwei Gao, Emil Karshalev, Liangfang Zhang, and Joseph Wang. Cell-like micromotors. *Accounts of Chemical Research*, 51(9):1901–1910, 2018.

[23] Lukas Schwarz, Mariana Medina-Sánchez, and Oliver G Schmidt. Hybrid biomicromotors. *Applied Physics Reviews*, 4(3):031301, 2017.

[24] Jinxing Li, Soracha Thamphiwatana, Wenjuan Liu, Berta Esteban-Fernández de Ávila, Pavimol Angsantikul, Elodie Sandraz, Jianxing Wang, Tailin Xu, Fernando Soto, Valentin Ramez, Xiaolei Wang, Weiwei Gao, Liangfang Zhang, and Joseph Wang. Enteric micromotor can selectively position and spontaneously propel in the gastrointestinal tract. *ACS Nano*, 10(10):9536–9542, 2016.

[25] Zhiguang Wu, Lei Li, Yiran Yang, Peng Hu, Yang Li, So-Yoon Yang, Lihong V Wang, and Wei Gao. A microrobotic system guided by photoacoustic computed tomography for targeted navigation in intestines *in Vivo*. *Science Robotics*, 4(32):eaax0613, 2019.

[26] Zhila Mohajeri Avval, Leila Malekpour, Farzad Raeisi, Aziz Babapoor, Seyyed Mojtaba Mousavi, Seyyed Alireza Hashemi, and Marjan Salari. Introduction of magnetic and supermagnetic nanoparticles in new approach of targeting drug delivery and cancer therapy application. *Drug Metabolism Reviews*, 52(1):157–184, 2020.

[27] Paniz Siminzar, Yadollah Omidi, Asal Golchin, Ayuob Aghanejad, and Jaleh Barar. Targeted delivery of doxorubicin by magnetic mesoporous silica nanoparticles armed with mucin-1 aptamer. *Journal of Drug Targeting*, 28(1):92–101, 2020.

[28] S K Libutti, G F Paciotti, and A A Byrnes. Phase I and pharmacokinetic studies of cyt-6091, a novel pegylated colloidal gold-rhtnf nanomedicine. *Clinical Cancer Research*, 16(24), 2010.

[29] Jonathan E Zuckerman, Ismael Gritli, Anthony Tolcher, Jeremy D Heidel, Dean Lim, Robert Morgan, Bartosz Chmielowski, Antoni Ribas, Mark E Davis, and Yun Yen. Correlating animal and human phase ia/ib clinical data with calaa-01, a targeted, polymer-based nanoparticle containing sirna. *Proceedings of the National Academy of Sciences*, 111(31):11449–11454, 2014.

[30] Sonke Svenson, Marc Wolfgang, Jungyeon Hwang, John Ryan, and Scott Eliasof. Preclinical to clinical development of the novel camptothecin nanopharmaceutical crlx101. *Journal of Controlled Release*, 153(1):49–55, 2011. Eighth International Nanomedicine and Drug Delivery Symposium.

[31] Neil Senzer, John Nemunaitis, Derek Nemunaitis, Cynthia Bedell, Gerald Edelman, Minal Barve, Robert Nunan, Kathleen F Pirollo, Antonina Rait, and Esther H Chang. Phase i study of a systemically delivered p53 nanoparticle in advanced solid tumors. *Molecular Therapy*, 21(5):1096–1103, 2013.

[32] Dirk Strumberg, Beate Schultheis, Ulrich Traugott, Christiane Vank, and Joachim Drevs. Phase i clinical development of atu027, a sirna formulation targeting pkn3 in patients with advanced solid tumors. *International Journal of Clinical Pharmacology and Therapeutics*, 50(1):76–78, 2012.

[33] Denise A Yardley, Lowell Hart, Linda Bosserman, Mansoor N Salleh, David M Waterhouse, Maura K Hagan, Paul Richards, Michelle L Desilvio, Janine M Mahoney, and Yasir Nagarwala. Phase ii study evaluating lapatinib in combination with nab-paclitaxel in her2-overexpressing metastatic breast cancer patients who have received no more than one prior chemotherapeutic regimen. *Breast Cancer Research & Treatment*, 137(2):457–464, 2013.

[34] Lobo Christopher, Lopes Gilberto, Baez Odalys, Castrellon Aurelio, Ferrell Annapoorna, Higgins Connie, Hurley Erin, Hurley Judith, Reis Isildinha, and Richman Stephen. Final results of a phase ii study of nab-paclitaxel, bevacizumab, and gemcitabine as first-line therapy for patients with her2-negative metastatic breast cancer. *Breast Cancer Research & Treatment*, 123(2):427–435, 2010.

[35] A Gennari, Z Sun, U Hasler-Strub, M Colleoni, M J Kennedy, R Von Moos, J Cortés, M J Vidal, B Hennessy, and J Walshe. A randomized phase ii study evaluating different maintenance schedules of nab-paclitaxel in the first-line treatment of metastatic breast cancer: final results of the ibcsg 42-12/big 2-12 snap trial - sciencedirect. *Annals of Oncology*, 29(3):661–668, 2018.

[36] M Johannsen, U Gneveckow, L Eckelt, A Feussner, and A Jordan. Clinical hyperthermia of prostate cancer using magnetic nanoparticles: Presentation of a new interstitial technique. *International Journal of Hyperthermia*, 21(7): 637–647, 2005.

[37] Akihiko Matsumine, Katsuyuki Kusuzaki, Takao Matsubara, Ken Shintani, Haruhiko Satonaka, Toru Wakabayashi, Shinichi Miyazaki, Katsuya Morita, Kenji Takegami, and Atsumasa Uchida. Novel hyperthermia for metastatic bone tumors with magnetic materials by generating an alternating electromagnetic field. *Clinical Experimental Metastasis*, 24(3):191–200, 2007.

[38] Klaus Maier-Hauff, Frank Ulrich, Dirk Nestler, Hendrik Niehoff, Peter Wust, Burghard Thiesen, Helmut Orawa, Volker Budach, and Andreas Jordan. Efficacy and safety of intratumoral thermotherapy using magnetic iron-oxide nanoparticles combined with external beam radiotherapy on patients with recurrent glioblastoma multiforme. *Journal of Neuro-Oncology*, 103(2):317–324, 2011.

[39] Joshua M Stern, Viktor V Kibanov Solomonov, Elena Sazykina, Jon A Schwartz, and Glenn P Goodrich. Initial evaluation of the safety of nanoshell-directed photothermal therapy in the treatment of prostate disease. *International Journal of Toxicology*, 35(1):38, 2016.

[40] Ben Wang, Kostas Kostarelos, Bradley J Nelson, and Li Zhang. Trends in micro-/nanorobotics: Materials development, actuation, localization, and system integration for biomedical applications. *Advanced Materials*, 2020.

[41] Hui Xie, Mengmeng Sun, Xinjian Fan, Zhihua Lin, Weinan Chen, Lei Wang, Lixin Dong, and Qiang He. Reconfigurable magnetic microrobot swarm:

Multimode transformation, locomotion, and manipulation. *Science Robotics*, 4(28):eaav8006, 2019.

[42] Sandhya Rani Goudu, Immihan Ceren Yasa, Xinghao Hu, Hakan Ceylan, Wenqi Hu, and Metin Sitti. Biodegradable untethered magnetic hydrogel milli-grippers. *Advanced Functional Materials*, 30(50):2004975, 2020.

[43] Changyong Gao, Zhihua Lin, Daolin Wang, Zhiguang Wu, and Qiang He. Red blood cell-mimicking micromotor for active photodynamic cancer therapy. *ACS Applied Materials & Interfaces*, 11(26), 2019.

[44] Qing Xia, Yongtai Zhang, Zhe Li, Xuefeng Hou, and Nianping Feng. Red blood cell membrane-camouflaged nanoparticles: A novel drug delivery system for antitumor application. *Acta Pharmaceutica Sinica B*, 2019.

[45] Jiangfan Yu, Dongdong Jin, and Li Zhang. Mobile paramagnetic nanoparticle-based vortex for targeted cargo delivery in fluid. In *2017 IEEE International Conference on Robotics and Automation (ICRA)*, 2017.

[46] Jiangfan Yu and Li Zhang. Reconfigurable colloidal microrobotic swarm for targeted delivery. In *2019 16th International Conference on Ubiquitous Robots (UR)*, 2019.

[47] Hui Xie, Xinjian Fan, Mengmeng Sun, Zhihua Lin, Qiang He, and Lining Sun. Programmable generation and motion control of a snakelike magnetic microrobot swarm. *IEEE/ASME Transactions on Mechatronics*, 24(3):902–912, 2019.

[48] Xiaozhen, Liu, Shengliang, Yingpeng, Wan, Jia-Xiong, Chen, Shuang, Tian, and Zhongming, Huang. Biodegradable π-conjugated oligomer nanoparticles with high photothermal conversion efficiency for cancer theranostics. *ACS Nano*, 13(11):12901–12911, 2019.

[49] Johan Karlsson, Hannah J Vaughan, and Jordan J Green. Biodegradable polymeric nanoparticles for therapeutic cancer treatments. *Annual Review of Chemical and Biomolecular Engineering*, 9(1):annurev–chembioeng–060817–084055, 2018.

[50] Byung-Wook Park, Jiang Zhuang, Oncay Yasa, and Metin Sitti. Multifunctional bacteria-driven microswimmers for targeted active drug delivery. *ACS Nano*, 11(9):8910–8923, 2017.

[51] Jiangfan Yu, Ben Wang, Xingzhou Du, Qianqian Wang, and Li Zhang. Ultra-extensible ribbon-like magnetic microswarm. *Nature Communications*, 9(1):3260, 2018.

[52] H-W Huang, Fazil Emre Uslu, Panayiota Katsamba, Eric Lauga, Mahmut S Sakar, and Bradley J Nelson. Adaptive locomotion of artificial microswimmers. *Science Advances*, 5(1):eaau1532, 2019.

[53] Juan Jiang, Shi jin Yang, Jian cheng Wang, Li juan Yang, Zhen zhong Xu, Ting Yang, Xiao yan Liu, and Qiang Zhang. Sequential treatment of drug-resistant tumors with rgd-modified liposomes containing sirna or doxorubicin. *European Journal of Pharmaceutics and Biopharmaceutics*, 76(2):170–178, 2010.

[54] Jitendrakumar Patel, Jitendra Amrutiya, Priyanka Bhatt, Ankit Javia, Mukul Jain, and Ambikanandan Misra. Targeted delivery of monoclonal antibody conjugated docetaxel loaded plga nanoparticles into egfr overexpressed lung tumor cells. *Journal of Microencapsulation*, page 1, 2018.

[55] Fengtong Ji, Dongdong Jin, Ben Wang, and Li Zhang. Light-driven hovering of a magnetic microswarm in fluid. *ACS Nano*, XXXX(XXX), 2020.

[56] Zhengxin Yang, Lidong Yang, and Li Zhang. Autonomous navigation of magnetic microrobots in a large workspace using mobile-coil system. *IEEE/ASME Transactions on Mechatronics*, 26(6):3163–3174, 2021.

[57] Lidong Yang and Li Zhang. Large-workspace and high-resolution magnetic microrobot navigation using global-local path planning and eye-in-hand visual servoing. In *2020 IEEE 16th International Conference on Automation Science and Engineering (CASE)*, 2020.

[58] Xinjian Fan, Mengmeng Sun, Lining Sun, and Hui Xie. Ferrofluid droplets as liquid microrobots with multiple deformabilities. *Advanced Functional Materials*, 30(24), 2020.

[59] Lidong Yang, Jiangfan Yu, and Li Zhang. Statistics-based automated control for a swarm of paramagnetic nanoparticles in 2-d space. *IEEE Transactions on Robotics*, 36(1):254–270, 2020.

[60] Wang, Xiaopu, Chengzhi, Schurz, Lukas, De, Marco, Carmela, Chen, and Xiangzhong. Surface-chemistry-mediated control of individual magnetic helical microswimmers in a swarm. *ACS Nano*, 12(6):6210–6217, 2018.

[61] Jiangfan Yu, Dongdong Jin, Kai-Fung Chan, Qianqian Wang, Ke Yuan, and Li Zhang. Active generation and magnetic actuation of microrobotic swarms in bio-fluids. *Nature Communications*, 10(1):5631, 2019.

[62] Zhang, Hao, Wang, Tingting, Qiu, Weibao, Han, Yaobao, Sun, and Qiao. Monitoring the opening and recovery of the blood-brain barrier with noninvasive molecular imaging by biodegradable ultrasmall cu2-xse nanoparticles. *Nano Letters*, 2018.

[63] Hongyue Zhang, Zesheng Li, Changyong Gao, Xinjian Fan, Yuxin Pang, Tianlong Li, Zhiguang Wu, Hui Xie, and Qiang He. Dual-responsive biohybrid neutrobots for active target delivery. *Science Robotics*, 6(52):eaaz9519, 2021.

[64] Kanat Dukenbayev, Ilya V Korolkov, Daria I Tishkevich, Artem L Kozlovskiy, Sergey V Trukhanov, Yevgeniy G Gorin, Elena E Shumskaya, Egor Y Kaniukov,

Denis A Vinnik, Maxim V Zdorovets, Marina Anisovich, Alex V Trukhanov, Daniele Tosi, and Carlo Molardi. Fe3o4 nanoparticles for complex targeted delivery and boron neutron capture therapy. *Nanomaterials*, 9(4), 2019.

[65] Bolla, Pradeep, Kumar, Rodriguez, A Victor, Kalhapure, S Rahul, and Kolli. A review on ph and temperature responsive gels and other less explored drug delivery systems. *Journal of Drug Delivery Science and Technology*, 46:416–435, 2018.

[66] Dirk Schmaljohann. Thermo- and ph-responsive polymers in drug delivery. *Advanced Drug Delivery Reviews*, 58(15):1655–1670, 2006.

[67] Yang Zheng, Lei Wang, Lin Lu, Qian Wang, and Brian C. Benicewicz. Ph and thermal dual-responsive nanoparticles for controlled drug delivery with high loading content. *ACS Omega*, 2(7):3399–3405, 2017.

[68] Qianqian Wang and Li Zhang. External power-driven microrobotic swarm: From fundamental understanding to imaging-guided delivery. *ACS Nano*, 15(1):149–174, 2021.

[69] Wang Ben, Zhang Yabin, and Zhang Li. Recent progress on micro- and nanorobots: Towards in vivo tracking and localization. *Quantitative Imaging in Medicine & Surgery*, 8(5):461–479, 2018.

[70] Xian Wang, Tiancong Wang, Guanqiao Shan, Junhui Law, Changsheng Dai, Zhuoran Zhang, and Yu Sun. Robotic control of a magnetic swarm for on-demand intracellular measurement. In *2020 IEEE International Conference on Robotics and Automation (ICRA)*, pages 11385–11391. IEEE, 2020.

[71] Chen Shen, Xiaoxiong Wang, Zhixing Zheng, Chuang Gao, Xin Chen, Shiguang Zhao, and Zhifei Dai. Doxorubicin and indocyanine green loaded superparamagnetic iron oxide nanoparticles with pegylated phospholipid coating for magnetic resonance with fluorescence imaging and chemotherapy of glioma. *International Journal of Nanomedicine*, pages 101–117, 2019.

[72] Harel Nagar and Yael Roichman. Deep penetration fluorescence imaging through dense yeast cells suspensions using airy beams. *Optics Letters*, 44(8):1896–1899, 2019.

[73] Lingchen Meng, Xibo Ma, Shan Jiang, Guang Ji, Wenkun Han, Bin Xu, Jie Tian, and Wenjing Tian. High-efficiency fluorescent and magnetic multimodal probe for long-term monitoring and deep penetration imaging of tumors. *Journal of Materials Chemistry B*, 7, 2019.

[74] Xiaohua Feng, Fei Gao, and Yuanjin Zheng. Magnetically mediated thermoacoustic imaging toward deeper penetration. *Applied Physics Letters*, 103(8), 2013.

[75] Hayit Greenspan, Bram van Ginneken, and Ronald M Summers. Guest editorial deep learning in medical imaging: Overview and future promise of an exciting new technique. *IEEE Transactions on Medical Imaging*, 35(5):1153–1159, 2016.

[76] Maribel Torres-Velázquez, Wei-Jie Chen, Xue Li, and Alan B McMillan. Application and construction of deep learning networks in medical imaging. *IEEE Transactions on Radiation and Plasma Medical Sciences*, 5(2):137–159, 2021.

[77] Fernando Soto, Jie Wang, Rajib Ahmed, and Utkan Demirci. Medical micro/nanorobots in precision medicine. *Advanced Science*, 7(21):2002203, 2020.

[78] Ajay Vikram Singh, Mohammad Hasan Dad Ansari, Peter Laux, and Andreas Luch. Micro-nanorobots: important considerations when developing novel drug delivery platforms. *Expert Opinion on Drug Delivery*, 16(11):1259–1275, 2019.